Tropical Diseases

Tropical Diseases

A Practical Guide for Medical Practitioners and Students

Yann A. Meunier, MD

(with contributions from Michael Hole,
Takudzwa Shumba, and B. J. Swanner)

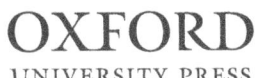

OXFORD
UNIVERSITY PRESS

Oxford University Press is a department of the University of Oxford.
It furthers the University's objective of excellence in research, scholarship,
and education by publishing worldwide.

Oxford New York
Auckland Cape Town Dar es Salaam Hong Kong Karachi
Kuala Lumpur Madrid Melbourne Mexico City Nairobi
New Delhi Shanghai Taipei Toronto

With offices in
Argentina Austria Brazil Chile Czech Republic France Greece
Guatemala Hungary Italy Japan Poland Portugal Singapore
South Korea Switzerland Thailand Turkey Ukraine Vietnam

Oxford is a registered trademark of Oxford University Press in the UK
and certain other countries.

Published in the United States of America by
Oxford University Press
198 Madison Avenue, New York, NY 10016

© Oxford University Press 2014

All rights reserved. No part of this publication may be reproduced, stored in a
retrieval system, or transmitted, in any form or by any means, without the prior
permission in writing of Oxford University Press, or as expressly permitted by law,
by license, or under terms agreed with the appropriate reproduction rights organization.
Inquiries concerning reproduction outside the scope of the above should be sent to the
Rights Department, Oxford University Press, at the address above.

You must not circulate this work in any other form
and you must impose this same condition on any acquirer.

Library of Congress Cataloging-in-Publication Data
Meunier, Yann A., author.
Tropical diseases : a practical guide for medical practitioners and students / Yann A.
Meunier ; with contributions from Michael Hole, Takudzwa Shumba & B.J. Swanner.
  p. ; cm.
Includes bibliographical references and indexes.
ISBN 978–0–19–999790–9 (alk. paper)
I. Hole, Michael, author. II. Shumba, Takudzwa, author.
III. Swanner, B. J., author. IV. Title.
[DNLM: 1. Tropical Medicine. 2. Travel. WC 680]
RC961
616.9'883—dc23
2013020453

Contents

Book Introduction xi
About the Main Author xiii
About the Contributing Authors xv
Acknowledgments xvii
Disease and Patient Introduction xix

Part One: Parasitic Diseases

(A) Adult Parasite Location	1
Blood and Lymphatic Systems	1
Filariasis (Lymphatic)	1
Leishmaniasis (Visceral, or Kala-Azar, or Dum Dum Disease)	4
Malaria (Blackwater Fever)	7
Trypanosomiasis (African, or Sleeping Sickness)	15
Trypanosomiasis (American, or Chagas disease)	19
Digestive Tract	22
Amebiasis	22
Intestinal Amebiasis	22
Liver Amebiasis	24
Ameboma	25
Ancylostomiasis (or Hookworm Infection)	27
Ascariasis	30
Balantidiasis (or Balantidiosis)	32
Distomatosis (Biliary/Liver, or Biliary/Liver Fluke Infection)	32
Distomatosis (Intestinal)	37
Giardiasis (Beaver Fever)	39
Schistosomiasis (Intestinal)	40
Strongyloidiasis	46
Trichuriasis (Whipworm Infection)	49
Lungs	49
Paragonimiasis (or Lung Fluke Infection)	49
Nails and Hair	52
Candidiasis (or Moniliasis)	52
Dermatophytosis	52

Pediculosis Capitis (or Head Lice)	53
Pthiriasis (or Crabs)	54
Tinea Capitis (or Head Ringworm)	54

Sexual Organs — 55
Candidiasis (or Moniliasis)	55
Trichomoniasis	56

Skin and Integumentary System — 58
Candidiasis (or Moniliasis)	58
Dermatophytosis	58
Dracunculiasis (Guinea Worm Disease, Guinea Worm Infection, or Dracontiasis)	59
Leishmaniasis (Cutaneous)	63
Leishmaniasis (Mucocutaneous)	67
Loiasis (or African Eyeworm)	70
Malasseziosis (or Pityriasis Versicolor)	73
Myiasis (or Tumba Fly)	73
Onchocerciasis (or River Blindness)	76
Pediculosis Corporis (or Body Lice)	80
Scabies (or Norwegian Itch)	80
Tinea Nigra Palmis and Plantaris	82
Tungiasis	82

Urinary Tract — 85
Schistosomiasis (Urinary)	85

(B) Parasitic Dead Ends and Larval Diseases — 89
Angiostrongyliasis	89
Cenurosis	91
Cysticercosis	91
Gnathostomiasis	94
Hydatidosis	96
Larva Migrans (Cutaneous, or Creeping Eruption)	99
Linguatulosis	100
Porocephalosis	100
Sparganosis	101
Toxocariasis (Toxocarosis, Visceral Larva Migrans or Roundworm Infection)	103
Trichinosis (or Trichinellosis)	104

Part Two: Deep Fungal Diseases

Basidiobolomycosis	107
Blastomycosis (North American or Gilchrist Disease or Chicago Disease)	109

Blastomycosis (South American or Lutz-Splendore-Almeida Disease)	110
Chromomycosis	113
Coccidioidomycosis (or Posadas-Wernicke, or Posadas-Rixford Disease)	115
Conidiobolomycosis	118
Histoplasmosis (African)	120
Histoplasmosis (American or Darling Disease)	123
Lobomycosis (or Jorge Lobo Disease)	127
Mycetoma (or Madura Foot)	129
Pythiosis	132
Rhinosporidiosis	134
Scytalidiosis	136

Part Three: Bacterial, Chlamydial, and Prion Diseases

Bacterial Diseases	**139**
Anthrax	139
Bartonellosis (or Carrion Disease)	141
Bejel (or Endemic Syphilis)	143
Buruli Ulcers (or Bairnsdale, Daintree, Mossman, or Searls Ulcer, or Mycoburuli Ulcers)	144
Chancroid (or Soft Chancre or Ulcus Molle)	146
Cholera	146
Diphtheria	152
Gonorrhea (or Clap)	153
Granuloma Inguinale (or Donovan Disease)	155
Leprosy (or Hansen Disease)	159
Leptospirosis (or Weil Disease or Nanukayami Fever)	162
Melioidosis (or Whitmore Disease)	163
Meningococcal Meningitis	167
Pertussis (or Whooping Cough)	170
Pinta (or Carate)	171
Plague (or Black Death)	174
Pneumococcal Disease	177
Salmonellosis (Typhoid Fever or Enteric Fever and Paratyphoid Fever)	182
Salmonellosis (*Salmonella* gastroenteritis)	187
Shigellosis	188
Syphilis (or Hard Chancre)	190
Tuberculosis	192
Yaws (Pian, Parangi, Paru, or Frambesia Tropica)	195

Chlamydial Diseases	**196**
Lymphogranuloma Venereum (or Nicholas-Favre-Durand Disease)	196
Trachoma (or Granular Conjunctivitis or Egyptian Ophthalmia)	199
Urethritis and Cervicitis	201
Prion Disease	**202**
Variant Creutzfeldt-Jakob Disease	202

Part Four: Viral Diseases

Common Diseases	**205**
Dengue Fever (or Breakbone Fever)	205
Hepatitis	209
Herpes Simplex (or Cold or Fever Sore)	215
HIV/Aids	216
Influenza (or Flu)	225
Measles	227
Poliomyelitis (or Polio)	229
Yellow Fever (or Black Vomit)	232
Rare Diseases	**235**
Arboviral Diseases	235
Arenaviral Diseases	237
Bunyaviral Diseases	239
Coronaviral Disease	242
Filoviral Diseases	243
Flaviviral Diseases	245
Paramyxoviral Diseases	246
Reoviral Diseases	247
Rhabdoviral Diseases	249
Togaviral Diseases	250

Part Five: Tropical Health Hazards

Animal-Induced Diseases	**253**
Bees and Hymenoptera	253
Butterflies	254
Cats	256
Centipedes	260
Dogs	260
Fish	265
Fleas	266
Jellyfish, Sea Anemones, and Physaliae	269

Leeches	269
Lice	270
Mollusks	274
Muraenae (or Moray Eels)	274
Rats	275
Scorpions	276
Snakes	277
Spiders	278
Ticks	279
Trombiculidae	282
Exotic Food Poisoning	**284**
Ciguatera	284
Ichthyosarcotoxisms (Other)	287
Fish Poisoning	287
Mushroom Poisoning	288
Heat-Related Illnesses	**290**
Heat Asthenia (or Tropical Anhidrotic Asthenia)	290
Heat Exhaustion	290
Heat Stroke	291
Miliaria (or Prickly Heat)	292
Travelers and Tropical Diseases	**292**
Precautions to Take Before, During and after Traveling	294
Traveler's Diarrhea (or Turista)	297
Antibiotic Resistance	**299**
Addendum	**303**
Differential Diagnosis	303
International Generic and Brand Names of Drugs	306
Contraindications for Drugs	314
List of FDA-Approved Vaccines	333
List of Vaccines Available in France	336
Link to Major International Health-Care Organizations	338

Map and Table Index 339
Patient Cases Index 341
Disease Index 343
Symptom Index 347
Meaning of Abbreviations 367
References 369
Index 379

Book Introduction

The face of medicine is changing faster than ever at the onset of the 21st century. For health professionals, challenges are multifold. Rare viral diseases have emerged. Through migrations and tourism people are increasingly exposed to old diseases, which, for some, present new problems. We assigned ourselves six purposes, while creating a unique and convenient reference tool for medical practitioners:

- To propose a clinically convenient classification of parasitic diseases, according to the adult or final stage of the parasite location in the human body
- To provide geographic distribution maps which aid the fast finding of disease origin and infection risk
- To approach each disease systematically with succinct historical background, geographic distribution, main symptoms, treatment, and prevention (given the tremendous gap between the gold-standard tests for parasitic diseases and what is currently available in most hospitals, we intentionally left out the laboratory diagnostic aspect)
- To create an awareness of potential global risks of tropical diseases and present means of prevention at the individual level
- To illustrate the text with vignettes of clinical examples, gathered from global medical practice, aimed at making theory come to life
- To embrace clarity and simplicity in an era of rapidly increasing complexity and sophistication

We have included a differential diagnosis list for diarrhea, fever, pruritus, and splenomegaly. Medication names are given according to the international common denomination. Treatments are based on experience and take into account factors such as greatest efficacy and fewest adverse reactions, geographic availability, and cost in developing countries. Unfortunately, the gold-standard therapeutic options are not available in every community around the world. To help medical practitioners observe their duty of primum non noncere, we have included a list of contraindications of all the medications cited in the book. Also, we have listed all the FDA-approved vaccines and those available in France and given a link to international health-care organizations. For easy reference, we have opted for an alphabetical order throughout the text.

We emphasize practicality and therefore efficiency in our recommendation of optimal diagnostic and curative approaches in as many health-care settings as possible.

For historical and mnemonic reasons, we mention the common names of diseases. In an effort to honor the researchers who worked passionately to bring tropical diseases out of obscurity and ignorance, we have identified many of them also by these pioneers' names.

Yann Meunier

About the Main Author

Yann Meunier, MD, studied medicine at Paris V University, at the Federal University of Rio de Janeiro, and at George Washington University. He holds specialty degrees in emergency medicine from Paris XII University and tropical diseases from Paris VI University.

He was a general practitioner in France, New Caledonia, Nigeria, and Singapore, where he was a physician of reference for fifteen embassies, various consulates, and a high commission. He was chief medical officer for Chevron Oil in Papua New Guinea and resident physician for Allucam in Cameroon, for Electricité de France in China, and for Spie-Batignolles and Schlumberger in Nigeria. He led corporate missions for Conoco Oil and Total Oil in Angola, a timber consortium in Congo, Bosch in Gambia and Egypt, Club Med in Haiti, International SOS in Thailand, the French Foreign Affairs Ministry in Turkey, USAID in Senegal, and a nonprofit organization in China.

He was assistant professor in tropical diseases and public health at Paris V University and Paris VI University and adjunct assistant professor of medicine at George Washington University.

He was also research manager for Hoffman LaRoche and export medical director for Delagrange drug companies in Paris, France.

At Stanford, Dr. Meunier was the director of international corporate affairs and business development for Stanford Hospital and Clinics and the director of the Stanford Health Promotion Network.

Currently, he is the CEO of HealthConnect International, a health-care consulting company based in Silicon Valley, CA, and advisor in the Medscholars Research Fellowships Program at Stanford University School of Medicine.

He is an honorary member of the Brazilian Academy of Medicine; an associate member of the Academy of Medicine, Singapore; a member of the International Academy of Fellows and Associates, Royal College of Physicians and Surgeons of Canada; and a fellow of the Australasian College of Tropical Medicine.

About the Contributing Authors

Michael Hole is an MD/MBA candidate at Stanford's Schools of Medicine and Business with scholarly concentrations in community and international health and development. He has founded and led several organizations that have built schools, clinics, orphanages, agricultural initiatives, and a hospital in Ecuador, Guatemala, Haiti, Malawi, Mexico, and Uganda. His recent research surrounds policy to reduce HIV/AIDS prevalence in sub-Saharan Africa, medical curriculums used to lower infant mortality rates in the developing world, and US policy affecting domestic child trafficking. Prior to medical school, he attended Butler University where he was named the institution's most outstanding student.

Takudzwa Shumba is a Zimbabwean medical student at the Stanford University School of Medicine with a scholarly concentration in health services and policy research. She holds a BS in molecular, cellular and developmental biology and an MPH with a concentration in global health, both from Yale University. She is interested in women's reproductive health, governance and health policy, medical education, and infectious disease. Her recent awards include a Wellesley College M.A. Cartland Shackford Medical Fellowship (2009–2010), Global Health Council's New Investigators in Global Health Fellowship (2010), and an American Association of University Women International Fellowship (2010–2011). She is currently involved in implementation of the NIH/Fogarty Medical Education Partnership Initiative with the University of Zimbabwe College of Health Sciences.

BJ Swanner received his B.A. in Geography with an emphasis in Geographic Information Systems (GIS) from the University of California Los Angeles. He is currently employed as a GIS Manager for Epic Land Solutions. where he leads a team of GIS analysts and geospatial software designers. He is the co-founder of the Fellowship for International Service and Health (FISH), a 501(c)3 organization dedicated to providing medical aid to the underserved and hands on medical experience to undergraduate students. He has also worked with a number of other non-profit organizations focusing on international development and has provided mapping and GIS services around the developing world. He is currently developing a low-cost, unmanned aerial vehicle to gather high-resolution aerial imagery for use in surveying and GIS.

Acknowledgments

We would like to thank the following persons:

Marc Gentilini, MD
Professor emeritus in infectious and tropical diseases,
  Pitié-Salpêtrière Hospital, Paris
Former president of the French Academy of Medicine
Former chair of the French Red Cross
President of the Water Academy

Luis Felippe de Queiros Mattoso, MD
Member of the Brazilian Academy of Medicine
Professor of radiology, "Universidade do Estado de Rio de Janeiro"

Paul Wise, MD, PhD
Richard E. Berhman Professor of Child and Health Society
Center for Health Policy/Center for Primary Care
  and Outcomes Research director
Core faculty member, Stanford University

Oscar Salvatierra, Jr., MD
Professor of surgery and pediatrics, active emeritus
Advising dean, Stanford University Medical Center,
  Stanford University School of
Medicine

George W. Rutherford, MD, AM
Salvatore Pablo Lucia Professor of Epidemiology,
  Preventive Medicine, Pediatrics and History
Vice chair, Department of Epidemiology and Biostatistics
Director, Prevention and Public Health Group,
  Global Health Sciences, University of California San Francisco

B. J. Swanner
Created the design and made all the maps in the book. We thank
  him for his great work. It has been a pleasure working with him.

Zach Wright
We are indebted to Mr. Wright for his efforts to organize
  and facilitate the submission of this book for publication.

Disease and Patient Introduction

In the later part of the 20th century and the early 21st, some historic diseases have gained attention. The ancient calamities of plague, cholera, and yellow fever have struck again, conjuring mental images of desolation.

Other diseases of old, such as tuberculosis and malaria, present new challenges to the medical and scientific world. The mainstays of treatment have begun to fail, and new threats have emerged such as counterfeit drugs. At the individual level, they can result in complications and death. At the collective level, devastating epidemics of these diseases may loom on the horizon if current efforts to eradicate them are not sustainable, as we have witnessed in the past with other illnesses.

New forms of old diseases have been appearing steadily. A new type of meningitis invaded the African continent. It also struck Brazil in 1974, where fortunately it was rapidly controlled by the effectiveness of a well-coordinated vaccination campaign. Dengue fever has also emerged on the public scene, with epidemics sweeping through the West Indies, New Caledonia, Southeast Asia, Paraguay, and Brazil. The hemorrhagic and lethal form of the disease has conquered new territories. Poliomyelitis mass-vaccination campaigns have hit a problematic and ominous hurdle in Afghanistan.

The emergence of "mad cow disease" in Great Britain caused an upheaval in Europe's political and agricultural environment. In Asia, melioidosis has become an increased public health concern and has entered the Western medical world through drug addicts' needles. The treatment of sexually transmitted disease is more challenging than ever because of spreading resistance of germs to multiple antibiotics in developing countries.

Despite the advances of modern medicine, the 20th century has witnessed a double phenomenon. While the risk of contracting infectious diseases has been drastically reduced in the global north, they are still killing millions of people in the global south. Through increased sanitation, better personal and collective hygiene, improved socioeconomic conditions (nutrition and housing in particular), and the emergence of efficient and well-tolerated treatments (mainly in the form of antibiotics and vaccines), developed countries have virtually rid themselves of many disease vectors and causal agents that continue to afflict and threaten the developing world.

Regrettably, only a minority of people live in communicable disease–controlled environments. Most of the world's population tries to survive in precarious conditions.

In the latter part of the 20th century, new viral diseases crossed the north–south divide, causing a new wave of concern for affluent nations. These new diseases are terrifying to the public because (1) the infectious agents do not respect the poverty line and (2) people are more easily exposed to contamination with modern marketplace globalization.

People are also more mobile than ever, and their diseases accompany them. Growing business interest in developing countries of the intertropical zone and the quest for exotic existential experiences by tourists facilitate the extension of tropical diseases.

Two major trends of translocation can be distinguished:

From developed to developing countries: The duration varies from short to long term. Long-term residents include expatriates, exchange students, missionaries, and relief workers. Short-term visitors range from businesspeople to tourists (between 1995 and 2005, growth in travel and tourism reached 60% in Latin America, 75% in Africa, 141% in Southeast Asia and China, 194% in the Pacific, and 235% in the Middle East). This evolution was only temporarily slowed by the global economic crisis and the outbreaks of SARS and swine flu in the first part of the 21st first century.

From developing to developed countries: Migrations occur primarily for economic and political reasons. They are mainly intercontinental. Many people leave less developed areas of Asia, Africa, and South and Central America in pursuit of a better standard of living in the developed nations of Europe, Australia, New Zealand, and North America. But they are intracontinental as well. For example, in Asia, workers are pouring into rapidly developing regions where low-skill jobs are available. It is not uncommon in Kuala Lumpur and other major cities of Malaysia to have gas pumped by Bangladeshis, trash cleared by Indonesians, hotel rooms made up by Filipinos, restaurant meals served by Myanmar nationals, and suit measurements taken by Pakistanis. Because of these migratory trends, tropical and infectious diseases are becoming a growing global concern. In 2005, 191 million people in the world were migrants.

Tropical diseases are important for various other reasons. For example, they are linked to biodiversity and demographic growth. The latter plays an important role in their dissemination and poses many challenges to their control. In many tropical countries one can observe an epidemiologic transition to chronic diseases. These issues are dealt with in textbooks and are not included in this guide, whose main focus is on the diseases themselves. We hope that your understanding of them deepens by using this tool for practical and efficient diagnosis and treatment.

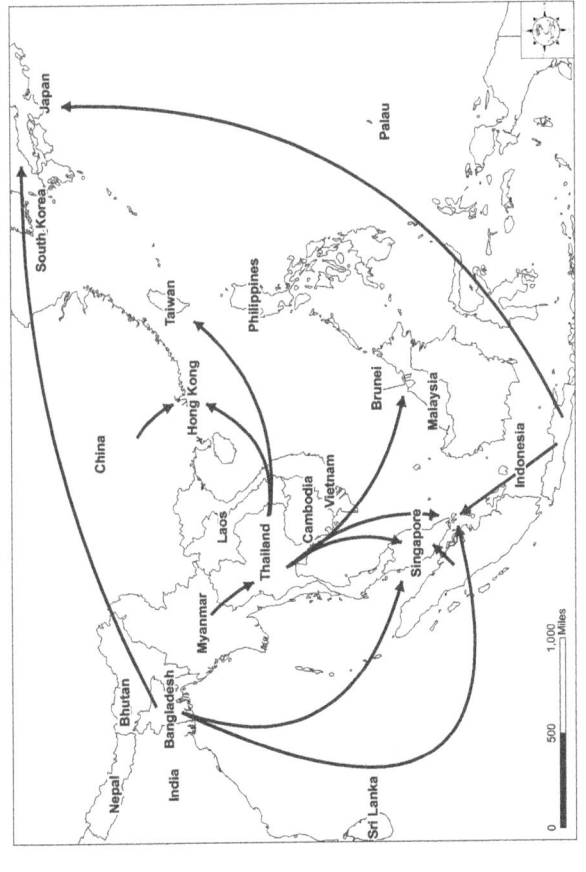

Intra-continental Migration of Workers in Asia

Disease and Patient Introduction

Part 1

Parasitic Diseases

Parasitic diseases are categorized (A) according to the adult or final stage location in the body and (B) as parasitic dead ends and larval diseases.

(A) Adult Parasite Location
- Blood and Lymphatic Systems
- Digestive Tract
- Lungs
- Nails and Hair
- Sexual Organs
- Skin and Integumentary System
- Urinary Tract

(B) Parasitic Dead Ends and Larval Diseases

(A) Adult Parasite Location

Blood and Lymphatic Systems

Filariasis (Lymphatic)

Wuchereria bancrofti, Brugia malayi, Brugia timori

Geographic Distribution

Lymphatic filariasis is a nematodosis endemic to many countries of the intertropical zone, including South and Central America, Africa, Asia, and Oceania. In 2013, according to the WHO, nearly 1.4 billion people in 73 countries worldwide are threatened by lymphatic filariasis. Over 120 million people are infected, with about 40 million disfigured and incapacitated by the disease.

Main Symptoms

Three to 20 months after being bitten by an infected *Culex*, *Aedes*, or *Anopheles* mosquito, symptoms appear in two distinct phases, sometimes with complications.

Acute

Scrotum lymphangitis and funiculitis, orchitis (often followed by a chylous hydrocele), fever (known as Fiji fever), fatigue, sometimes delirium, acute centrifugal lymphangitis (with inflammation of one or more lymphatic vessels) in the limbs or deep in the thorax with intense chest pain, and axillar or inguinal edema can occur. Acute adenitis can be isolated or accompanied with lymphangitis. Secondary bacterial infections with *Streptococcus* are common.

Chronic
Hydrocele, chronic orchiepididymitis, adenopathies, adenolymphocele, varicose lymphatic vessels, elephantiasis, and chyluria can occur.

Complications
Tropical pulmonary eosinophilia is due to *Wuchereria bancrofti* and *Brugia malayi*. Symptoms include paroxysmal cough, dyspnea, malaise, fever, and weight loss.

Treatment
- D.E.C. is a microfilaricide drug, which is partially macrofilaride in the treatment regimens indicated below.
- D.E.C. should not be prescribed during acute bouts of the disease. Treatment should start when acute symptoms have subsided.
- Tolerance warrants close monitoring, but good success rates can be expected.
- For acute periods of lymphangitis, broad-spectrum antibiotics are needed.
- Dosing:
  * D.E.C., 200 mg, po, bid, q12h, for adults and 6 mg/kg/day, po, for children, for 12 days, repeated 10 days later. Another possible regimen is 400 mg/day, po, 3 weeks in a row.
  * To avoid or minimize side effects, dosing should be increased slowly. For adults, start with 1/32 of a 100 mg tab, bid, q12h, then 1/16, bid, q12h, and so on until reaching 2 tabs, bid, q12h. For children the incremental proportion is identical.
- If lymphatic filariasis is diagnosed at the chronic stage, surgery may become necessary but is not always possible.

Preventive Measures
- Use insecticide-treated mosquito netting at night to prevent bites.
- Use insecticides to kill vectors.
- Use repellents containing DEET (15–30%). Be aware that they can only provide transitory protection.
- Treat clothes with insecticides containing permethrin.
- DEC, 500 mg, po, for 2 days, once a month, for adults for a lengthy stay (i.e., several months) in endemic areas.

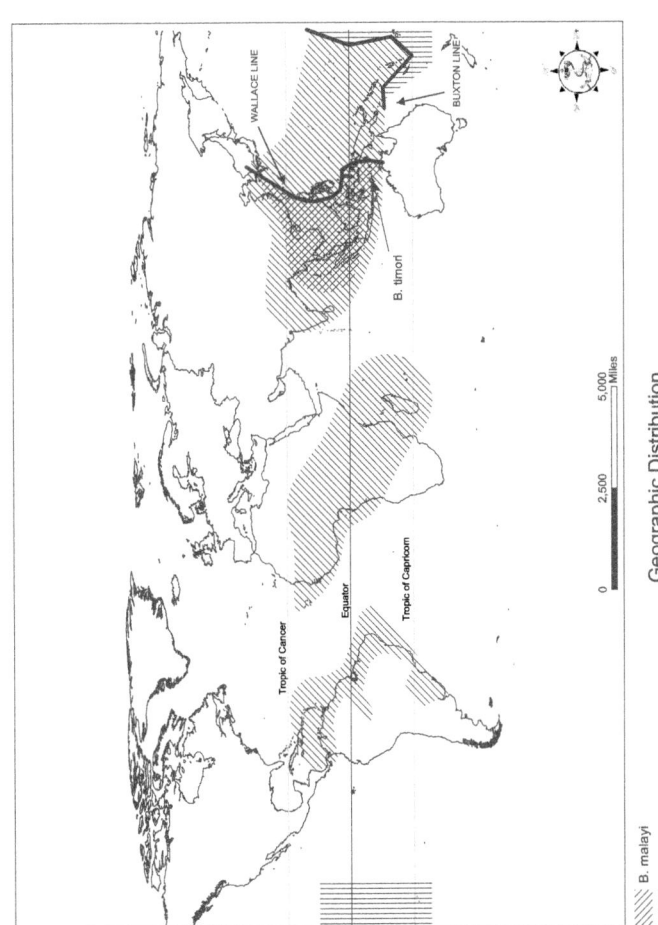

Geographic Distribution of Lymphatic Filariasis

- B. malayi
- W. bancrofti Periodic Nocturnal
- W. bancrofti Sub-Periodic Diurnal

Leishmaniasis (Visceral, or Kala-Azar, or Dum Dum Disease)

Leishmania donovani, L. infantum

Geographic Distribution

Kala-azar is a protozoosis. Foci of the disease have been identified in South America, Africa, the Mediterranean basin, the Middle East, India, and China. Visceral leishmaniasis is one of the most neglected parasitic diseases, and it affects the poorest populations. The disease is also known as Burdwan fever, Sirkari disease, Sahib's disease, kala-dukh, kala-jwar, or

Assam fever. Kala azar is endemic to 76 countries, putting approximately 200 million people at risk for infection. The Drug for Neglected Diseases Initiative estimates that there are 400,000 new cases each year with a mortality of 40,000. According to the WHO in 2013, 90% of all cases of kala azar occur in Bangladesh, Brazil, India, Nepal and Sudan.

Main Symptoms

One to 2 months after indirect infection by a bite of an infected female sand fly (genus *Phlebotomus* in the old world and genus *Lutzomya* in the new world), which sometimes creates a skin ulcer and leaves a scar, the following symptoms often occur: fever, fatigue, pallor, weight loss, hepatomegaly, splenomegaly (kala-azar produces the largest spleen enlargement of all tropical diseases), adenopathy, and diarrhea. Diffuse skin symptoms are present in more than 50% of cases in Sudan and 5–10% in India. Low-grade fever and subacute GI disorders have been described in US military personnel after the Gulf War. Mild forms of kala-azar have been observed in Brazil. Purpura may also appear in some cases. Without treatment, prognosis is poor in most patients.

Treatment

- Antimoniate of meglumine is the drug of choice except for pregnant women, patients with cardiac diseases, and in Northern Bihar, India. Tolerance warrants hospital monitoring. Success rates are high. An equivalent is sodium stibogluconate. Liposomal amphotericin B can also be used.
- Dosing:
  * Antimoniate of meglumine, 20 mg/kg, daily, IM (or slow IV), for adults and children, for 28 days (maximum: 3 g/day).
  * or Sodium stibogluconate, 20 mg/kg daily, IM (or slow IV), for adults and children, for 28 days (maximum: 850 mg/day)
  * Liposomal amphotericin, when available, has the highest therapeutic efficacy and safety profile. The dosing depends on the country, for example, in India and Kenya, 2 mg/kg, IV, on days 1–4 and day 10; and in Brazil, 2 mg/kg, slow IV, for 10 days (cumulated max dose: 6–40 mg/kg)

Preventive Measures

- People are not completely protected from kala-azar with usual netting because *Phlebotomus* sand flies can fly through the holes.
- Use insecticides to kill vectors.

- Use repellents containing DEET (15–30%). Be aware that they can only provide transitory protection.
- Treat clothes with insecticides containing permethrin.

Meiling was a 6-year-old Chinese girl admitted for fatigue, fever, and weight loss. Her clinical exam revealed a poor general condition: height 1.10 m (3.6 ft) and weight 17 kg (37.5 lb), with a 38.4°C (101.1-F) temperature. Her liver and spleen were enlarged and her lymph nodes, diffusely swollen. A complete blood count showed anemia, leukopenia, and thrombopenia. Her leishmaniasis serology came back positive. She was successfully treated with pentavalent antimony (Sb5+).

DID YOU KNOW THAT:
- Fever is the beacon sign of kala-azar (it is characteristically without a pattern and resists every nonspecific treatment).
- Splenomegaly is always present and prominent.
- Adenopathy appears late in the disease.
- Skin lesions are rare in children, unlike in adults (maculae or nodules).
- Without treatment, death is likely.

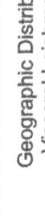

Geographic Distribution of
Visceral Leishmaniasis

Endemic Areas

Malaria (Blackwater Fever)

Plasmodium falciparum, Plasmodium vivax, Plasmodium ovale, Plasmodium malariae

Historical Background

In the 19th and early 20th centuries, malaria became a serious problem for European colonizers in most tropical areas. In West Africa, the disease killed so many English people that the region became known as "the white man's grave."

The malaria parasite was discovered in northern Africa by Alphonse Laveran in 1880. Later, three distinct species were identified: *Plasmodium falciparum*, *Plasmodium vivax*, and *Plasmodium malariae*. In 1898, the mode of transmission in birds was revealed by Ronald Ross, and 2 years later it was described in humans by Battista Grassi. *Plasmodium ovale* was discovered in 1922 by John William Watson Stephens. In 1948, Henry Edward Shortt and Percy Cyril Claude Garnham showed that some stages of the parasite's evolution take place in the liver, where *P. ovale*, *P. vivax*, and *P. malariae* lay dormant. In 1972, Tu Youyou discovered artemisinin in the leaves of *Artemisia annua* (annual wormwood). In the 21st century, it has become the basis for malaria treatment. In 2012, each minute one child (mostly from 6 months to 2 years of age) died of malaria. Two billion people (one-third of Earth's population) live in areas where malaria can be transmitted, and 1 billion carry or have carried the parasite at one time in their lives.

New Problems

The second half of the 20th century saw the emergence of strains of malaria parasites (mainly *P. falciparum*) resistant to chloroquine, which was the most commonly used drug for treatment of the disease. This phenomenon started in Southeast Asia and extended to East and West Africa and simultaneously to South America (mostly in the Amazonian basin).

While resistance spread geographically, it also evolved chemically including to other antimalarial drugs like quinine, sulfadoxine, pyrimethamine, and proguanil.

The discovery of mefloquine at the Walter Reed Institute in the late 20th century offered a glimmer of hope, although drug side effects are a concern, especially in children. Some parasites were found either to be naturally resistant or to mutate to become unaffected by the drug. Presently, the multidrug resistance of *P. falciparum* is progressing slowly but steadily. Some areas, like the borders between Thailand and Burma and Thailand and Cambodia, show high levels of resistance across the board (Fig. 1.1).

This disseminating resistance is of major concern epidemiologically because *P. falciparum* is by far the most common and the only lethal species. New treatment alternatives are urgently needed in order to increase efficiency and decrease the risk of resistance. The current antimalaria strategy recommends the use of combinations either of artemisinin derivatives (artemether + lumefantrine, artesunate-mefloquine, artesunate-amodiaquine, artesunate-sulfadoxine-pyrimethamine) or atovaquone and proguanil. There is some resistance to artemisinin. Although remarkable progress in the fight against the disease has been achieved through global initiatives like "roll back malaria," their long-term sustainability is uncertain. The risk of reinvasion by infected mosquitoes and/or contamination of local mosquitoes by human healthy carriers is constant in malaria-free areas, particularly tropical countries.

Geographic Distribution

Malaria is a protozoosis. In 2012, malaria was endemic to many tropical countries. It was notably absent from the following areas:

Americas: All the cities (except in the Amazon basin) and Antigua and Barbados, Dutch Antilles, Bahamas, Bermuda, Canada, Chile, Cuba, Dominica, United States, Guadeloupe, Grenada, Cayman Islands, Falkland Islands, Virgin Islands, Jamaica, Martinique, Puerto Rico, Saint Lucia, Trinidad and Tobago, Uruguay

Asia: All the cities (except in India) and Brunei, Guam, Hong Kong, Japan, Macao, Maldives, Mongolia, Singapore, Taiwan

Near and Middle East: All the cities and Bahrain, Israel, Jordan, Kuwait, Lebanon, Qatar

Oceania: All the cities and Australia, Fiji, Hawaii, Mariana Islands, Marshall Islands, Micronesia, New Caledonia, New Zealand, Easter Island, French Polynesia, Samoa, Tonga, Tuvalu, Wallis and Futuna, Kimbati, Cook Islands, Western Samoa, Niue, Nauru, Palau

In 2012, Kazakhstan was declared a malaria-free country by the WHO.

P. falciparum is widely spread. *P. vivax* can be found in northern Africa, Asia, and the Middle East. *P. ovale* and *P. malariae* exist in sub-Saharan Africa and Madagascar.

Main Symptoms

The initial phase is identical. The disease then evolves according to each species. The characteristic fever patterns are tertian fever for *P. vivax* and *P. ovale* and quartan fever for *P. malariae*.

Initial phase

Usually, 7–21 days (and up to 9 months for *P. vivax*) after being bitten by an infested female *Anopheles* mosquito (most often at night), fever, chills, sweating, arthralgia, myalgia, cephalgia, malaise, nausea, and sometimes emesis, diarrhea, and abdominal pain appear. A herpetic lesion may emerge on the lips. Icterus occurs with massive infestation. The fever may or may not have a typical pattern.

Typical fever patterns

Tertian fever
P. ovale and *P. vivax*

Fever starts abruptly, with chills, heat sensation, and sweating (in sequence). These symptoms last for about 10 h, ending with the patient experiencing a euphoric state. Bouts of fever happen every other day or every day (double tertian) and can recur up to 2 years after infection.

Quartan fever
P. malariae

Febrile bouts happen on days 1, 4, 7, 10, and so on. This form of malaria can emerge up to 20 years after initial infection.

Complications

Cerebral malaria

P. falciparum

Cerebral malaria has a clinical picture that includes any neurological sign associated with *P. falciparum* infection. Often, cerebral malaria is seen in a febrile comatose patient. Early neurological signs include mental confusion, localized or generalized convulsions, and hypo- or hypertonia. Additional symptoms may include icterus, intense diarrhea and emesis, acute diffuse pain, and renal failure. Other complications can occur, especially pneumonia.

Chronic or subacute malaria

P. vivax, *P. ovale*, and *P. malariae*

Paleness, dyspnea, edema of the lower limbs, heart murmur from anemia, and abdominal protrusion due to splenomegaly may appear. It is more common in children.

Severe malaria

According to the WHO, criteria for severe malaria include the following:

- Decreased consciousness
- Significant weakness such that the person is unable to walk
- Inability to feed
- Two or more convulsions per 24 h
- Hypotension (<70 mm Hg in adults or 50 mm Hg in children)
- Difficulty breathing
- Hypovolemic shock
- Kidney failure or hemoglobinuria
- Hemorrhage or hemoglobin <5 g/dl or hematocrit <15%
- Pulmonary edema
- Hypoglycemia (<2.2 mmol/l or 40 mg/dl)
- Acidosis or lactate levels >5 mmol/l
- Hyperparasitemia ($\geq$4% in the nonimmune poatient and $\geq$20% in the semi-immune patient
- Icterus (clinical or total bilirubin $\geq$50 mcmol/l)

When there is a neurological sign associated with a *P. falciparum* infection, it overlaps with cerebral malaria as defined by French tropical disease specialists.

Treatment

- Cerebral malaria: Intravenous quinine is now the second drug of choice. The first option should be artemether + lumefantrine. Artesunate suppositories can also be used, when necessary
- Prognosis of a coma: The shorter the duration, the better the outcome; but there is no link to parasitemia levels.
- In all forms of malaria, the origin of the disease and the parasite-resistance profile will determine the drug of choice. When the parasite comes from an area of multiple resistance, a combination of drugs is often necessary.

- In case of pregnancy, lactation, immunodepression, or allergies, individual adjustments must be made.
- Dosing
  * Quinine, 1.5–2 g, IV, over 4 h, q8h, for adults, and 25 mg/kg for children, then po, as soon as possible, for 3–10 days. It warrants hospital monitoring.
  * Artesunate, 2.4 mg kg, IV, followed by the same dose at 12 and 24 h, then once daily until the patient is able to take artesunate (2 mg kg/day) po, to complete 7 days.
  * When the IV route is unavailable, artesunate rectal suppositories can be used as follows:

In adults

Table 1.1 Artesunate suppositories: adult doses

In adults	
<40 kg: 10 mg/kg	40–59 kg: 400 mg
60–80 kg: 800 mg	>80 kg: 1,200 mg

In children

Table 1.2 Artesunate suppositories: children doses

In children	
5–8.9 kg: 50 mg	9–19 kg: 100 mg
20–29 kg: 200 mg	30–39 kg: 300 mg

Suppositories come in 50-mg, 100-mg, and 400-mg forms.

* Chloroquine: Children and adults should receive an initial dose of 10 mg/kg, po, followed 6–8 h later by 5 mg/kg, then 5 mg/kg on the following 2 days
* Other drugs:

Table 1.3 Malaria presumptive treatment regimens

Drug	Adult Dose	Pediatric Dose	Precautions
Atovaquone-proguanil Adult tab: 250 mg atovaquone + 100 mg proguanil. Pediatric tab: 62.5 mg atovaquone +25 mg proguanil.	4 tabs, once daily, po, for 3 days	Dose/day, po/3 days: 5–8 kg: 2 tabs 9–10 kg: 3 tabs 11–20 kg: 1 adult tab 21–30 kg: 2 adult tabs 31–40 kg: 3 adult tabs >41 kg: 4 adult tabs	Contraindication: creatinine clearance <30 ml/min Not recommended for people on atovaquone-proguanil prophylaxis Not for children <5 kg, pregnant women, women breast-feeding infants <5 kg
Artemether + lumefantrine 1 tab: 20 mg artemether + 120 mg lumefantrine	3 days/6 doses, po, for adults and children; 2nd dose 8 h after 1st then 1 dose twice/day for 2 days 5–<15 kg: 1 tab/dose 15–<25 kg: 2 tabs/dose 25–<35 kg: 3 tabs/dose ≥35 kg: 4 tabs/dose		Not for people on mefloquine prophylaxis Not for children <5 kg, pregnant women, and women breast-feeding infants weighing <5 kg

- Other oral combinations for treatment:
  - Artesunate + amodiaquine, target dose of 4 mg/kg/day artesunate and 10 mg/kg/day amodiaquine, once a day for 3 days, with a therapeutic dose range of 2–10 mg/kg/day artesunate and 7.5–15 mg/kg/day amodiaquine
  - Artesunate + mefloquine, target dose of 4 mg/kg/day artesunate given once a day for 3 days and 25 mg/kg of mefloquine either split over 2 days as 15 mg/kg and 10 mg/kg or over 3 days as 8.3 mg/kg/day once a day for 3 days. The therapeutic dose range is 2–10 mg/kg/dose/day of artesunate and 7–11 mg/kg/day of mefloquine
  - Artesunate + sulfadoxine-pyrimethamine, target dose of 4 mg/kg/day artesunate given once a day for 3 days and a single administration of 25/1.25 mg/kg sulfadoxine-pyrimethamine on day 1, with a therapeutic dose range of 2–10 mg/kg/day artesunate and 25–70/1.25–3.5 mg/kg sulfadoxine-pyrimethamine
  - Artesunate + tetracycline or doxycycline or clindamycin, artesunate (2 mg/kg once a day) plus tetracycline (4 mg/kg four times a day) or doxycycline (3.5 mg/kg once a day) or clindamycin (10 mg/kg twice a day). Any of these combinations should be given for 7 days.
- Since the map of resistance is constantly evolving, to know which drug(s) to take or recommend and the dosing, call the CDC malaria hotline: 855-856-4713.

Preventive Measures

- Some drugs can be taken prior to or upon entering a malaria endemic country. The drug choice has to take into account the following factors: (1) country of destination and its resistance pattern, (2) length of stay, (3) age, (4) allergies, (5) pregnancy, (6) lactation, (7) immunodepression, and (8) cost.
- Use mosquito nets coated with insecticides.
- Use insecticides to kill vectors.
- Use repellents containing DEET (15–30%). Be aware that they can only provide transitory protection.
- Treat clothes with insecticides containing permethrin.
- Avoid poor housing conditions and swampy areas.
- Since the map of resistance is constantly evolving, to know which drug(s) to take/recommend and the dosing, call the CDC malaria hotline: 855-856-4713.

Peter was a 35-year-old American civil engineer. We received his blood for testing from the neurology department, where he had been referred in a coma from the emergency department of the Versailles hospital near Paris. We only knew that he had been found unconscious in a park where he was picnicking alone. Computed tomographic scans, an electroencephalogram, a spinal tap, and biochemical and toxicological blood tests were not conclusive. An identification search was launched by the police because he was not carrying any particulars. A malaria screening was performed because the last stamp on his passport was from Thailand. From the time he first received medical attention, his passport was found, and his parasitological blood test came back positive for *Plasmodium falciparum*, 12 h had elapsed. He received IV quinine but died the next day.

Table 1.4 Malaria prophylaxis regimens

Drug	Usage	Adult Dose	Pediatric Dose	Precautions
Atovaquone + proguanil	Prophylaxis in all areas	Adult tab: 250 mg atovaquone + 100 mg proguanil hydrochloride; 1 adult tab po, daily	Pediatric tab: 62.5 mg atovaquone + 25 mg proguanil hydrochloride 5–8 kg: 1/2 tab daily >8–10 kg: 3/4 ped tab daily >10–20 kg: 1 ped tab daily >20–30 kg: 2 ped tabs daily >30–40 kg: 3 ped tabs daily >40 kg: 1 adult tab daily	Begin 1–2 days before travel and take at the same time each day and for 7 days after leaving malarious areas. Contraindicated if creatinine clearance <30 ml/min. Take with food or a milky drink. Not for children <5 kg, pregnant women, and women breast-feeding infants weighing <5 kg. Partial tab doses may need to be prepared by a pharmacist.
Chloroquine phosphate	Prophylaxis only in areas with chloroquine-sensitive malaria	300 mg base (500 mg salt) orally, once/week	5 mg/kg base (8.3 mg/kg salt), po, once/week; maximum adult dose 300 mg base	Begin 1–2 weeks before travel, take weekly on the same day of the week and for 4 weeks after leaving malarious areas. May exacerbate psoriasis.
Doxycycline	Prophylaxis in all areas	100 mg po, daily	≥8 years of age: 2.2 mg/kg up to adult dose of 100 mg/day	Begin 1–2 days before travel, take daily at the same time and for 4 weeks after leaving malarious areas. Not for children <8 and pregnant women.
Mefloquine	Prophylaxis in areas with mefloquine-sensitive malaria	Adult tab: 228 mg base (250 mg salt), po, once/week	≤9 kg: 4.6 mg/kg base (5 mg/kg salt), once/week >9–19 kg: 1/4 tab, once/week >19–30 kg: 1/2 tab, once/week >30–45 kg: 3/4 tab, once/week >45 kg: 1 tab, once/week	Begin ≥2 weeks before travel to malarious areas. Take weekly on the same day of the week and for 4 weeks after leaving malarious areas. Contraindicated in people (1) allergic to mefloquine or related compounds (quinine, quinidine); (2) with active depression, a recent history of depression, generalized anxiety disorder, psychosis, schizophrenia, other major psychiatric disorders; or (3) seizures. Not recommended for persons with cardiac conduction abnormalities.

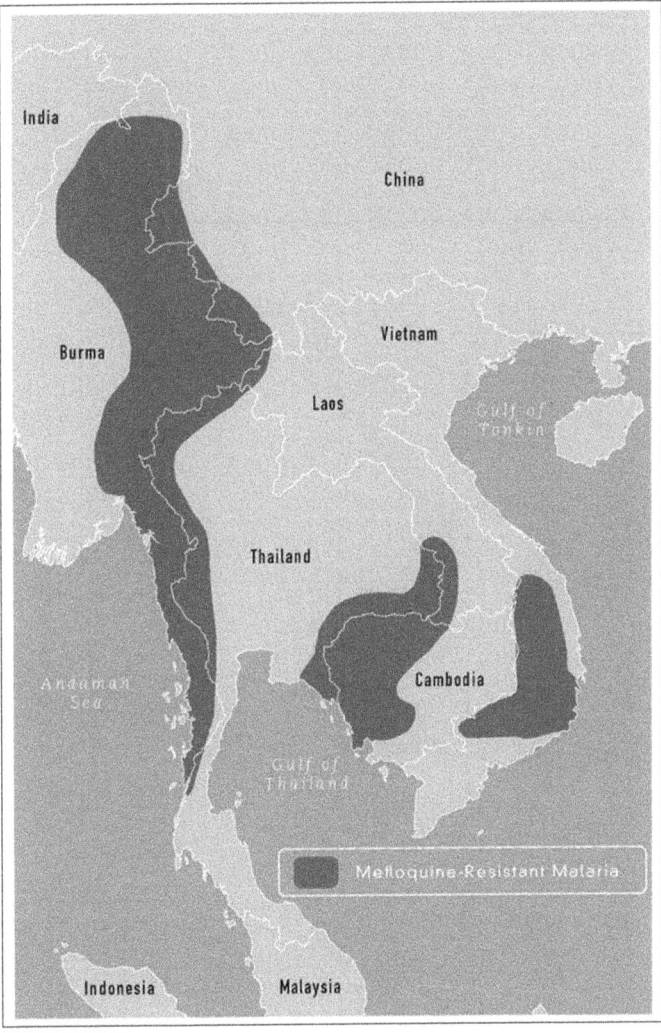

Figure 1.1 Mefloquine-resistant areas in Southeast Asia (from CDC).

DID YOU KNOW THAT:

- When living in a malaria endemic area and opting for "presumptive treatment" as a prophylactic scheme, take a full malaria treatment course at any early sign or symptom of malaria (fever with nausea, even muscle ache, joint pain, etc.) The drug of choice and dosing are the same as for normal treatment.
- Always adapt the curative or prophylactic treatment to the area of residence or destination (i.e., the drug regimen must be effective against resistant strains).
- Coma can be the first neurological symptom of cerebral malaria.

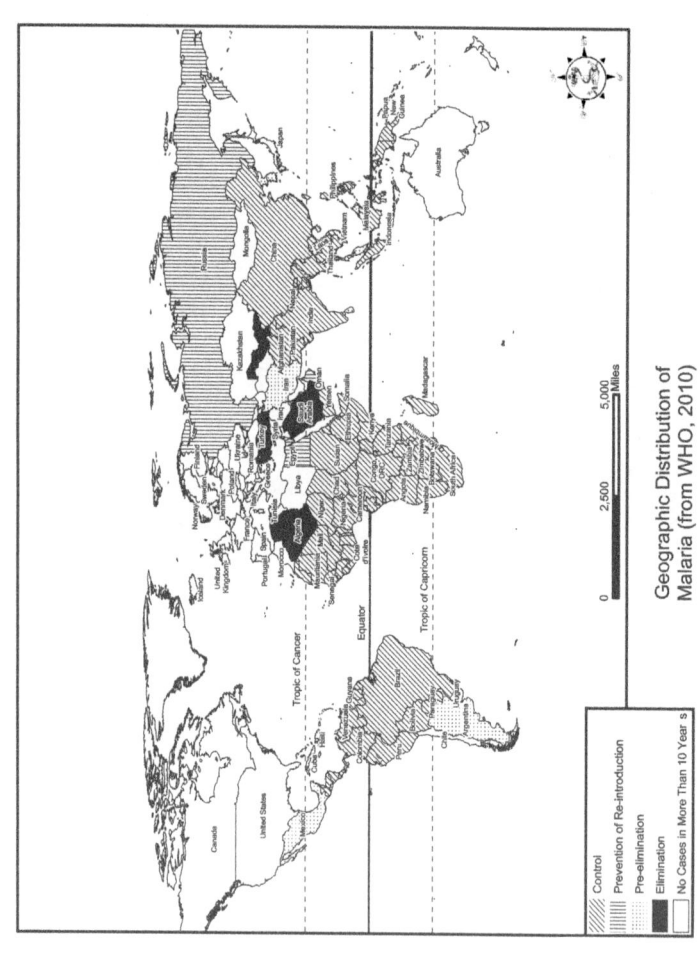

Trypanosomiasis (African, or Sleeping Sickness)

Trypanosoma brucei gambiense, Trypanosoma brucei rhodesiense

Historical Background

In 1901, *Trypanosoma gambiense* was first detected in the blood of an English soldier stationed in Gambia. A deadly epidemic broke out in Cameroon between 1924 and 1926 but was brought under control by Eugene Jamot and coworkers. With the multiple eradication campaigns of the 1960s, sleeping sickness became relatively rare in Africa.

Unfortunately, after independence, the disease reemerged as a public health threat because the postcolonial African states found themselves ill-equipped to combat it. Most African nations now rely on international programs sponsored by United Nations agencies to help them fight the disease effectively.

Geographic Distribution

Trypanosomiases are protozooses. Sleeping sickness caused by *T. brucei gambiense* is endemic to West Africa (hyperendemic areas include Cameroon, Gabon, Congo, and the Democratic Republic of Congo), while sleeping sickness induced by *T. brucei rhodesiense* is endemic to East Africa. According to the WHO in 2012, sleeping sickness occured in 36 sub-Saharan Africa countries. The people most exposed were in rural areas and *T. brucei gambiense* accounted for 95% of reported cases. In 2010 there were 7,139 new cases worldwide.

Main Symptoms

Five to 20 days (and sometimes many months) after a bite of an infected glossin or tsetse fly (which sometimes causes a skin ulcer with local adenopathy lasting for a few days), symptoms may appear in two phases:

Generalization

Typical adenopathy, mainly in the neck (in the posterior cervical area = Winterbottom's sign) and supraclavicular area; fever; hepatomegaly; splenomegaly; and trypanide skin lesions (erratic red patches on the torso and roots of the arms and legs) occur. Pruritus is common. Facial edema should evoke the disease.

Cerebral polarization

It occurs weeks to months after disease onset for *T. brucei rhodesiense* and 6 months to several years for *T. brucei gambiense*. Fever is the only persisting symptom from the first phase. The symptoms of this phase are more severe:

- *Neurological*:
  - *Sensory*: Deep hyperesthesia (e.g., when turning a key, known as Kerandel's sign), muscle cramps, paresthesia, neuralgia, or anesthesia
  - *Motor*: Palsy, seizures, tremor, choreic or athetosic movements, cerebellar incoordination, or extrapyramidal hypertonia
- *Psychiatric*: Mood swings, suicidal tendency, instinct perversion, or personality changes

- *Other symptoms*: Cephalgia, sluggishness, thirst disturbances, loss of libido, amenorrhea, sterility, and thyroid insufficiency
- *Final stages*: Patients becomes very confused and fall into a comatose state

Acute and subacute forms of the disease exist with *T. brucei gambiense*. Mild and asymptomatic forms have been described.

Treatment

- *Generalization phase*: Pentamidine is the drug of choice. Its tolerance warrants hospital monitoring, but high success rates can be achieved.
- *Cerebral polarization phase*: Melarsoprol is the drug of choice. Its tolerance warrants strict hospital monitoring. Success rates vary, with often partial efficacy on neurological signs. It can provoke a chemical meningitis, encephalopathy, and polyneuropathy.
- *Dosing*:
  * Pentamidine, 4 mg/kg/2 days, IM, 7–10 injections (maximum: 300 mg/injection and 48 h are needed between each injection), for adults and children
  * Melarsoprol, 3.6 mg/kg, IV, every other day with a series of three injections repeated two or three times and with 15 days between each series.

Preventive Measures

- Wear long sleeves and trousers (avoid blue or dark colors, which attract tsetse flies)
- Use insecticide-treated mosquito nets while napping during the day
- Use insecticides to kill vectors.
- Use repellents containing DEET (15–30%). Be aware that they can only provide transitory protection.
- Treat clothes with insecticides containing permethrin.

Gnossos was a 28-year-old Greek marine officer, bedridden in the emergency department of a Paris hospital. His past medical history revealed travel to the Ivory Coast 6 years prior, where he went bush hunting. There, he developed a few febrile bouts, which were treated with chloroquine. On his way back to Greece, he noticed enlarged lymph nodes on his neck and in his armpits. His family physician discovered an enlarged spleen, but no diagnosis was made and no treatment prescribed. His physical condition remained good for an entire year. Then, he was hospitalized in Athens for exploration of his persistent swollen lymph nodes, and biopsies showed atypical dysplasia.

A year later, he was hospitalized for 3 months in the United States, where no final diagnosis was reached. Although plagued with a skin rash, he generally felt good. Almost a year later, another lymph node biopsy performed in Greece yielded the same result. Gnossos then began to complain of fatigue with difficulty concentrating. At this point, he had also lost control of urination and defecation. A neurological checkup was performed, and steroids were prescribed. He fell gravely ill, and in the emergency department his bone marrow biopsy revealed *Trypanosoma gambiense*. He was then treated with melarsoprol, and his symptoms, with the exception of urinary incontinence, disappeared.

DID YOU KNOW THAT:
- After ruling out malaria, always think of trypanosomiasis when a patient coming from Africa presents with fever, especially when she or he comes from a hyperendemic area.
- Look for *T. gambiense* and *rhodesiense* in the blood, using triple centrifugation in particular, during the generalization phase.
- During the generalization phase, drugs eliminate all symptoms and have lesser side effects than during the cerebral polarization phase.

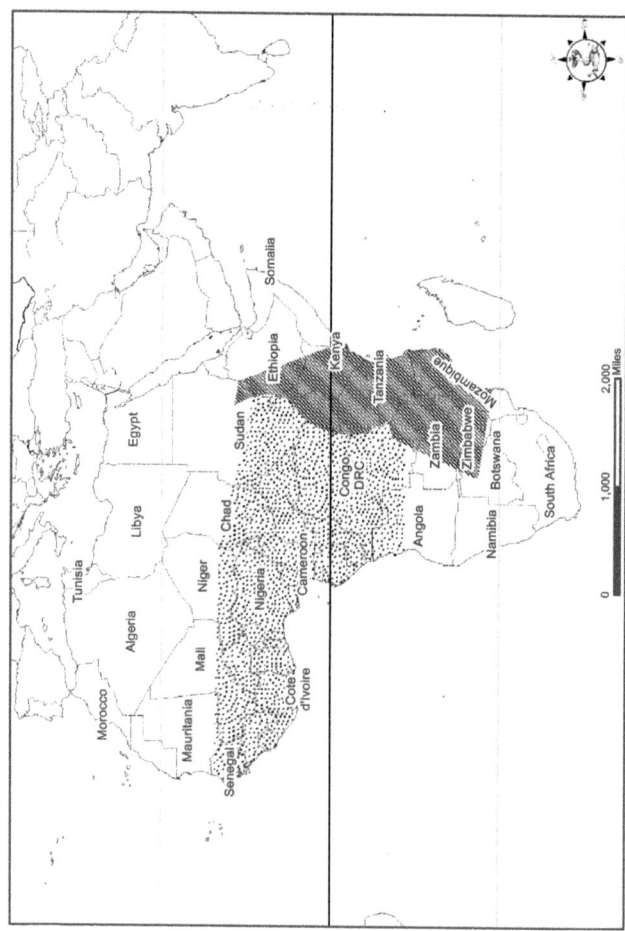

Geographic Distribution of
African Trypanosomiasis

▓ T. b. gambiense
▓ T. b. rhodesiense

Trypanosomiasis (American, or Chagas Disease)

Trypanosoma cruzi

Historical Background

In 1909, Carlos Chagas isolated *Trypanosoma cruzi*, a parasite he named to pay tribute to his mentor, Oswaldo Cruz. Later, he discovered the prominent aspects of the disease with the help of his coworkers, notably Astrogildo Machado and Cesar Guerreiro, who established the parasite serology. Awareness of the disease subsequently increased, and in the early 1930s its extension to other South American countries was proved by various researchers: Salvador Mazza in Argentina, Jose Francisco Torrealba and Felix Pifano in Venezuela, Rodolfo V. Talice in Uruguay, and Amador Neghme in Chile.

Geographic Distribution

Trypanosomiases are protozooses. American trypanosomiasis is endemic to 21 Latin American countries. According to the CDC most recent estimates, approximately 7.6 million people have Chagas disease with a mortality of 10–12,000 each year. In 2009, more than 30 million individuals remained at risk for infection.

Main Symptoms

Five to 12 days after being bitten at night by an infected triatoma (cockroach called "kissing bug" in the United States or "vinchuca", "chupon", "chinchorro", "bandola", or "pito" in Spanish-speaking countries and "chupão" or "barbeiro" in Brazil), 25–45 days after transfusion of tainted blood, or a few days after birth from a contaminated mother, the clinical picture evolves in four phases.

Invasion

In approximately 75% of cases, either palpebral edema with a preauricular adenopathy (Romana's sign) or a skin ulcer (chagoma) where the insect has bitten will appear. All symptoms heal spontaneously.

Acute

Symptoms include fever that can last up to 2 months, diffuse adenopathy, edema of the face and lower limbs persisting for many months, schizotrypanides (red plaques), and GI and respiratory disturbances. In rare cases, meningoencephalitis or tachycardia and myocarditis with acute cardiac failure can lead to death, which occurs in about 10% of Chagas disease cases. In neonates, the clinical picture is similar to the TORCH complex.

Latent

All symptoms of the acute phase completely regress. Most patients will enter the symptom-free latent phase of the disease, which will last from days to years.

Chronic

During the latent phase or (rarely) directly after the acute phase, the chronic phase begins. Some symptoms are more prominent than others depending on the geographical area of infection. Chronic cardiovascular problems such as angina, arrhythmia, cardiac failure, thrombosis, and embolism are frequent in

Brazil and Venezuela. Enlargement of organs (mega syndromes) can also occur. It involves the esophagus, stomach, small and large bowels, or bladder. This is common in Brazil but rare in Chile and Argentina. In some cases, Chagas disease causes chronic encephalopathy.

Treatment

- *Acute phase*: Nifurtimox or benznidazole offers high success rates with good tolerance.
- *Dosing*:

Table 1.5 Drug regimens for the treatment of Chagas disease in acute phase

Drug	Age	Regimen
Benznidazole	<12 years	10 mg/kg/day, po, in two divided doses, q12h, for 60 days
	≥12 years	5–7 mg/kg/day, po, in two divided doses, q12h, for 60 days
Nifurtimox	≤10 years	15–20 mg/kg/day, po, in three divided doses, for 90 days
	11–16 years	12.5–15 mg/kg/day, po, in three divided doses, for 90 days
	≥17 years	8–10 mg/kg/day, po, in three divided doses, for 90 days

- *Chronic phase*: Surgery of dilated organs is sometimes necessary.

Preventive Measures

- Sleep in rooms with clean concrete walls and floors. Triatomas nest in dirt wall holes and come out at night to feed on mammalian blood.
- Control blood donations by screening donors.
- Gentian violet, alone or combined with ascorbic acid and light, inactivates *T. cruzi* in donor blood. Long-term toxicity is an issue.
- Use insecticides in wall and floor crevices.

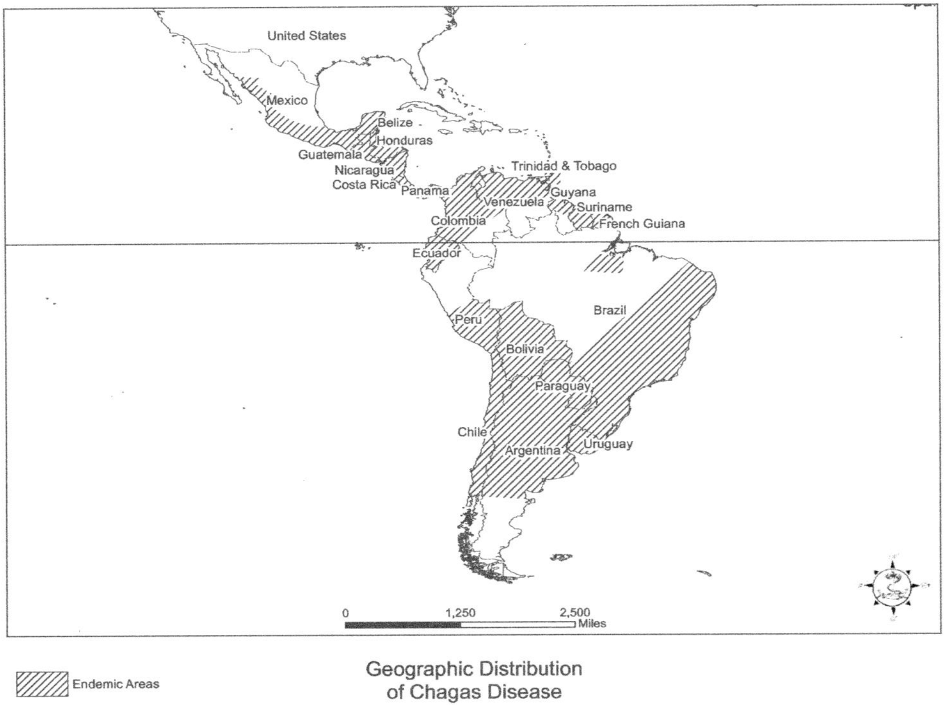

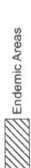

Geographic Distribution
of Chagas Disease

Endemic Areas

Digestive Tract

Amebiasis

Entamoeba histolytica

Historical Background

The amebiasis parasite, as a cause of diarrhea, was first identified in Russia in 1875 by Fedor Loesch. Later, Robert Koch and Stephanos Kartulis were able to describe the role of *Entamoeba histolytica* in some dysenteric syndromes. Heinrich Quincke and Ernst Roos discovered the amebic cyst and subsequently the mode of transmission of the disease. In the 20th century, Peter G. Sargeaunt and coworkers differentiated between invasive and noninvasive forms of *E. histolytica*, leading to today's knowledge of the parasite.

There are three forms of the disease, according to the parasite location: it can (1) invade the small bowel and stay there (*intestinal amebiasis*) or migrate (2) to the liver (*liver amebiasis*) or (3) to the large bowel (*ameboma*). Rarer manifestations with cardiac, pulmonary, or brain involvement can also occur.

Geographic Distribution

Amebiasis is a protozoosis, and it exists almost everywhere in the world. However, it is endemic only to the intertropical zone. According to the WHO, in some areas the disease reaches a prevalence of 50% in the general population. It is estimated to cause more than 100,000 deaths annually.

Intestinal Amebiasis

Main Symptoms

The amebic parasite is transmitted indirectly by the ingestion of contaminated food or water or directly by oro-anal sex with an infected partner. The following symptoms may be experienced days to years after infection: abdominal cramps and pain (mainly in the lower right and left quadrants), tenesmus, diarrhea (with blood and mucus in the stools), bloating, fatigue, and weight loss. There is no or very low grade fever.

Treatment

- Two types of drugs must be used:
  - *First*: Metronidazole or derivatives (such as tinidazole, secnidazole, or ornidazole). The latter are more convenient because they significantly shorten the course of treatment, which results in better compliance. Metronidazole and derivatives have very high success rates.
  - *Second*: Luminal amebicides such as diloxanide furoate, iodoquinol, paromycin, or tiliquinol/tilbroquinol. They destroy the cysts, thereby preventing a resurgence of the disease in the host and stopping transmission to others. Luminal amebicides offer good tolerance and very high success rates.

- Dosing:

Table 1.6 Nitro-imidazole regimens for the treatment of amebiasis

Drug	Dose	Duration
Metronidazole	A: 1.5–2 g/day, po C: 30 mg/kg/day	7–14 days
Tinidazole	A: 1.5–2 g/day, po C: 30 mg/kg/day, po	3–5 days
Ornidazole	A: 1.5 g/day, po C: 30 mg/kg/day, po	5 days
Secnidazole	A: 2 g/day, po C: 30 mg/kg/day, po	1–5 days

A = adults; C = children.

* Iodoquinol, 650 mg, po, tid, q8h, for 20 days for adults; 10–13 mg/kg, po, divided in three doses, q8h (maximum of 2 g/day), for 20 days for children
* or Tilliquinol/tilbroquinol, 1.2 g, po, daily (2 × 300 mg caps, bid, q12h) for 10 days for adults
* or Paromomycin, 8–11 mg/kg, po, tid, q8h, for 7 days for adults; 25–35 mg/kg, for 7 days for children
* or Diloxanide furoate, 500 mg, po, tid, q8h, for 10 days for adults; 7 mg/kg, po, tid, q8h, for 10 days for children

Preventive Measures

In endemic areas

- Avoid ice cubes and ice cream.
- Boil or filter tap water or only drink from encapsulated water bottles.
- Only eat fruits which need to be peeled.
- Avoid salads and uncooked vegetables or wash them with water sterilized with potassium permanganate.

Everywhere
- Systematically wash hands before meals.
- Do not engage in oro-anal sex with casual partners.

Henrik was a 32-year-old singer who had never left Denmark. He was homosexual and had had relations with over 150 partners in the past year.

After experiencing diarrhea and abdominal pain, he decided to visit a physician. His past medical history revealed various STDs. A parasitological stool examination showed cysts of *Entamoeba histolytica*. He was successfully treated with secnidazole and tilbroquinol.

DID YOU KNOW THAT:
- Amebiasis is hyperendemic in men who have sex with men in large cities (e.g., 30–50% in New York City vs. 4% in the general population in 2001).
- The main risk factor for transmission is oro-anal contact in this population.
- Intestinal amebiasis is not clinically different in homosexual males. However, amebic liver abscesses appear to be rarer.

- *E. histolytica* is often associated with other parasites and/or bacteria in homosexuals.
- Shigellosis and salmonellosis are also endemic in this population.
- For homosexual males who do not travel to tropical countries, prevention is based on avoiding anilingus with casual partners.
- Amebiasis is associated with gay bowel syndrome.

Liver Amebiasis

Main Symptoms

Weeks or years after infection, with or without previous symptoms of intestinal amebiasis, the following symptoms often appear: abdominal pain (usually in the right upper quadrant) radiating to the right shoulder (described as feeling like a suspender) and high fever. The severity of the disease warrants hospital monitoring.

Treatment

- Please see above for intestinal amebiasis.
- Surgical open drainage is indicated in patients who fail to respond to conservative methods and those with complicated amebic abscess (e.g., secondary infection or peritonitis with perforation).

Preventive Measures

- Please see above for intestinal amebiasis.

Andrew was a 55-year-old Canadian minister who traveled back and forth to Cameroon. He started to experience fever, cough, and pain in the left upper quadrant of his abdomen. Two weeks later, he sought medical attention and received an unsuccessful antibiotic regimen. The abdominal pain then shifted from the left side to the right upper quadrant. His past medical history did not reveal amebic dysentery. The patient's physical exam showed tenderness and enlargement of the liver. Blood tests revealed hyperleukocytosis, an accelerated erythrocyte sedimentation rate, and a positive amebic serology. He was successfully treated with secnidazole and tilbroquinol.

DID YOU KNOW THAT:

- Fever, abdominal pain, and very often a stay in a tropical area suggest amebic liver abscess.
- Treatment must be started early to prevent rupture of the abscess in the abdominal or pleural cavity.
- Treatment must always include a luminal amebicidal drug to prevent relapse and disease spread.
- Amebic liver abscesses can occur without a previous episode of amebic diarrhea.

Ameboma

Main Symptoms

Years after contamination, constipation and/or an isolated abdominal mass resulting from an ameboma (usually located in the cecum or sigmoid colon) can appear.

Treatment

- Please see above for intestinal amebiasis.
- Surgical ablation is indicated in patients who fail to respond to medications.

Preventive Measures

- Please see above for intestinal amebiasis.

Geographic Extent of Amebiasis

— Northern Extent
--- Southern Extent

Ancylostomiasis (or Hookworm Infection)

Necator americanus, Ancylostoma duodenale

Geographic Distribution

Ancylostomiasis is a nematodosis. It is endemic not only to the intertropical zone but also around the Mediterranean basin and in vast areas of subtemperate Asia. According to the CDC in 2013, an estimated 576–740 million people in the world are infected with hookworm.

Main Symptoms

Walking barefoot on infested soil triggers infection almost immediately. One may experience a rash and pruritus where larvae break through the skin.

Ten to 14 days after penetration of a parasite, a productive cough may appear (mainly in the evening), with odynophagia and odynophonia. After 20–30 days, symptoms evolve into stomach pain, nausea, emesis, diarrhea, and weight loss. Hookworm-induced intestinal blood loss can cause anemia in young children and pregnant women (with pale skin, white nails, dyspnea, tachycardia, and edema of the face, lower limbs, or genitalia). Nail alterations can also occur as a result of iron deficiency.

Treatment

- Mebendazole, or flubendazole, or albendazole have very high success rates with good tolerance.
- Dosing:
  * Mebendazole or flubendazole, 100 mg, po, bid, q12h, for 3 days, for adults and children
  * *or* Albendazole, 400 mg, po, once for adults and 10 mg/kg, once, for children
- Given the efficacy and tolerance of current drugs, systematic treatment of people (particularly children) living in highly endemic areas is recommended every 5–10 years.

Preventive Measures

- Wear proper shoes that cover the skin.
- Do not walk barefoot on grass, especially around swimming pools.
- Avoid unsupervised beaches.

Dieter was a 41-year-old German dentist who, after experiencing a loss of appetite, nausea, occasional vomiting, and heartburn, decided to have his condition evaluated. He mentioned a trip he had taken to Martinique 6 weeks earlier, where he stayed at different hotels and walked barefoot around swimming pools. His parasitological examination showed eggs of *Necator americanus*. He was prescribed albendazole, and his condition resolved.

DID YOU KNOW THAT:
- Some patients never experience the skin symptoms of ancylostomiasis (itching on the feet) that appear immediately after larvae penetrate.

- Anemia, a classical complication of ancylostomiasis, can be seen only in pregnant women and children.
- The differentiation between *Ancylostoma duodenale* and *Necator americanus* species bears no consequence on treatment.
- Prevention of ancylostomiasis is as simple as wearing proper shoes that cover the skin.

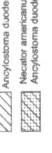

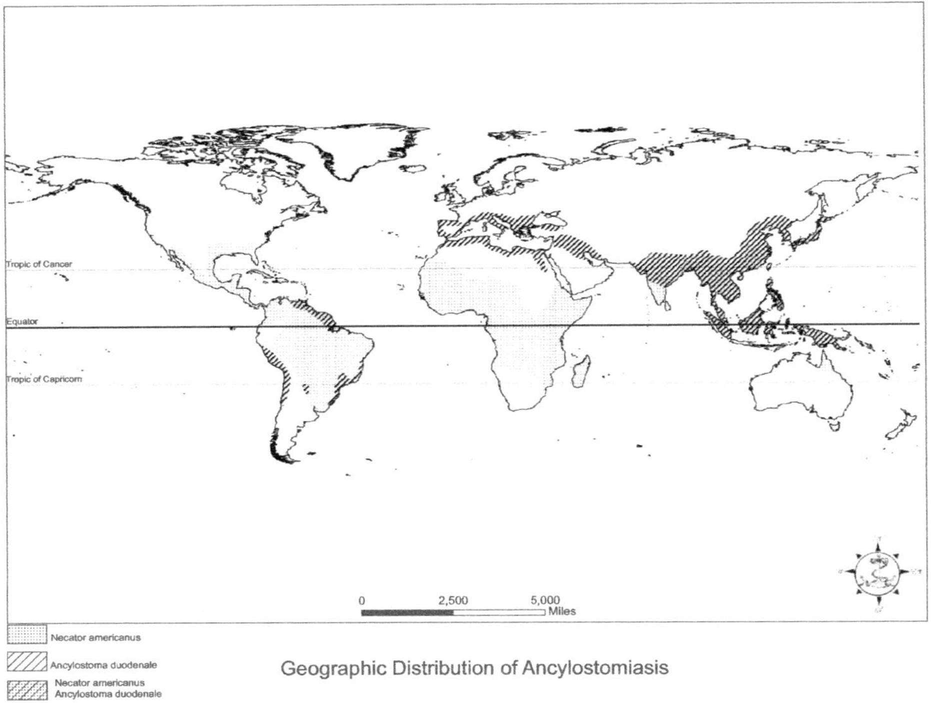
Tropic of Cancer
Equator
Tropic of Capricorn
0
2,500
5,000
Miles
Necator americanus
Ancylostoma duodenale
Necator americanus
Ancylostoma duodenale

Geographic Distribution of Ancylostomiasis

Ascariasis

Ascaris lumbricoides

Geographic Distribution

Ascariasis is a nematodosis that can be found almost anywhere but is more prevalent in the intertropical zone as a result of hygienic, climatic, socioeconomic, and agricultural factors (such as the use of human feces as fertilizer in far eastern Asia). According to the CDC in 2013, an estimated 807–1,221 million people in the world are infected with *A. lumbricoides*.

Main Symptoms

Approximately 10 days after indirect infection by ingestion of contaminated food or water symptoms may appear. They include a low-grade fever and/or dry cough and Loeffler syndrome (pulmonary infiltrate + eosinophilia). Up to 2 months after contracting the disease, one may experience abdominal pain, nausea, emesis (occasionally containing an adult worm, in heavy infections), and diarrhea. Complications are rare, but an adult parasite may migrate to the liver (causing hepatitis), the gallbladder (causing cholecystitis), or the appendix (causing appendicitis) or even perforate the peritoneum (causing peritonitis). Intestinal obstruction occurs with massive worm infection.

Treatment

- Albendazole, pyrantel, mebendazole, and flubendazole have very high success rates and good tolerance.
- Dosing:
  * Albendazole, 400 mg, once, po, for adults, and 200 mg, once, po, for children
  * *or* Pyrantel, 10 mg/kg, po, once, for adults and children
  * *or* Mebendazole/flubendazole, 100 mg, po, bid, q12h, for 3 days, for adults and children
- Some complications may require surgery.
- Given the efficacy and tolerance of current drugs, systematic treatment of people (particularly children) living in highly endemic areas is recommended every 5–10 years.

Preventive Measures

- Boil or filter tap water or drink only from encapsulated water bottles.
- Only eat fruits which need to be peeled.
- Avoid salads and uncooked vegetables, or wash them with water sterilized with potassium permanganate.
- Systematically wash hands before meals.

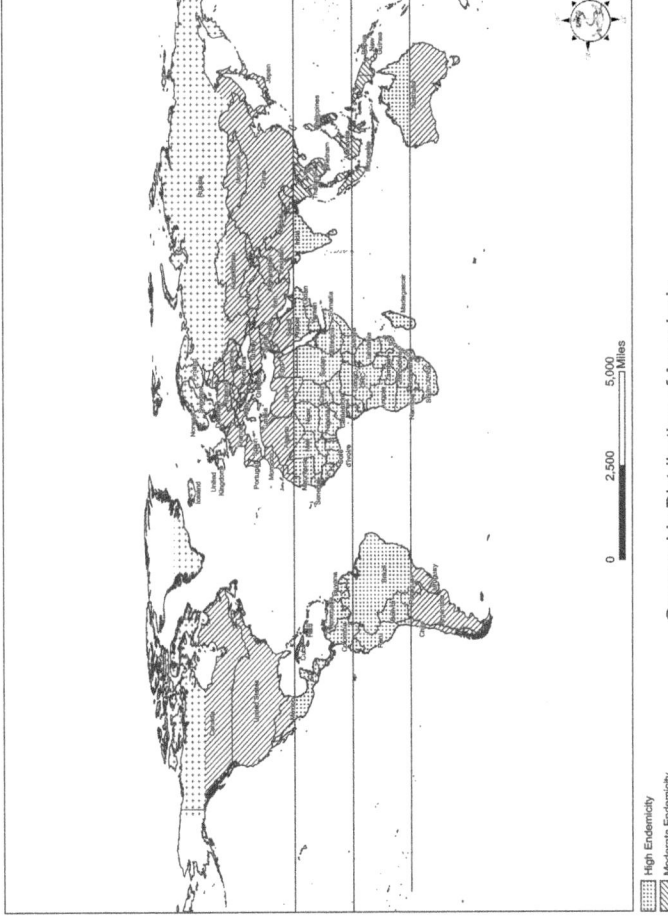

Geographic Distribution of Ascariasis

Balantidiasis (or Balantidiosis)

Balantidium coli

Geographic Distribution

Balantidiasis is a ubiquitous protozoosis, which is more frequent in hot-climate countries like Brazil and Mexico and in the Middle East. Pigs may be the primary parasite reservoir.

Main Symptoms

Transmission occurs by ingesting contaminated water or eating poorly cooked pork sausages. Asymptomatic infections are frequent. Symptoms mimic amebic dysentery with diarrhea (watery, bloody, mucoid), nausea, emesis, abdominal pain, anorexia, weight loss, cephalgia, and dehydration. Chronic forms have been reported. Complications include intestinal hemorrhage or perforation, appendicitis, and liver abscess. Cases of chronic colitis due to *Balantidium coli* have been described.

Treatment

- Tetracyclines, 500 mg, po, qid, for adults and older children for 10 days is very efficient. For infants and children 8 years of age and younger, tetracyclines are contraindicated because they can permanently stain teeth.
- Volume replacement and electrolyte repletion in patients with severe diarrhea.
- Surgery: appendectomy or drainage of a liver abscess, when necessary.

Preventive Measures

- Boil or filter tap water or drink only from encapsulated water bottles.
- Cook pork sausages thoroughly.

Distomatosis (Biliary/Liver or Biliary/Liver Fluke Infection)

Fascioliasis

Fasciola hepatica, *Fasciola gigantica* (in tropical areas)

Geographic Distribution

Cases of fascioliasis have been reported in Africa, Europe, Hawaii, the mainland United States, the West Indies, the Middle East, China, and Siberia. Reports estimate that as many as 2.4–17 million people worldwide may be infected with fascioliasis. Among areas where human fascioliasis is hyperendemic, the Northern Bolivian Altiplano shows the highest prevalence, reaching of up to 72%–100% in some communities.

Main Symptoms

The disease evolves in two phases according to the parasite cycle.

Larval invasion

One to 4 weeks after indirect infection by drinking infested water or eating infested watercress or dandelion, the following symptoms may appear: fever, right upper quadrant or epigastric pain (irradiating upward or backward), allergies (like urticaria or asthma), and moderate icterus. Occasionally, various but very transient neurological symptoms may occur.

Worm maturity

Approximately 3 months after infection, the symptoms often include abdominal pain in the right upper quadrant, hepatomegaly, fever, hepatic colic, angiocholitis bouts, and icterus. The clinical picture may mimic that of a gallbladder lithiasis.

Treatment

- Triclabendazole is efficient but can trigger allergic reactions, abdominal pain, and even hepatic colic when dead flukes are ousted. It should be taken with meals.
- 2-Dehydroemetine can be used. However, its many side effects necessitate strict monitoring in a hospital. High success rates are obtained during the larval invasion phase.
- Dosing:
  * Triclabendazole, 10 mg/kg/day, po, for adults and children, for 1 or 2 days
  * DHE, 1 mg/kg/day, S/C, for 10 days
- Antispasmodics and antihistaminics to control triclabendazole side effects, if needed

Preventive Measures

- Cook aquatic plants.
- Filter or boil drinking water or drink only from encapsulated water bottles.
- Do not eat watercress or dandelion coming from suspect sources.

Ekashai was a 34-year-old Thai business manager of a drug company. He was taken into the emergency ward of a hospital for fever and acute pain in the right upper quadrant of his abdomen. It was found that he had spent the previous month in China. His clinical exam revealed a temperature of 40°C (104°F) and a tender abdominal right side with a slightly enlarged liver. His parasitological stool examination was negative, but the distomatosis serology came back positive. He was successfully treated with triclabendazole.

DID YOU KNOW THAT:

- Fascioliasis symptoms usually appear 1–4 weeks after infection.
- At the larval invasion and worm maturity stages triclabendazole is very efficient.
- At the adult stage, after treatment with triclabendazole, elimination of dead worm fragments can trigger allergic reactions and cause abdominal pain.
- DHE is efficient only at the larval invasion stage.
- During DHE treatment, the following must be monitored: reflexes, blood pressure, and electrocardiogram.
- Serious side effects of DHE include sensitive or motor polyneuritis and myocarditis.
- Prevention of fascioliasis is based on avoiding eating suspicious raw food (all dandelion or watercress) in endemic areas.

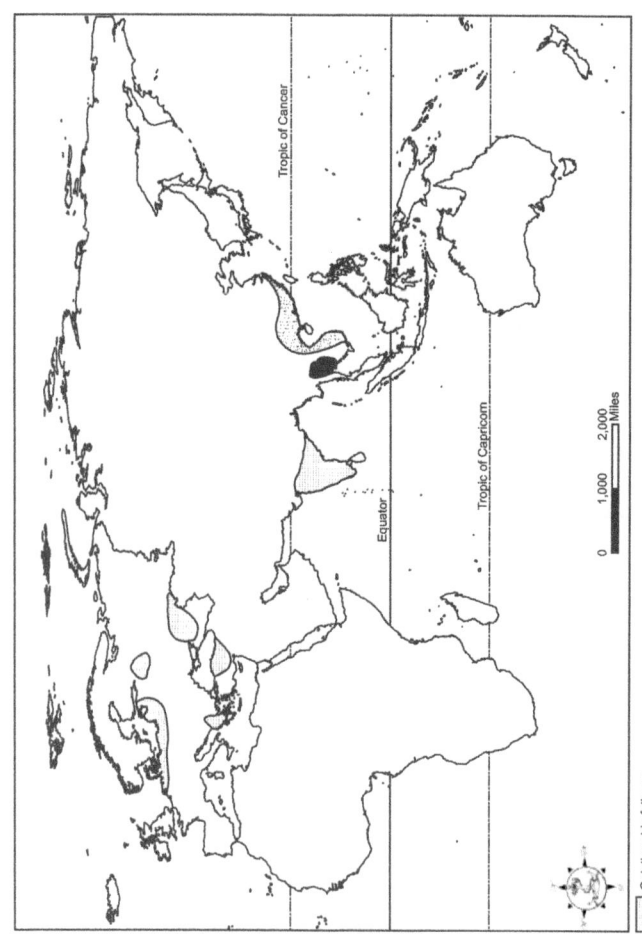

Geographic Distribution of Opisthorchiasis

Opisthorchiasis

Clonorchis sinensis, Opistorchis felineus, Opistorchis viverrini

Geographic Distribution

Clonorchis sinensis can be found only in the Far East (China, Japan, Korea, Taiwan, and the Indochinese peninsula). *Opistorchis felineus* exists in Asia (mainly in India), Russia, and Central Europe. *Opistorchis viverrini* is present in Cambodia, Laos, Thailand and Vietnam. Prevalence rates of 24–90% have been reported for *O. viverrini* from villages in Thailand and 40–80% in Laos. For *C. sinensis* in China it varies from <1 to 57%. In 2013, it is estimated that worldwide over 23 million people are infected with *O. felineus* or *O. viverrini* (including 15 million in China) and 35 million people by *C. sinensis* with 600 million at risk for the latter.

Main Symptoms

The disease is contracted by eating contaminated freshwater fish (either raw or marinated in vinegar). At least 1 month after ingestion, the following symptoms may appear: abdominal pain (usually in the right upper quadrant), diarrhea, constipation, asthenia, allergies (like urticaria and asthma-like dyspnea), icterus, hepatomegaly, hepatic colic, angiocholitis, angiocholecystitis, and fever.

The main complication is liver cirrhosis, which occurs when patients have experienced multiple reinfections and are harboring numerous worms. Occasionally, a worm may migrate into the pancreatic duct and cause pancreatitis. In heavy infections, complications include chronic angiocholitis bouts, recurring icterus, and liver cirrhosis. Death occurs from liver failure, digestive hemorrhage, or concomitant infection. Opisthorchiasis is a risk factor for cholangiocarcinoma, which can develop after 20–30 years of chronic infection.

Treatment

- Praziquantel offers good tolerance and high success rates.
- Dosing:
  * Praziquantel, 75 mg/kg/day, po, divided in three doses, for adults and children, for 1–2 days

Preventive Measures

- Cook all fish

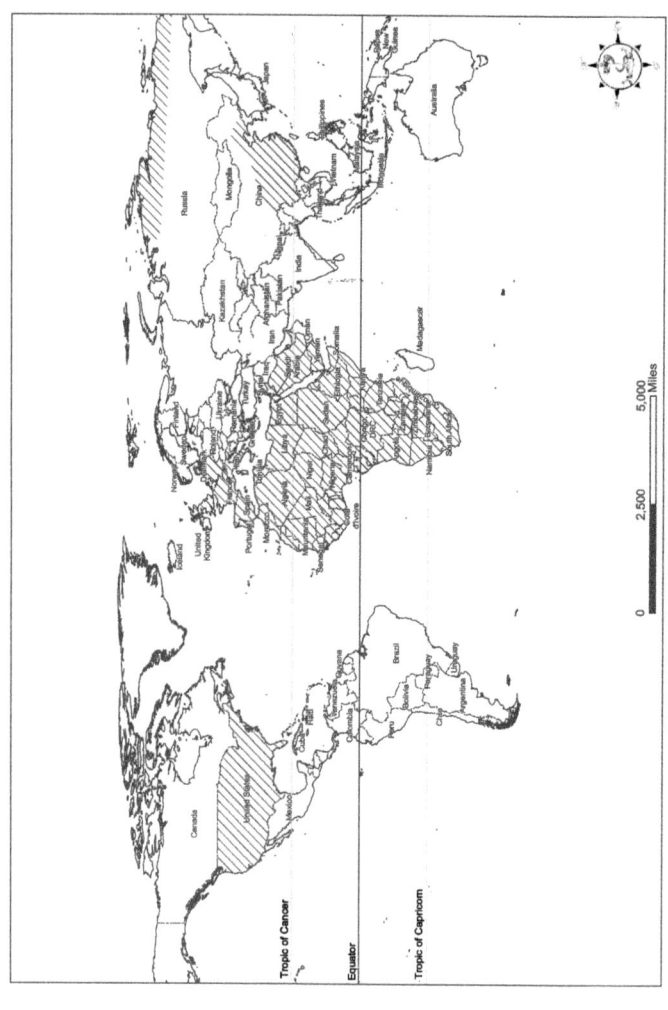

Geographic Distribution of Fascioliasis

Distomatosis (Intestinal)

Fasciolopsis burki, Heterophyes heterophyes, Metagonimus yokogawai

Geographic Distribution

Intestinal distomatosis exists almost everywhere in the world. However, it is more frequent in the intertropical zone, particularly in Asia (China and Vietnam for *F. burki*, and Southeast Asia, Japan, Korea and India for *M. yokogawai*. *H. heterophyes* can be found in the Far East and also in Egypt, Tunisia, and Peru

Main Symptoms

Ingestion of the following contaminated food is the means of contamination:

- *F. burki*: water chestnut (*Trapa natans*), bamboo shoots, caltrops
- *Metagonimus yokogawai* and *Heterophyes heterophyes*: raw fish or fish marinated in vinegar and contaminated water

Infection by a few worms does not cause any disturbances. However, when hundreds of them inhabit the small bowel, symptoms will appear. Two to 3 months following infection, one may experience watery, yellowish diarrhea (5–10 bowel movements per day) and abdominal pain. In chronic cases, weight loss, asthenia, and carential edema of the face and lower extremities are common. Cardiac and neurological complications (egg emboli in the brain) may occur with *H. heterophyes*. Myocarditis can cause sudden death.

Treatment

- Praziquantel is the drug of choice, offering good success rates and tolerance.
- Dosing:
  * Praziquantel, po, 40 mg/kg, once, for adults and children

Preventive Measures

- Filter or boil drinking water or drink only from encapsulated water bottles.
- Cook aquatic plants.
- Cook fish.

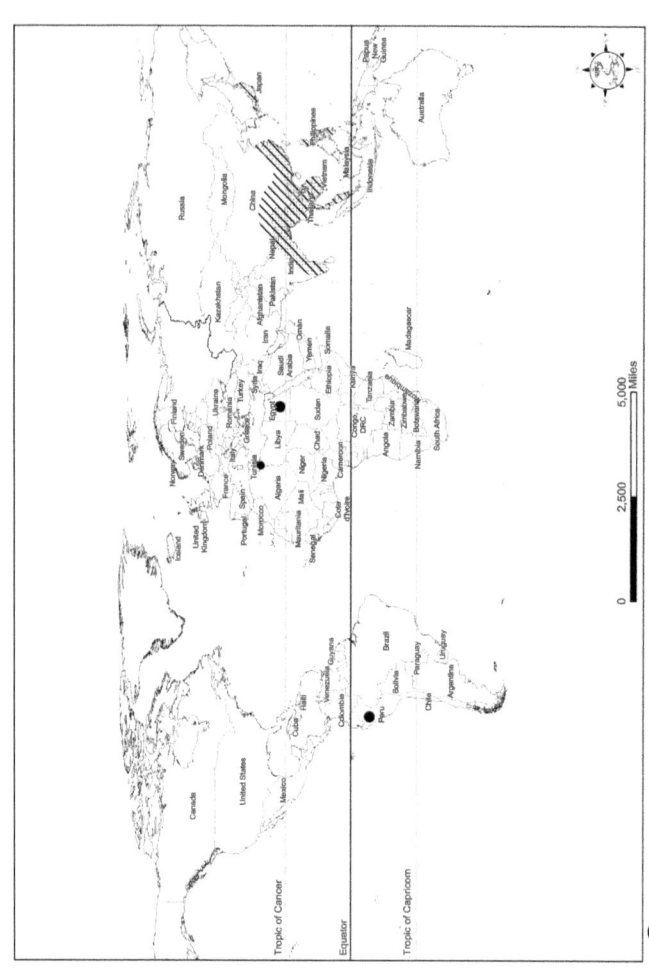

Giardiasis (Beaver Fever)

Giardia lamblia (or G. duodenalis or G. intestinalis)

Historical Background

Many outbreaks of giardiasis have gained media attention in the United States and Europe. With the focus shifting to more deadly infections, the disease has faded into the background. It is a public health concern in developing countries. According to the CDC in 2012, giardia infected nearly 2% of adults and 6% to 8% of children in developed countries, whereas approximately 33% of people in developing countries have had giardiasis.

Geographic Distribution

Giardia is a protozoan that can be found almost everywhere; however, it is highly endemic to the intertropical zone because of local climatic, hygienic, and socioeconomic conditions.

Main Symptoms

From days to years after indirect infection by ingestion of soiled food or water or direct contamination by oro-anal sex with an infected partner, the following symptoms may appear: abdominal pain, diarrhea or soft stools, flatulence, eructation, pyrosis, burning sensation when defecating, nausea, and anorexia. In children it can cause a malabsorption syndrome, leading to stunted growth. In immunocompromised people giardiasis can be deadly. Immunosuppression and male homosexuality are risk factors.

Treatment

- Intakes of metronidazole or derivatives 2 weeks apart treat giardiasis effectively, with rare side effects. All members of the same household must be treated to ensure eradication of the parasite in the close environment, particularly if there is contact with pregnant women or immunocompromised individuals.
- Dosing:
  * Metronidazole, 750 mg (250 mg, tid, q8h), po, daily for adults and 25 mg/kg, po, daily for children (divided in three doses, q8h), both for 5 days
  * *or* Tinidazole, 2 g/day, po, for adults and 50 mg/kg, po, for children, both once
  * *or* Albendazole, 400 mg, once a day, po, for adults, for 5 days, if nitroimidazoles are contraindicated

Preventive Measures

In endemic areas

- Avoid ice cubes and ice cream.
- Boil or filter tap water or drink only from encapsulated water bottles.
- Only eat fruits which need to be peeled.
- Avoid salads and uncooked vegetables, or wash them with water sterilized with potassium permanganate.

Everywhere
- Systematically wash hands before meals.
- Do not engage in oro-anal sex with casual partners.

Craig was a 33-year-old Canadian traveling in Vietnam. After experiencing bloating, gas, and soft stools, he decided to seek medical attention. He presented with occasional nausea, burping, heartburn, and alternating diarrhea and constipation. His physical exam was benign, but a parasitological stool examination revealed cysts of *Giardia lamblia*. He was successfully treated with tinidazole.

DID YOU KNOW THAT:
- A parasitological stool examination should be repeated if negative because *G. lamblia* appears only intermittently in the stools.
- For this reason, presumptive treatment based on symptomatology and epidemiology alone is a valid option.
- Treating all household members simultaneously decreases the risk of relapse.
- Prevention is based on fecal hygiene, systematically washing hands prior to eating, and practicing safe sex.

Schistosomiasis (Intestinal)

Schistosoma mansoni, S. japonicum, S. mekongi, S. intercalatum, S. guineensis

Historical Background

Intestinal schistosomiasis originated in Africa. Slaves exported the disease to South America and the West Indies. In 1852, Theodore Bilharz discovered and described *Schistosoma haematobium*. Patrick Manson depicted the eggs of *Schistosoma mansoni* in 1904. During the same year, Fijiro Katsurada found *Schistosoma japonicum* in Japan. *Schistosoma mekongi* was identified in Laos in 1978.

Geographic Distribution

S. mansoni is endemic to Brazil, Africa, and the West Indies. *S. japonicum* and *S. mekongi* are located in the Far East. *S. intercalatum* is endemic to the south of the Democratic Republic of the Congo and *S. guineensis* to the rest of the Democratic Republic of the Congo, the Republic of the Congo, Gabon, Cameroon, the Central African Republic and Angola. According to the WHO, at least 243 million people required treatment for schistosomiasis in 2011 in more than 75 developing countries. In 2013, nearly 800 million are at risk for contracting the disease, which kills an estimated 280,000 individuals annually.

Main Symptoms

Intestinal schistosomiasis can be divided into four phases according to the parasite cycle.

Penetration

Immediately after contact with contaminated water, skin eruption and pruritus may appear and last from a few hours to 2 days. With *S. mansoni*, these symptoms are called *piquina* in Puerto Rico and with *S. japonicum*, *kabure* in Japan.

Invasion

Four days after infection, one may observe allergic reactions such as urticaria with fever, cephalgia, arthralgia, myalgia, transient edemas, cough, dyspnea, and diarrhea. This clinical picture is also known as "safari fever" or "Katayama fever."

Worm maturity

Months after infection, the following symptoms can often be seen: diarrhea, abdominal pain, and rectal pain. Skin symptoms include elevated, nonpruriginous papules around the umbilicus or on the thorax.

Chronic phase

Symptoms and signs appear after years in heavy infections. They include splenomegaly, hepatomegaly, portal hypertension, and cirrhosis.

Complications

Complications can be divided in two categories.

Evolution of the chronic phase

Rupture of esophageal varices, liver failure, and right ventricular failure can occur.

Erratic migrations

Adult worms or their eggs can migrate to the brain (mainly with *S. mansoni* and *S. japonicum*), inducing tumor-like symptoms, transverse myelitis, medulla compression, or seizures.

Treatment

- Oxamniquine (for *S. mansoni*) and praziquantel (for all schistosomal species) offer good efficacy and tolerance.
- Dosing:
  * Oxamniquine, 15–30 mg/kg, po, once for adults and 15–20 mg/kg, po, once for children
  * *or* Praziquantel, po, 40–75 mg/kg for one day divided in three doses, for adults and children
- Delay treatment 1–2 months after infection in case of Katayama fever
- Surgery for complications

Preventive Measures

- Avoid freshwater baths in endemic areas (controlled swimming pools and seawater are safe).

Stephen was a 32-year-old Irish chemical engineer who began to experience erratic abdominal pain and irregular bowel movements. He sought medical attention. The history of his disease revealed that 6 months earlier he had gone swimming in a river during a holiday in northeastern Brazil. His parasitological stool examinations showed eggs of *Schistosoma mansoni*. He was successfully treated with praziquantel.

DID YOU KNOW THAT:
- Generally, intestinal schistosomiasis symptoms are minor and appear at least 3 months after contamination from skin contact with infested water.
- Liver complications (cirrhosis and portal hypertension) do not occur in mild infections.
- Treatment is very efficient with few side effects using praziquantel or oxamniquine.
- Prevention is based on avoiding skin contact with freshwater in uncontrolled endemic areas.

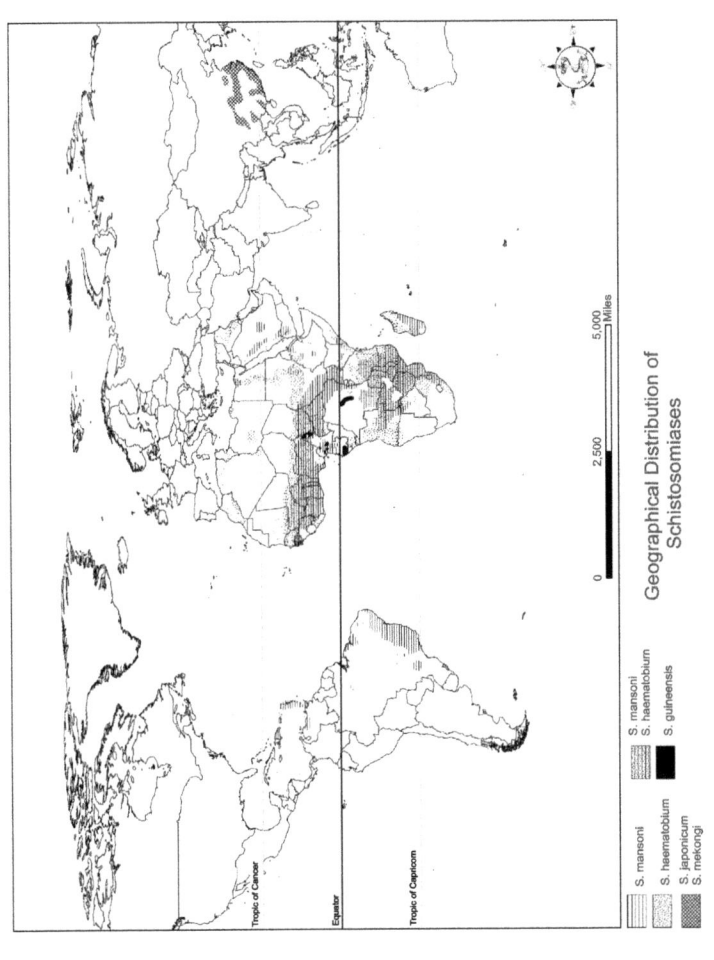

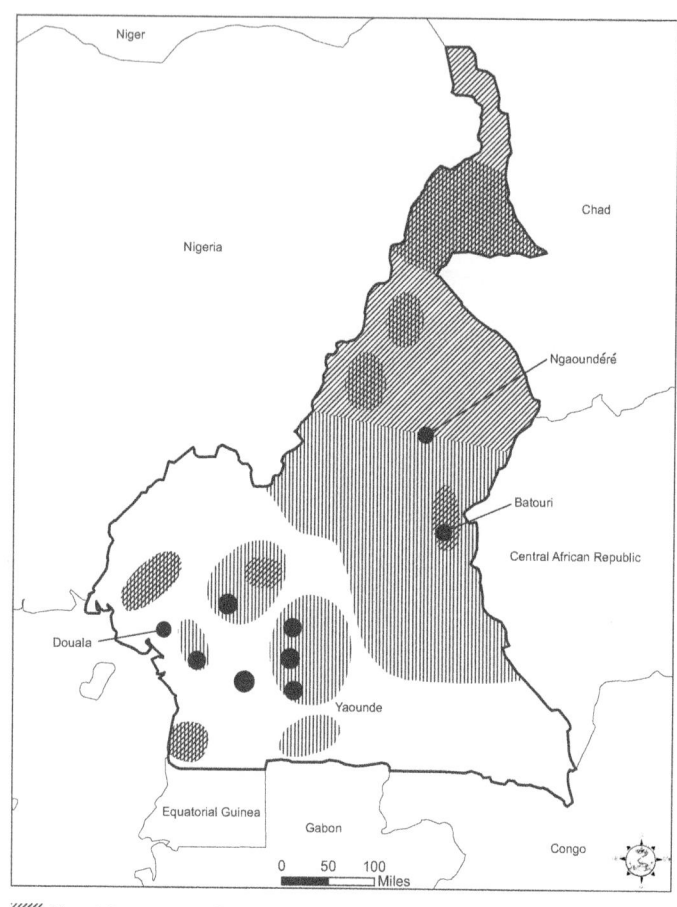

S haematobium
S mansoni
S intercalatum

Geographic Distribution of Schistosomiases in Cameroon

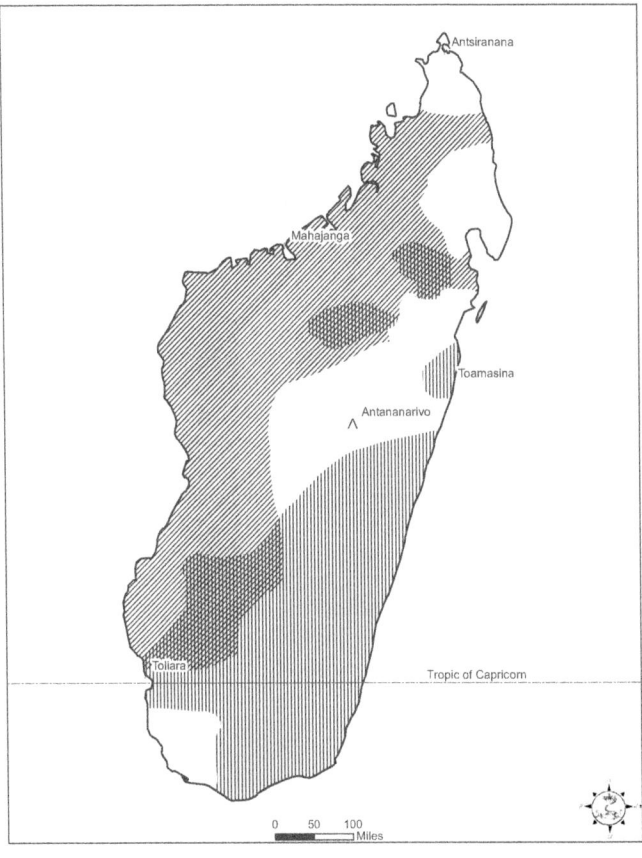

S. haematobium
S. mansoni

Geographic Distribution of Schistosomiases in Madagascar

Strongyloidiasis

Strongyloides stercoralis

Geographic Distribution

Strongyloidiasis is a nematodosis. Its geographic distribution is very similar to that of ancylostomiasis. It is endemic mainly to the intertropical zone. According to the WHO in 2013, an estimated 30–100 million people are infected with the disease worldwide. Precise data on prevalence are unknown in endemic countries.

Main Symptoms

Skin eruption and pruritus (localized to the feet, where the larvae penetrate) appear almost simultaneously with infection. A few days later, a cough, asthma-like dyspnea, and rhinorrhea may occur. About 1 month after infection, many patients experience gastralgia or abdominal pain and diarrhea (or bouts of diarrhea alternating with constipation). Other symptoms include larva currens, a rare skin manifestation consisting of a transient red line stemming from the anus, on the waist or on the torso. Symptoms due to strongyloidiasis can appear many years after contamination. Some British soldiers stationed in Asia during World War II presented symptoms of the disease up to 30 years after their exposure. In organ-transplanted/immunodepressed patients or patients undergoing therapy including corticosteroids (≥1 mg/kg and ≥1 month), hyperinfection can occur. Larvae multiply rapidly and migrate to the brain. This form of the disease is associated with a high risk of mortality. Exceptionally larvae may infect a host via the oral cavity. Transmammary transmission is possible.

Treatment

- Ivermectin is well tolerated and has high success rates.
- Dosing:
  * Ivermectin, 200 µg/kg, po, once for adults and children. It should be repeated the next day in massive infections.
- In hyperinfections, treatment can be prolonged for days. Sometimes the S/C form of ivermectin must be used for faster and better results.
- Given the efficacy and tolerance of ivermectin, systematic treatment of people (particularly children) living in highly endemic areas is recommended every 5–10 years except where strongyloidiasis and lymphatic filariasis and/or loiasis can be found simultaneously.

Preventive Measures

- Wear proper shoes that cover the skin.
- Do not walk barefoot on grass, especially around swimming pools.
- Avoid unsupervised beaches.
- Treat risk patients presumptively with ivermectin before any immunosuppressive event (organ transplant, immunosuppressive therapy, corticosteroid therapy).

Rupert was a retired 65-year-old Dutch engineer who began to experience cyclical itchy skin lesions on his chest every 2–3 h. Occasionally, he had heartburn, bloating, gas, diarrhea, and abdominal cramps. His past history disclosed a trip to Malaysia 20 years earlier. A complete blood count revealed eosinophilia. The parasitological stool exam (including a Baermann concentration method) showed larvae of *Strongyloides stercoralis*. He was successfully treated with ivermectin.

DID YOU KNOW THAT:
- Strongyloidiasis is endemic to the intertropical zone.
- The main skin symptom is a larva currens syndrome which is pathognomonic of strongyloidiasis, occurring mainly on the buttocks, lower back, and sometimes the abdomen or chest.
- The cycle of *S. stercoralis* both perpetuates the contamination through autoinfection and is responsible for the very late appearance of symptoms in rare cases.
- Prevention is based on wearing shoes that cover the skin.

Geographic Distribution of Strongyloidiasis

Trichuriasis (Whipworm Infection)

Trichuris trichiura

Geographic Distribution

Trichuriasis is a nematodosis found almost everywhere but more prevalently in the intertropical zone due to hygienic, climatic, socioeconomic, and agricultural factors (such as the use of human feces as fertilizer in far eastern Asia). Its geographic distribution and prevalence are very similar to that of ascariasis (please see the map, page 31)

Main Symptoms

The mode of contamination is the same as that for ascariasis. Symptoms appear mainly in children and frequently when a patient's worm load is heavy, as a result of multiple reinfections. Abdominal pain, diarrhea (with mucus and blood in the stools), tenesmus, and rectal prolapse may occur.

Treatment

- Mebendazole or flubendazole provides very high success rates with good tolerance. Albendazole is a good alternative.
- Dosing:
  * Mebendazole or flubendazole, 100 mg, po, bid, q12h, for 3 days for adults and children
  * Albendazole, 400 mg, po, once for adults; 200 mg, po, once for children under 2 years of age.
- Given the efficacy and tolerance of current drugs, systematic treatment of people (particularly children) living in highly endemic areas is recommended every 5–10 years.

Preventive Measures

- Boil or filter tap water or drink only from encapsulated water bottles.
- Only eat fruits which need to be peeled.
- Avoid salads and uncooked vegetables, or wash them with water sterilized with potassium permanganate.
- Systematically wash hands before meals.

Lungs

Paragonimiasis (or Lung Fluke Infection)

In Asia: *Paragonimus westermani*, *Paragonimus heterotremus*, *Paragonimus miyazakii*, *Paragonimus skrjabini*
   In Africa: *Paragonimus africanus*, *Paragonimus uterobilateralis*
   In America: *Paragonimus hellicotti*, *Paragonimus rudis*

Geographic Distribution

Paragonimiasis is a distomatosis that can be found in many countries, but it is more frequent in Asia (Indonesia, Japan, Korea, China, the Philippines, and Laos).

In 2013, it is estimated that 20 million people are infected by paragonimiasis worldwide, and more than 290 millions are at risk for contracting the disease.

Main Symptoms

One month to 2 years after indirect infection by eating contaminated raw crabs, shrimps, or crayfish, symptoms appear including cough, hemoptysis, chest pain, and a low-grade fever. It can mimic TB.

The disease slowly progresses to chronic respiratory and right cardiac failure. Erratic locations of the worm are common in the abdominal muscles, peritoneum, liver, urogenital tract, and mainly brain (causing meningitis, seizures, paralysis, visual deficiencies, and altered consciousness).

Treatment

- Praziquantel is efficient and well tolerated.
- Dosing:
  * Praziquantel, 75 mg/kg/day, divided in three doses, po, for 2–3 days for adults and children

Preventive Measures

- Cook crabs, shrimps, or crayfish prior to eating.

Geographic Distribution of Paragonimiasis

● Endemic Areas

Nails and Hair

Candidiasis (or Moniliasis)

Candida albicans

Geographic Distribution

Candidiases and dermatophytoses are mycoses. Hair and nail fungi thrive on the moist and humid air of the intertropical zone.

Main Symptoms

Candida albicans can cause nail lesions, starting at their base, turning the surrounding skin red, and coating it with a whitish film. Nails become yellow only when a secondary bacterial infection occurs.

Treatment

- Cut the damaged nail.
- Itraconazole po + ketoconazole or econazole in cream, lotion, or spray form used locally can effectively treat nail candidiasis and dermaphytosis.
- Dosing, for adults:

Table 1.7 Itraconazole pulse regimens for the treatment of candidiasis onyxis

Site	W 1	W 2, 3, 4	W 5	W 6, 7, 8	W 9
Toenails	Pulse 1 200 mg, po, bid	No treatment	Pulse 2 200 mg, po, bid	No treatment	Pulse 3 200 mg, po, bid
Fingernails	Pulse 1 200 mg, po, bid	No treatment	Pulse 2 200 mg, po, bid		
W = week(s).					

- Dosing for children: 5 mg/kg/day, divided, bid (max: 10 mg/kg/day or 600 mg/day). To be taken with food.
- Because of the length of treatment, itraconazole can be fatally hepatotoxic; therefore, liver enzymes must be monitored on a monthly basis.
- Broad-spectrum antibiotics clear up secondary bacterial infections.

Preventive Measures

- Wear sandals and avoid thick socks.
- Use air conditioning at night.
- Dry hands and feet well.

Dermatophytosis

Caused by fungi of the genera *Microsporum*, *Trichophyton*, and *Epidermophyton*

Main Symptoms

Dermatophytic onyxis affects the outer border of the nails, which progressively become yellow, thick, brittle, and laminated. There is no surrounding inflammation.

Treatment and Prevention

- Same as above for candidiasis.

Pediculosis Capitis (or Head Lice)

Pediculus humanus capitis

Geographic Distribution

Pediculoses are ectoparasitoses. Although head lice are commonly found in all areas of the world, the intertropical zone accounts for the majority of cases because of poor local hygienic and socioeconomic conditions. They are more common in children.

Main Symptoms

A few days after contact with infected people's head wear or scalp, itching begins. It is worse behind the ears and in the occipital area. Bacterial secondary infections (with pus production) frequently appear as a result of scratching, associated with posterior cervical adenopathy. Eczema-like skin lesions can often be found in the nape and on the shoulders.

Treatment

- Permethrin 1% cream rinse has been used successfully. Benzyl alcohol solution is a newer alternative.
- Dosing:
  * Benzyl alcohol lotion, apply to the scalp and hair for 10 min and then rinse it off with water; 7 days later repeat the treatment; not for children younger than 6 months.
- See treatment for scabies (page 81).
- Broad-spectrum antibiotics clear up secondary bacterial infections.

Preventive Measures

- Basic body hygiene.
- Do not wear suspicious head wear.
- Wash all clothing properly.
- Avoid head-to-head (hair-to-hair) contact during all activities.
- Do not share clothing.
- Do not share combs, brushes, or towels.
- Do not lie on beds, couches, pillows, carpets, or stuffed animals that have recently been in contact with an infected person.

Pthiriasis (or Crabs)

Phtirius pubis

Geographic Distribution

Phtiriasis is an ectoparasitosis. Pubic lice are prevalent in the intertropical zone due to poor local hygienic and socioeconomic conditions.

Main Symptoms

A few days after sexual contact with an infected partner, pubic itching occurs. Sometimes, it affects other areas, such as the groin, thighs, chest, axillae, beard, eyebrows, or eyelashes. These involvements help to differentiate from head and body louse infection. Papules may form around bite sites.

Treatment

- Permethrin 1% cream rinse or pyrethrins with piperonyl butoxide shampoo or mousse.
- Apply to the affected areas and wash off after 10 min.
- Treat eyelashes by applying petrolatum jelly up to five times a day, for 5–7 days. Alternatively, recommend physostigmine ophthalmic ointment 0.25%, applied to the lashes four times daily, for 3 consecutive days.
- Treat sexual partner(s).
- Clothing and bed linens must be washed.
- Check for other STDs.

Preventive Measures

- Know the health status of your sex partner(s).
- Practice strict personal hygiene

Tinea Capitis (or Head Ringworm)

Caused by fungi from the genera *Microsporum* and *Trichophyton*

Geographic Distribution

Tineas are mycoses. Tinea capitis is frequently found in the intertropical zone, where the hot and humid climate accelerates fungal growth. Poor hygiene also causes parasites to multiply rapidly.

Main Symptoms

Four forms have been described.

Large plaques

Human

Very contagious, causing school outbreaks in black Africa and Asia. The plaques are microsporic.

Animal

Can be transmitted from animals (mainly dogs and cats) to humans but not from contaminated humans to healthy humans. It occurs predominantly in children. The disease starts with a pink plaque growing and becoming progressively grayish. It is well defined, squamous, and dry. Two or 3 plaques appear secondarily and may merge. Hair is broken 3–4 mm from the base. Healing at puberty without residual alopecia is the rule but only for males.

Small plaques
Only human. Secondary infections may occur. Alopecic plaques are trichophytic, small, ill-defined, numerous, and covered with dandruffs. Healthy and sick hair coexist in the same area.

Favus
Due to *Trichophyton schoenleini*. It has become rare but could be easily found in northern Africa. The disease starts with erythematous maculae, which evolve to gray or yellow cupulas, "smelling like mice," and lying on an inflammatory base. Hair falls, and alopecia is irreversible.

Purulent tineas
Fungi come from the soil and are carried by animals. Therefore, the disease affects mainly breeders. Scalp inflammation is pronounced with elevated, purulent, oozing, and painful plaques covered with pustules called "kerions."

Treatment
- Get rid of head wear.
- Itraconazole po is effective + selenium sulfide or ketoconazole shampoo 2%, which reduces fungal spread.
- Dosing:
  * Itraconazole, 200 mg, po, bid, q12h, for adults, and 5 mg/kg, po, bid, q12h, for children, in one to three pulses, both for 4 or 8 weeks (see candidiasis page 58)

Preventive Measures
- Keep hair, skin, and clothing clean and dry.
- Strict personal hygiene

Sexual Organs

Candidiasis (or Moniliasis)

Candida albicans

Geographic Distribution
Candidiases are mycoses. Although found all over the world, they are more frequent in tropical countries with local climatic conditions conducive to fungal growth (heat and humidity).

Main Symptoms

In women
Burning, pruritus, and redness of the vulva, vagina, and/or cervix. A thick, whitish, odorless, cottage cheese–appearing vaginal discharge is common but can be minimal. Dyspareunia may be reported. Symptoms often begin just before menses.

They are commonly associated with pregnancy, oral contraceptives, or postmenopause. The disease can be sexually transmitted, but most frequently it is not.

In men

Usually no symptoms, but if balanitis is found, the patient should be tested for diabetes.

In men and women, risk factors include heat, moisture, tight clothing, diabetes, broad-spectrum antibiotics, corticosteroids, immunosuppressants, and AIDS.

Treatment

- Miconazole, one 200 mg vaginal suppository, or terconazole, one 80 mg vaginal suppository, both for 3 days, or terconazole, 150 mg, po, once
- For balanitis and recurring vulvo vaginitis itraconazole po or ketoconazole po is necessary
- Dosing:
  * Itraconazole, 200–400 mg/day, administered after the main meal, for adults, for 3 days
  * or Ketoconazole, 200–400 mg, daily, for adults, and 7 mg/kg, daily, for children, both for 14 days
- Treat sexual partner(s), if appropriate
- Check for other STDs, if appropriate

Preventive Measures

- Practice strict personal hygiene.
- Wear loose clothing.
- Use air conditioning.
- Use specific and not broad-spectrum antibiotics, as much as possible.
- Control diabetes.
- Use condoms during sexual activities with a new partner(s).
- Use only water-based lubricants.
- Avoid sharing towels or underclothing.
- Wash before and after intercourse.
- Urinate after intercourse.

Trichomoniasis

Trichomonas vaginalis

Geographic Distribution

Trichomoniasis is a protozoosis common in tropical countries because of poor hygiene and socioeconomic conditions.

Main Symptoms

Trichomoniasis is an STD.

In women

Vaginal, yellowish, foul-smelling (musty) discharge is rare (seen in only 12% of patients). It may be purulent, frothy, or bloody. Vaginal pruritus, burning, or soreness may occur, with inflammation and infection of the urethra, bladder, or Skene's ducts. In rare cases, the cervix and fallopian tubes are involved. Dyspareunia and lower abdominal pain can be experienced. Complications include postcoital bleeding and pelvic inflammatory disease.

In men

Urethritis, rarely accompanied with dysuria, and discharge. Usually, the disease remains dormant. Testicular or lower abdominal pain has been occasionally reported. Exceptional cases of balanitis, cystitis, or prostatitis have been described.

Treatment

- Ornidazole, tinidazole, secnidazole, or nimorazole is very effective. Women are also prescribed metronidazole *or* derivatives intravaginally.
- Dosing:
  * Tinidazole or nimorazole, 2 g, po, once
  * *or* for women, one intravaginal tinidazole ovule, daily, for 3 days
- Treat sexual partner(s).
- Check for other STDs.

Preventive Measures

- Use condoms during sexual intercourse.
- Use only water-based lubricants.
- Avoid sharing towels or underclothing.
- Wash before and after intercourse.
- Urinate after intercourse.

Evelyn was a 28-year-old flight attendant who consulted for "vaginal, musty discharge and itching." Her exam disclosed a frothy, yellowish, and smelly discharge. Direct microscopic examination revealed the presence of flagellated pyriform protozoa identified as *Trichomonas vaginalis*. She was treated successfully with tinidazole.

DID YOU KNOW THAT:

- A microscopic exam should always be requested for abnormal vaginal discharge.
- A presumptive treatment can be started before the lab test result and adjusted later.
- Local treatment alone (without oral medication) can cause relapse.
- The sexual partner(s) should be treated simultaneously.
- Sexual intercourse should be discontinued for 4–5 days post-treatment.
- Alcohol should be avoided with metronidazole and derivatives (they can cause nausea and emesis).
- Other side effects of metronidazole and derivatives include sleepiness (be careful while driving for 24 h after intake).
- Treatment is easy and very efficient, with metronidazole derivatives necessitating a single oral intake.

Skin and Integumentary System

Candidiasis (or Moniliasis)

Candida albicans

Geographic Distribution

Candidiases are mycoses that are found more frequently in the intertropical zone because *C. albicans* thrives in hot and moist environments, conducive to fungal growth.

Main Symptoms

On the skin

A red lesion appears in a fold in the groin (tinea cruris), between the buttocks, under the breasts, at the corner of the mouth, in the axillae, or occasionally between the toes or fingers or in the umbilicus.

In the mouth

The disease is also called "thrush." It appears as a red lesion covered with a white film inside the cheeks, on the back of the tongue, on the gingivae and/or palate, in the pharynx, or in the larynx. The oral cavity and the tongue can also be inflamed. The tongue becomes completely red, loses its taste buds, and occasionally turns black.

Treatment

- *Skin lesions*: Econazole or miconazole in cream, lotion, or spray form, prn
- *Oral lesions*: Use nystatin (suspension) or miconazole (gel)
- Dosing:
  * *Nystatin*: For infants, 2 ml (200,000 units), qid, q6h, in the mouth. Use dropper to place one-half dose on each side and avoid feeding for 5–10 min. For premature and low–birth weight infants, 1 ml, qid, is effective. For children and adults, 4–6 ml (400,000–600,000 units), qid, q6h, in the mouth, one-half dose on each side, keep in the mouth as long as possible before swallowing. Continue treatment 48 h after symptoms have disappeared.
- Gentian violet is very active on thrush. Apply bid, as many days as needed.

Preventive Measures

- Practice strict personal hygiene.
- Sleep in an air-conditioned room.
- Dry skin well after a bath or shower.
- Avoid tight clothing.

Dermatophytosis

Caused by many fungi belonging to the following genera: *Microsporum*, *Trichophyton*, and *Epidermophyton*

Geographic Distribution

Dermatophytoses are mycoses frequent in the intertropical zone with local climatic conditions (heat and moisture) conducive to fungal growth. The most common is *Trichophyton rubrum*.

Main Symptoms

Some of the frequent clinical manifestations of these skin parasites include the following:

- Tinea barbae (*Trichophyton verrucosum*, *Trichophyton mentagrophytes*, *Trichophyton rubrum*, *Trichophyton megninii*) affects the beard, creating alopecia.
- Tinea circinata or tinea corporis (body ringworm) appears as red, scaly skin maculae, bordered by small blisters which grow centrifugally with a red-colored, raised border and a clearer center. The border may look scaly. The eruption may occur on the arms, legs, face, or other exposed body areas.
- Hebra's marginatum eczema emerges as red skin lesions under the axilla, which can become itchy. It is also called "tinea cruris" (jock itch) when it affects often symmetrically the groin skinfolds, sparing the scrotum. The latter's main differential diagnosis is erythrasma, which is a bacterial disease caused by *Corynebacterium minutissimum* not responding to antifungal treatments.
- Tinea pedis (feet ringworm) and tinea manuum cause itching, burning, and stinging in the webs between the toes (athlete's foot) or on the palms of the hands or soles of the feet.
- Tokelau is indigenous to Southeast Asia, Oceania, and Central America. It is similar to a tattoo made of lines forming irregular and parallel circles on the skin.

Treatment

- Econazole spray (or dry powder) is very effective, with ketoconazole or itraconazole po.
- Dosing:
  * Ketoconazole, 200–400 mg/day, for adults, as many days as needed. For children, 3.3–6.6 mg/kg/day
  * Itraconazole, 200–400 mg, daily, for adults, prn
- Ketoconazole can be hepatotoxic, and liver enzymes must be monitored on a monthly basis. The same precaution must be taken for long treatments with itraconazole.
- Broad-spectrum antibiotics are used for secondary bacterial infections.

Preventive Measures

- Practice strict personal hygiene.
- Avoid prolonged exposure to moist and hot milieus (use air conditioning).
- Avoid wearing thick socks and closed shoes.

Dracunculiasis (Guinea Worm Disease, Guinea Worm Infection, or Dracontiasis)

Dracunculus medinensis

Geographic Distribution

Dracunculiasis is a filariasis that used to be endemic to Africa, India, Pakistan, Saudi Arabia, Iran, Israel, some Arab Emirates, and south Syria. After a mass eradication program led by the WHO and the Carter foundation over several years, in 2012 the last countries reporting the 542 cases of dracunculiasis worldwide were Ethiopia, Ghana, Mali, and Sudan with 96% of cases occurring in South Sudan.

Main Symptoms

Nine to 14 months after drinking contaminated water, one experiences the following symptoms: pruritus and a blister at the site where the worm will eventually come out. Without edema, the worm can be felt under the skin. A few days later, fever, asthma-like dyspnea, nausea, and emesis occur. After the blister bursts, the worm slowly leaves the body, in about 4–6 weeks. In approximately 75% of cases, the adult worms are located in the lower limbs. Secondary bacterial infections can occur. Often parasites become stuck inside the body, where they die and calcify. Complications arise if the worm migrates into the face, joints, tongue, neck, shoulders, breast, genitalia, lungs, or peritoneum. Acute medullar compressions by Guinea worms have been described.

Treatment

- Slowly roll the worm around a stick at the exit site (a few centimeters every day).
- Antibiotics are necessary if a secondary infection occurs.
- Nonsteroidal anti-inflammatory drugs help to relieve the pain.
- Tetanus immunization must be updated.

Preventive Measures

- Boil or filter all drinking water or drink only from encapsulated water bottles in endemic areas.

Salif was a 33-year-old Malian living in France and a father of 4 children he had left in his native country. He came to consultation for pain when walking and lower leg swelling. He had gone back to see his children 13 months earlier. The disease had lasted for 1 week, manifested by edema of the left internal malleolus and right calf with bilateral leg pain. Five days after his visit, Salif noted two blisters above the left malleolus and in the lower third of his right calf. Both ruptured, oozing a serous fluid. The next day, two whitish, thread-like worms appeared at these locations. He was successfully treated by rolling the worm on a wooden stick and careful antisepsis of his wounds.

DID YOU KNOW THAT:
- The diagnosis of dracunculiasis is purely clinical.
- Complications are rare:
  - Arthritis caused by migration of the worm locally (which can become purulent if it penetrates the joint space)
  - Other erratic migrations, which are particularly severe in the medulla

- Parasitic dead ends are frequent with calcified worms detected on routine X-rays.
- There is no specific drug treatment for dracunculiasis.
- Prevention is easy by filtering or boiling drinking water.
- If eradicated, dracunculiasis will be the second disease after smallpox that has been successfully eliminated by international efforts.

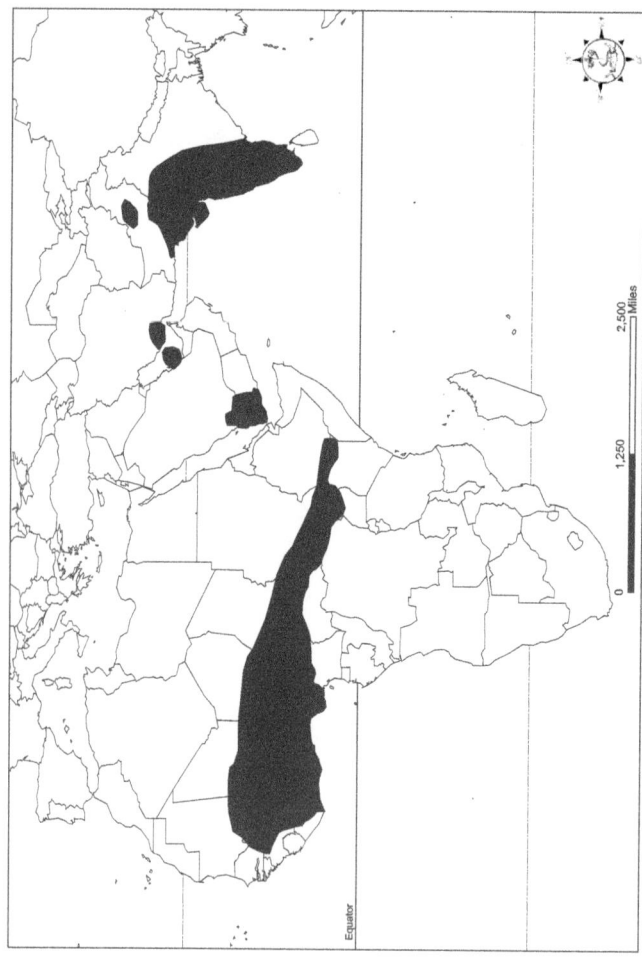

Geographic Distribution of Dracunculiasis (Historically)

Endemic Areas

Leishmaniasis (Cutaneous)

(1) Localized
   In the Old World: *Leishmania tropica, Leishmania major*
   In the New World: *Leishmania brasiliensis guyanensis, Leishmania brasiliensis, Leishmania mexicana mexicana, Leishmania peruviana*
(2) Diffuse
   Leishmania mexicana pifanoi, Leishmania mexicana amazonensis, Leishmania aethiopica

Geographic Distribution

Cutaneous leishmaniasis is endemic to Central and South America, Africa, the Mediterranean basin, and the Middle East. According to the WHO in 2013, 90% of cutaneous leishmaniasis cases occur in Afghanistan, Brazil, Iran, Peru, Saudi Arabia and Syria.

Main Symptoms

(1) Localized
   (a) *Old World*
      The disease is also known as "Aleppo boil," "Baghdad boil," "Biskra button," "Delhi boil," "Jericho boil," "Kandahar sore," "Lahore sore," "Nile boil," or "Oriental sore." Two to 4 months after being bitten by an infested phlebotomine sand fly, the following symptoms appear:

      - Dry form (urban areas)

      One or more skin lesions on the face or limbs, initially a red plaque (a flat or more often raised patch becoming ulcerated and covered with a crust, about 2–3 cm in diameter). The lesions may itch but are never painful, and they usually heal spontaneously within a few months. Scaring leaves non aesthetic marks. Secondary bacterial infections are frequent.

      - Wet form (rural areas)

      It evolves faster and has bigger, more numerous, more ulcerating and more inflammatory lesions than the dry form. It remains pain-free when not complicated by the merging of lesions or secondary bacterial infections. It heals spontaneously in 6–8 months. Scaring is significant. After infection, a temporary immunological protection against the disease is acquired by the patient and will last for years.

      - Sporadic and recurring forms have been described

   (b) *New World*
      The female mosquito vector of the parasite belongs to the genus *Lutzomya*. In the new world bay sore, or *ulcera dos chicleros* as it is sometimes referred to, is a somewhat rare form of cutaneous leishmaniasis. It often affects one ear with lesions, which become chronic. *Uta*, another form of the disease, is mainly found in children and can cause nose and mouth mutilation. *Buba* occurs in Guiana, and *ulcera de Bejuco* in Panama.

(2) Diffuse
Diffuse cutaneous leishmaniasis closely mimics the symptoms of lepromatous leprosy with diffuse papules (large or small, flat or raised, hypopigmented or reddish) and nodules. It is fatal without treatment.

Treatment

Three approaches are possible according to the parasite species, aspect, number and location of lesions, and association with cartilage involvement and/or lymphangitis.

1. No treatment
2. Local treatment: Glucantime
- Dosing:
  * Intralesional glucantime (at the base of the lesion): 1–2 ml, every 48 h, 2–10 times
3. Systemic treatment: Sodium antimony gluconate (SB5+), IV or IM. The former is better tolerated, but both warrant hospital monitoring.
- Dosing:
  * SB5+, 20 mg/kg, IV or IM, until the lesions are healed and for at least 4 weeks, for adults and children
- High success rates can be expected.
- Secondary bacterial infections can be controlled with broad-spectrum antibiotics.
- Update tetanus immunization.

Preventive Measures

- Use insecticides to kill vectors.
- Use repellents containing DEET (15–30%). Be aware that they can only provide transitory protection.
- Treat clothes with insecticides containing permethrin.
- Phlebotomine sand flies can fly through the holes of usual mosquito nets, which renders them ineffective.

Hercules was a 19-year-old Belgian mechanic who was concerned about an ulcer-like skin lesion that had appeared on his right forearm. The symptoms had started about 2 months earlier when he was in French Guiana, with a blister bursting, widening, and deepening progressively. The blister was now covered with a crust and oozing pus. His clinical exam revealed enlarged lymph nodes along the right arm without fever. Hercules mentioned that he had captured a three-toed sloth, which he had handled for several days while traveling along the Maroni River. The liquid under the crust was examined and showed *Leishmania tropica*. It healed completely with erythromycin and local antiseptic care.

DID YOU KNOW THAT:
- The incubation period of cutaneous leishmaniasis can be longer than 4 months.
- The parasitic search in the dermal oozing rarely isolates the leishmaniae, even after an antibiotic treatment.

- Leishmaniasis has various reservoir animals including rodents and the three-toed sloth in French Guiana.
- Serology is not very useful for the diagnosis of cutaneous leishmaniasis because it comes back negative most of the time, particularly in the Old World form of the disease.
- The prognosis is always favorable, with spontaneous healing but often non-aesthetic scars.
- Particularly when the lesion is on the face, intradermal injections of antimonials around the ulceration can stop its progression.

Geographic Distribution of Cutaneous
Leishmaniasis due to L. tropica and L. aethiopica

Endemic Areas

Leishmaniasis (Mucocutaneous)

Leishmania braziliensis braziliensis in the Amazon basin
L. panamensis
L. donovanii in Sudan
L. tropica, L. major in northern Africa

Geographic Distribution

In Latin America mucocutaneous leishmaniasis is endemic from Costa Rica to Argentina. It is also present in Africa (in Sudan and Chad). According to the WHO in 2013, 90% of mucocutaneous leishmaniasis occurs in Bolivia, Brazil and Peru.

Main Symptoms

Two to 4 months after a bite by an infected phlebotomine sand fly, a skin ulcer appears where the insect has bitten. The disease then spreads to other parts of the skin or to mucous membranes, after the first lesion has healed completely. Up to 30 years later, the disease, also called *espundia*, can affect the cartilage of the nose, mouth, esophagus, and larynx as well as soft tissues, which often get secondarily infected. The lesions are extremely painful and cause mutilation, with death occurring at advanced stages due to pneumonia and malnutrition.

Treatment

- Liposomal amphotericin B is the drug of choice, although its low tolerance warrants hospital monitoring.
- Dosing:
    * Amphotericin B, total dose 25–50 mg/kg, IV, for adults, and 1–1.4 mg/kg/day, IV, for children, until slit-skin smears are negative and for at least 4 weeks
- Broad-spectrum antibiotics are used for secondary bacterial infections.
- Update tetanus immunization.

Preventive Measures

- Use insecticides to kill vectors.
- Use repellents containing DEET (15–30%). Be aware that they can only provide transitory protection.
- Treat clothes with insecticides containing permethrin.
- Sand flies can fly through the holes of usual mosquito nets; therefore, one must be aware that using them does not protect against leishmaniases.

Geographic Distribution of Cutaneous and
Muco-cutaneous Leishmaniases in the New World

Endemic Areas

Geographic Distribution of Cutaneous and
Muco-cutaneous Leishmaniases in the Old World

Loiasis (or African Eyeworm)

Loa loa

Geographic Distribution

Loiasis is a filariasis that is present in some countries of western and central Africa: Nigeria, Cameroon, Central African Republic, Democratic Republic of Congo, Congo, Equatorial Guinea, Gabon, and Angola. The CDC estimated that in 2010 between 3 and 13 million people in West and Central Africa were infected with loiasis.

Main Symptoms

At least 3 months after a bite by an infected *Chrysops* fly, a pruritus frequently appears on the arms, torso, face, or shoulders. In heavy infections the presence of an adult worm of *Loa loa* is sometimes evident, moving very slowly under the skin (felt and described as a shoelace) or directly visible under the conjunctiva. Temporary but recurring edema of the extremities, particularly the hands and wrists, is common. Complications include neurological symptoms (meningitis, encephalitis, paralysis), cardiac involvement (endocarditis), and nephropathies. Most infected people are asymptomatic, with a positive serologic immune response to the infection as the only evidence of the disease.

Treatment

- DEC is the drug of choice. Doses must be appropriately adjusted to the parasite load in the blood. Good success rates are the norm.
- Lysis of microfilariae in the blood can trigger fever, cephalgia, nausea, arthralgia, pleural effusion, and encephalitis.
- Encephalitis post-treatment can also occur with ivermectin, particularly in very high microfilaremia (>30,000 microfilariae/ml).
- Treatment of patients with positive microfilaremia must be supervised.
- Treatment with ivermectin before DEC reduces microfilaremia when it is high and treatment risky.
- According to the worm load of the patient, antihistamines and corticosteroids are given with DEC to treat or prevent allergic reactions.
- Dosing:
  * DEC, 200 mg, bid, q12h, po, for adults, and 6 mg/kg, daily, po, divided in two doses, for children, both for 21 days
  * To avoid or minimize side effects, dosing should be increased slowly. For adults, start with 1/32 of a 100 mg tab, bid, then 1/16, bid, q12h, and so on until reaching 2 tabs, bid (400 mg/day). For children, the incremental proportion is identical.
  * Ivermectin, 400 µg/kg, po, once, for adults and children

Preventive Measures

- Use insecticides to kill vectors.
- Use repellents containing DEET (15–30%). Be aware that they can only provide transitory protection.

- Treat clothes with insecticides containing permethrin.
- DEC can be taken on a weekly basis (100 mg, po) or twice a week (50 mg, po).

Ingrid was a 40-year-old Swedish nurse working in Cameroon. She came in for medical consultation after experiencing swelling of her wrists and ankles accompanied with a skin rash. Her symptoms had started 6 months earlier when she noticed that her bracelet was feeling tight. She then found that the swelling was occurring erratically on the other wrist and bilaterally on the ankles. Ingrid said that she sometimes observed red spots on her skin (1–2 cm in diameter), which would disappear after a few hours. Although the clinical exam was completely normal, the filariasis serology came back positive. She was successfully treated with DEC.

DID YOU KNOW THAT:
- Transmission of loiasis occurs through a mosquito (*Chrysops*) bite, most often during the hottest hours of the day.
- The incubation period varies from a few weeks to many months.
- Swellings are elastic, cold, transient, painless, and migratory (they are known as Calabar edemas after the city in Cross-River State, coastal southeastern Nigeria).
- Sometimes the adult worm can be seen crawling in the eyes (more likely as the parasite load increases).
- Progressively increasing doses of DEC are recommended for treatment.
- Prevention is very difficult.

Geographic Distribution of Loiasis

Malasseziosis (or Pityriasis Versicolor)

Malassezia sp.

Geographic Distribution
Malasseziosis is a mycosis that is highly prevalent in the intertropical zone, with local climate conditions (heat and moisture) conducive to fungal growth.

Main Symptoms
Hypopigmented maculae that will not tan or, in some patients, brownish hyperpigmented maculae appear in areas of predilection on the torso, chest, neck, or limbs. There is no associated itching or pain.

Treatment
- The cream, lotion, or spray version of econazole, or ketoconazole, or miconazole is very effective and well tolerated.
- Dosing:
  * Apply twice a day for 2–3 weeks, for adults and children.

Preventive Measures
- Use air conditioning at night.
- Keep the skin dry.
- Do not lie directly on beach sand.
- Avoid sharing towels, T-shirts, and underwears with strangers.

Tracy was a 20-year-old British girl who noticed white spots on her tanned back after spending a 2-week holiday in Phuket, Thailand. She had a microscopic exam (scotch test) that revealed spores of *Malassezia furfur*. She was successfully treated with econazole spray.

DID YOU KNOW THAT:
- Tinea versicolor is very common in the intertropical zone.
- Treatment duration should not be less than 2 weeks in tropical countries.
- Clothes and bedsheets must be changed to avoid relapse.
- Seasonal change is often enough to get rid of the fungus in winter in temperate climates.
- Prevention is based on keeping the skin dry and ventilated as much as possible.

Myiasis (or Tumba Fly)

Mainly *Cordylobia anthropophaga* in Africa and *Dermatobia hominis* in South America

Geographic Distribution
Myiasis is an ectoparasitosis that is endemic to Africa and South America.

Main Symptoms

Infection occurs upon skin contact with fly eggs found on towels, bedsheets, underwear, T-shirts, or floors. In Africa the symptoms appear after a few days, whereas in South America it takes about 6 weeks for them to emerge. They include pruritus at the site of penetration, followed by a very painful boil-like skin nodule with a black head. After about 1 week, the larva (or maggot) spontaneously leaves the body. Individuals usually harbor multiple parasites. The disease is also known as "Cayor worm" in Africa, *torcel* in Venezuela, and *berne* in Brazil.

Treatment

- The larva is killed by applying ether. It is then removed by pressure or with a scalpel incision.
- Secondary bacterial infections are treated with broad-spectrum antibiotics.
- Update tetanus immunization.

Preventive Measures

- Iron all clothes carefully.
- Machine dry clothes if possible (instead of on an outdoor wire).

Farouk was a 24-year-old Lebanese civil engineer who lived in Abidjan, Ivory Coast. He sought medical advice for what he described as "maggots in his testes." The symptoms began 2 days earlier in his hotel room with very painful and throbbing, boil-like lesions on his scrotum. His girlfriend had left him, thinking his condition was an STD and horrified by the vision of "worms" coming out of this area. Farouk mentioned that a few days prior to the incident he was at a beach where he sat naked on a towel. The clinical exam revealed multiple nodules on both testes, which were hot and tender. Each nodule had one central black spot. Parasites, deadened by ether, were extracted by pressure and identified as *Cordylobia anthropophaga*. Erythromycin and paracetamol were prescribed, and his tetanus immunization was updated.

DID YOU KNOW THAT:
- Myiasis is endemic to Africa as well as South America.
- Pain is the prominent symptom.
- Treatment is based on physical extraction of the parasite (an incision is often necessary).
- Antibiotics are frequently needed.
- Tetanus immunization must be updated.

Geographic Distribution of Myiasis

Dermatobia hominis
Cordylobia anthropophaga

Onchocerciasis (or River Blindness)

Onchocerca volvulus

Geographic Distribution

Onchocerciasis is a filariasis present in 6 countries in Latin America, the Middle-East (Yemen), and Africa (especially in the Volta basin: Senegal, Guinea, Sierra Leone, Ivory Coast, Ghana, Benin, Togo, Nigeria, Mali). According to the WHO in 2013, at least 25 million people are infected with *O. volvulus* worldwide; including 300,000 who are blind and 800,000 with some visual impairment. Approximately 123 million people are at risk for becoming infected with the parasite. More than 99% of infected people live in sub-Saharan Africa.

Main Symptoms

After a bite by an infected *Simulium* black fly, the following symptoms appear:

- *Cutaneous syndrome*
  Pruritus, which can be intense (known as *craw-craw* in Africa), affecting mainly the lower torso, buttocks, thighs, and pretibial areas. It produces hyperpigmented plaques and lymphedema (orange skin). Later, hypopigmentation occurs (leopard skin) as well as lichinification (lizard skin). Symptoms involve more the upper parts of the body in Latin America than in Africa. In particular, *mal morado* is found in the elderly with a maculopapular eruption on the face, neck, arms, and pectoral region accompanied with a mauvish depigmentation. In Yemen, *sowda* affects mainly the lower limbs with pruritus and dark skin. These symptoms evolve faster than in Africa.
- *Cystic syndrome*
  Onchocercomas, which are cystic collections of adult parasites (macrofilariae)
- *Ocular syndrome*
  Its frequency is proportional to the duration and intensity of infection. Microfilariae can be found in the anterior chamber of the eye. Other symptoms include keratitis (leading to an onchocercosis pannus), iridocyclitis, chorioretinitis (leading to Hissette-Ridley type of lesions), and post–optic nerve atrophy.
- *Other symptoms*
  Adenopathy (known as "hanging groin" in Africa) and diffuse onchodermatitis.

Treatment

- Ivermectin for microfilariae
- Dosing:
  * Ivermectin, 150–200 µg/kg, po, once, for adults and children
- Nodulectomy for macrofilariae

Preventive Measures

- Use insecticides to kill vectors.
- Use repellents containing DEET (15–30%). Be aware that they can only provide transitory protection.
- Treat clothes with insecticides containing permethrin.
- Stay away from bodies of running water in endemic areas.

Angela was a 28-year-old mother of a premature child who came to consultation for itching all over her body. She had been living in Togo, where her husband had worked for 2 years. The itching started about a month earlier, first on her lower back, then on the buttocks and thighs. It was worse at night, and she therefore took sleeping pills. Her clinical exam revealed scratching lesions with hyperpigmented areas and slightly hypopigmented scars. Her filarial serology came back positive, and the skin biopsy showed microfilariae of *Onchocerca volvulus*. She was successfully treated with ivermectin.

DID YOU KNOW THAT:
- Ocular lesions of onchocerciasis and the cutaneous cysts occur late in the course of the disease.
- If onchocerciasis is suspected but the skin biopsy is negative and the serology questionable, a skin test using Nivea cream with 1% DEC should be performed. It provokes a typical erythema in patients with onchocerciasis called Mazzotti's reaction.
- Ivermectin is a more efficient and better-tolerated treatment than DEC.
- Prevention of onchocerciasis is very difficult.

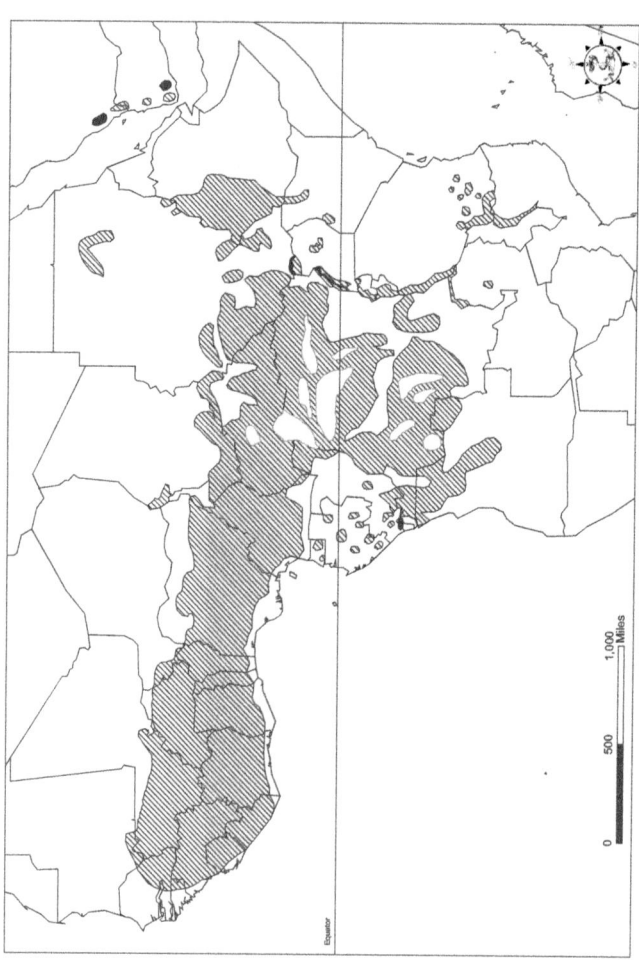

Geographic Distribution of Onchocerciasis in Africa and in the Arabic Peninsula

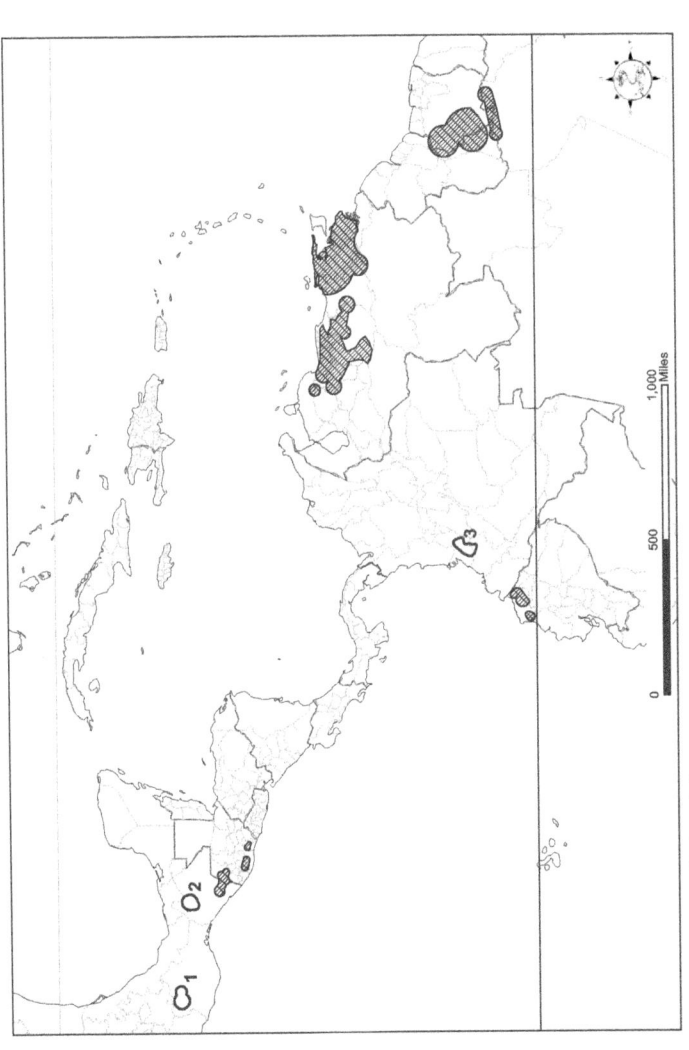

Geographic Distribution of Onchocerciasis in Latin America

Pediculosis Corporis (or Body Lice)

Pediculus humanus corporis

Geographic Distribution

Pediculoses are ectoparasitoses. Body lice are predominantly found in the intertropical zone because of poor local hygienic and socioeconomic conditions.

Main Symptoms

A few days after contact with contaminated clothes, by lying on contaminated beds or touching infected people, body lice can induce itching, particularly in covered skin areas around the lower back, shoulder blades, and thighs. Maculae or papules can be seen around the bite site. In chronic infections leukomelanoderma can occur. Secondary bacterial infections with pus (from scratching) are common.

Treatment

- Malathion lotion 0.5% is very active.
- Broad-spectrum antibiotics can treat secondary bacterial infections.
- Clothes and bed linen should be machine-washed at high temperature or removed and destroyed, if it is not possible.
- Insecticide should be spread on the bed and mattresses.

Preventive Measures

- Personal body hygiene prevents secondary bacterial infections.

Scabies (or Norwegian Itch)

Sarcoptes scabei

Geographic Distribution

Scabies is an ectoparasitosis that exists everywhere in the world but is more frequently found in the intertropical zone due to poor local hygiene and housing conditions. Canine or feline scabies can be transmitted to humans, on whom they cannot reproduce. They die usually in a couple of weeks after exposure. However, symptoms will persist if the affected animals continue to infect people.

Main Symptoms

A few days after contact (including sexual) with an infected person or after touching contaminated bedsheets or clothes, the following indicates a scabies infection: Diffuse pruritus (worse at night), with 3 dermatological characteristics:

- Skin blisters/vesicles or tiny lumps
- Parasitic burrows under the skin appearing between the fingers or toes and on the wrists, heels, palms, armpits, or waist
- Chancres and/or red bumps on the penile glans and shaft

The two latter are typical of scabies. Secondary bacterial infections are common due to scratching. Hyperkeratosis without pruritus can be observed in debilitated, cachectic, and immunodepressed patients. These infected people are extremely contagious.

Treatment

- A lindane or benzyl benzoate (10%) treatment involves one overnight application and has very high success rates. Infants or pregnant women cannot use lindane. Permethrin (5%) is an effective alternative. It also requires two applications.
- Other treatments include malathion and ivermectin (see below).

Table 1.8 Treatments for scabies and head lice		
Permethrin	Cover whole area, including fingernails. Apply weekly, prn.	S.R.: 90–100% following a single application
Lindane	Cover whole area, including fingernails. Apply over 2 successive days.	S.R.: 84–91% from a single application, 96% when applied for 6 h or more.
Malathion	Cover whole area, including fingernails. Apply a single dose, then repeat in 7–9 days as needed.	S.R.: ≥90%
Ivermectin	12 mg, po, for adults and 200 µg/kg for children	S.R.: >90%, may have to repeat dose 1 week later
S.R. = success rates.		

- The entire exposed household must be treated for scabies because it is highly contagious. Linens should be machine-washed at high temperature and bedsheets sprayed with appropriate insecticides to prevent a recurrence of disease.
- Treat sexual partner(s).
- Check for other STDs when there was sexual contact.
- Use broad-spectrum antibiotics for secondary bacterial infections.

Preventive Measures

- Practice strict body hygiene.
- Avoid locations with poor hygiene.
- Know the health status of sexual partner(s).

Rachel was an 18-year-old Melanesian girl living on the island of Lifou, New Caledonia. She came for consultation complaining of "itching under her armpits and between her fingers." The story of the disease revealed that she had recently adopted a kitten from a cousin. The animal roamed freely on the mats where her whole family spent a lot of time. Her clinical exam showed the typical burrows of scabies in her axillae and between her fingers. She and her siblings were treated successfully with benzyl benzoate.

DID YOU KNOW THAT:
To maximize the chances of success for scabies treatment:

- Take a bath or shower prior to applying the product.

- Wash the entire body with soap, then rinse.
- Before the skin dries, apply benzyl benzoate (10%) all over the body.
- Reapply the product 10 min later, targeting the skinfolds.
- Allow to dry.
- Wash again 24 h later.

Tinea Nigra Palmis and Plantaris

Exophalia werneckii

Geographic Distribution

Tineas are mycoses. Tinea nigra can be found in South America, Southeast Asia, and very rarely Africa.

Main Symptoms

Brown, nonscaling, nonpruritic maculae on the palms of the hands or on the soles of the feet. They can simulate a nevus planus or melanoma.

Treatment

- Benzoic or undecenoic acid cream, bid, as many days as needed

Preventive Measures

- Body hygiene

Tungiasis

Tunga penetrans

Geographic Distribution

Tungiasis is an ectoparasitosis that is prevalent in Africa, Madagascar, the West Indies, and Central and South America. Other names for the disease include *nigua*, *pio*, *bicho de pie*, and *pique*. Other names for *Tunga penetrans* include chigoe flea, jigger, nigua, and sand flea.

Main Symptoms

Four to 5 days after penetration of one or two parasites under the skin (generally on the side of a toenail, the soles of the feet, or around the malleoli), pain appears in the area. It will worsen and be at its peak when the flea reaches its final size of a pea. The area is surrounded with edema, and lesions usually become infected.

Treatment

- The parasite is surgically removed after being killed by local application of ether.
- Secondary bacterial infections require broad-spectrum antibiotics.
- Update tetanus immunization.

Preventive Measures

- Wear proper shoes.
- Avoid unsupervised beaches.

Kerry was an 18-year-old New Zealander who experienced pain in her right big toe after coming back from trekking in South America, where she wore sandals most of the time. Her clinical exam revealed a nodule the size of a pea centered under her right big toenail. The whole toe was very tender. A parasite was extracted by incision and identified as *Tunga penetrans*. Her tetanus immunization was updated and the lesion area cleaned. No antibiotics were needed.

DID YOU KNOW THAT:

- Tungiasis is endemic to Africa, Madagascar, the West Indies, and Latin America.
- Usually one or two *Tunga penetrans* parasites only can be found in the same patient.
- Treatment involves surgical extraction of the parasite.
- Tetanus immunization should be updated.
- Prevention consists of wearing appropriate footwear that protects the skin.

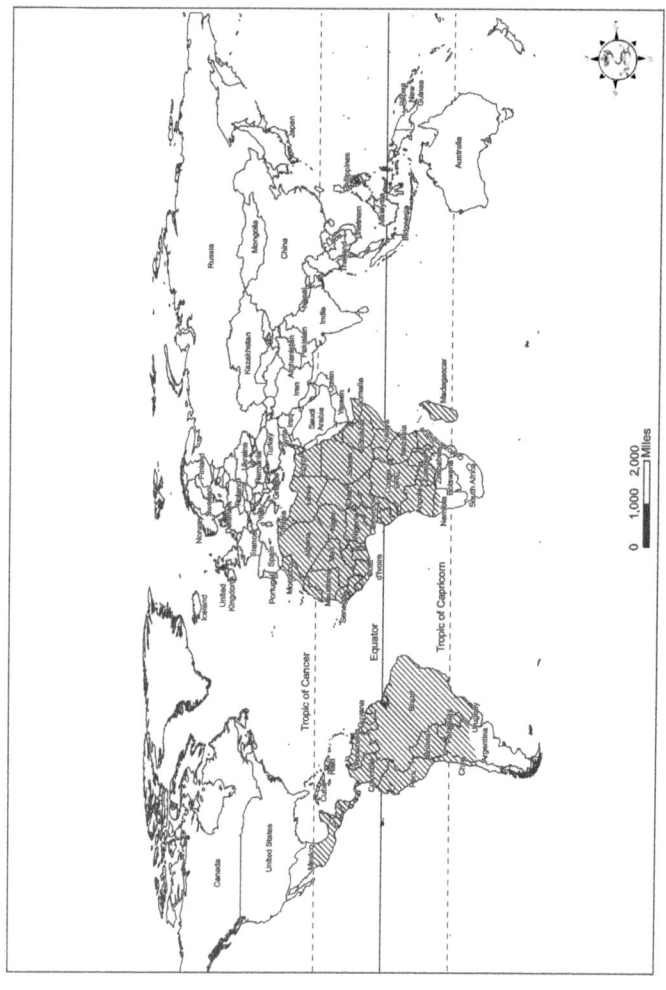

Geographic Distribution of Tungiasis

Urinary Tract

Schistosomiasis (Urinary)

Schistosoma haematobium

Historical Background

The first mention of urinary schistosomiasis can be traced back to Egypt (1500 b.c.e.), where some mummies were found with calcified bladders, which is characteristic of the disease. During the Middle Ages, Arabic doctors reported observing blood in the urine of caravaneers traveling through the Sahara Desert.

Geographic Distribution

S. haematobium can be found in Africa and the Middle East. In 2013, 37 sub-Saharan countries are endemic for urinary schistosomiasis. The 5–15 age group has the highest prevalence and intensity of infection. More than 100 million people are infected with the parasite in Africa.

Main Symptoms

Phases 1 and 2 are identical to those of intestinal schistosomiasis (see above, "Schistosomiasis [Intestinal]"). In phase 3, however, the following symptoms are likely to appear: hematuria, dysuria (with suprapubic pain), and polyuria. Skin symptoms encompass ulcerated granulomas on the genitalia. Early complications include acute cystitis, urinary tract higher infections, and vesical lithiasis. Late complications can be chronic cystitis, small and calcified bladder, renal failure, and genital involvement leading to sterility. Urinary schistosomiasis is a risk factor for bladder cancer.

Treatment

- Oxamniquine and praziquantel offer good efficacy and tolerance.
- Dosing:
  * Oxamniquine, 15–30 mg/kg, po, once, for adults, and 15–20 mg/kg once, for children
  * *or* Praziquantel, 40–60 mg/kg, po, once, for adults and children
- Surgery for renal pyonephrosis or ureteral/vesical lithiasis
- Extracorporeal shock wave lithotripsy for kidney stones

Preventive Measures

- Avoid freshwater baths in endemic areas (controlled swimming pools and seawater are safe).

Jens was a 25-year-old German student working in Ngo, Mali, on an agricultural project involving rice paddies. After experiencing blood in his urine, erratic burning upon urination, and a constant pain above his pubis, he sought medical attention. In his past medical history he had never had gonorrhea. The urine microscopic exam showed eggs of *Schistosoma haemotobium*. Cytoscopy exhibited parasitic granulomas. He was successfully treated with praziquantel.

DID YOU KNOW THAT:
- Hematuria is often the first symptom of urinary schistosomiasis.
- Complications such as cystitis or acute pyelonephritis (which can become chronic), happen only after years of disease evolution.
- Bladder cancer is a complication of urinary schistosomiasis, which is rare in sub-Saharan Africa but more common in Egypt.
- Treatment with praziquantel is very efficient and well tolerated.
- Avoiding skin contact with freshwater in uncontrolled endemic areas is the best means of prevention.

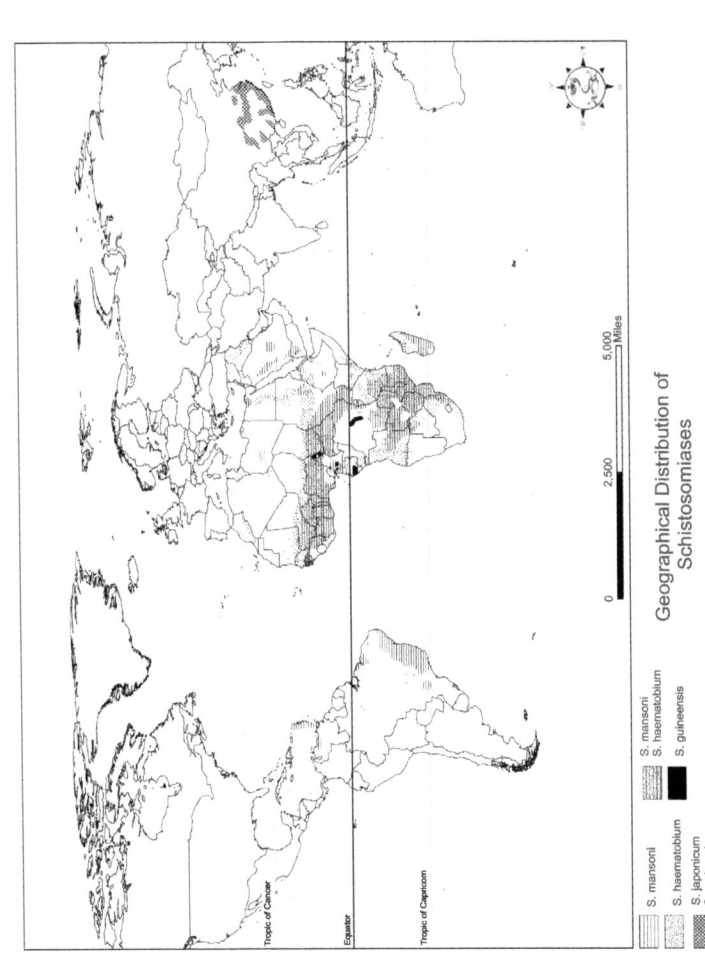

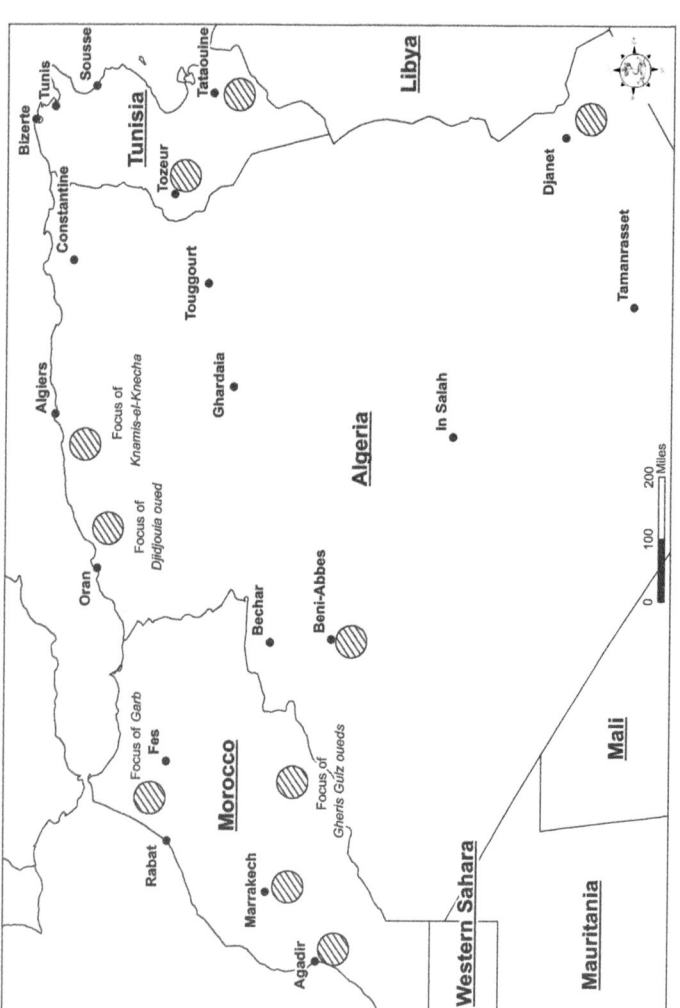

Geographic Distribution of Urinary Schistosomiasis in Northern Africa

(B) Parasitic Dead Ends and Larval Diseases

Parasitic dead-ends and larval diseases are diseases where the adult parasite is trapped and dies in the human body or the parasitic cycle cannot be completed to the adult stage.

Angiostrongyliasis

Angiostrongylus cantonensis

Geographic Distribution

Angiostrongyliasis is endemic to Southeast Asia (Thailand and Malaysia, in particular), Australia, Tahiti, New Caledonia, Vanuatu, and Hawaii. Various other countries have reported it. It affects primarily young children. The natural final host of the parasite is a rat.

Main Symptoms

The disease can be contracted by eating contaminated uncooked snails, slugs, crabs, shrimps, fish, or leafy vegetables or via dirty fingers.

One to 3 weeks after infection, the following symptoms and conditions may appear: severe cephalgia, fever, neck stiffness, nausea and emesis, meningoencephalitis, and multiple neurological symptoms (motor or sensory). The cranial nerves most involved are III, IV, VI, VII, and VIII. In days or weeks, complete healing usually occurs. Rare complications include facial palsy, diplopia, and impaired motor or sensory abilities. Death rarely ensues.

Treatment

- Symptomatic

Preventive Measures

- Always wash hands before eating.
- Avoid eating raw food, particularly snails, slugs, crabs, shrimps, fish, and leafy vegetables in endemic areas.

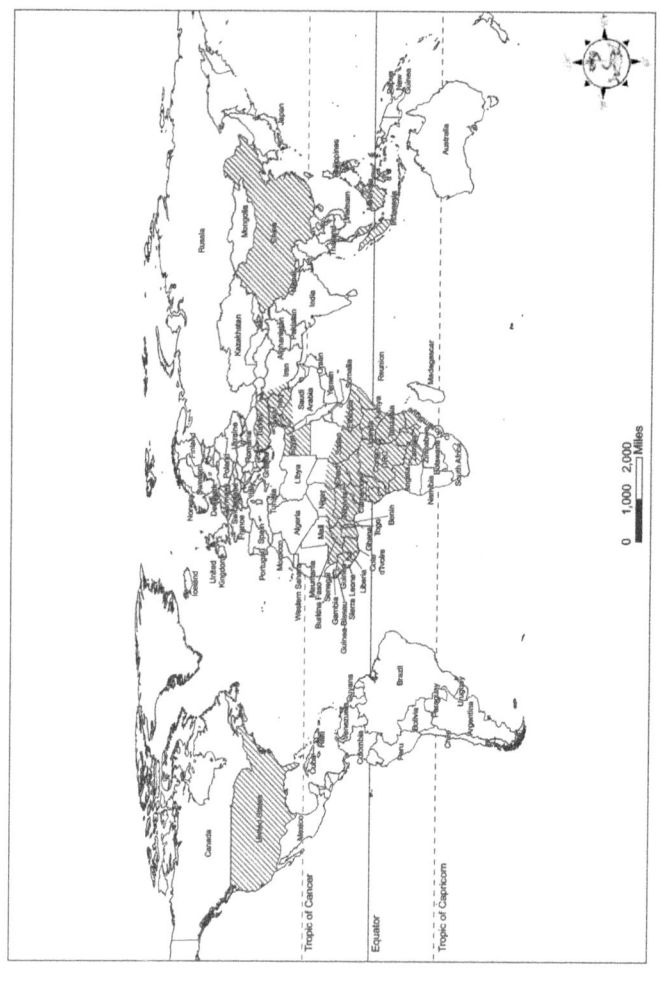

Geographic Distribution of Angiostrongyliasis

////// Endemic Areas

Cenurosis

Multiceps sp.

Geographic Distribution

Cenurosis is a rare disease, which occurs mainly in sub-Saharan Africa. Intermediary hosts carrying the parasite at its larval stage include sheep, rabbits, hares, rodents (central Africa), and primates (East Africa). The final host of the parasite at its adult stage is usually a dog but occasionally can be a wild predator.

Main Symptoms

Humans get infested by accidentally ingesting eggs shed by dogs or wild predators. Two forms of the disease have been identified according to the parasite location.

Subcutaneous

This form is due most frequently to the larva of *Multiceps serialis* and results in a subcutaneous nodule.

Cerebral

This form is due to the larva of *Multiceps multiceps*, which causes symptoms similar to those of a brain tumor, varying with the parasite's location in the brain. Vision, hearing, and balance can be affected.

Treatment

- Surgery aims at extracting the parasite, when possible. Sometimes, lesions are located at the base of the brain and invade surrounding tissues in all directions, making operations impossible.

Preventive Measures

- Avoid contact with dogs in endemic areas.

Cysticercosis

Cysticercus cellulosae

Geographic Distribution

Cysticercosis is endemic where pigs are infested by tapeworms, mainly in central Europe, Mexico, Peru, Chile, Africa, Madagascar, Reunion Island, and India. It is rare in Muslim countries and where religious or other beliefs ban the eating of pork. The natural final host of the parasite is a porcine.

Main Symptoms

Infection occurs either through dirty fingers, from eating food contaminated by tapeworm (but only *Taenia solium*) eggs, or by self-infection (i.e., when a segment of worm moves back from the small intestine to the stomach by reverse peristalsis).

Three to 4 months after larval entry through the stomach wall, the following symptoms may appear, according to the parasite location.

Muscles

Usually, there are no symptoms (it is the most common form of the disease).

Skin

Small, painless nodules appear under the skin.

Eyes

Exophthalmia with strabismus and diplopia as well as iritis, blepharitis, and retinitis can occur. Papilledema is the most frequent sign of cysticercosis. It can be found in 28% of cases.

Brain

Seizures (most frequent symptom, present in about 50% of cases), intense cephalgia (second most frequent symptom, present in about 44% of cases), nausea, emesis, progressive amaurosis, altered mental condition, and chronic meningitis can occur.

Treatment

- Praziquantel and albendazole offer good tolerance but have moderate success rates.
- Dosing:
  * Praziquantel, 50 mg/kg, po, daily, for 10–15 days for adults and children
  * *or* Albendazole, 15 mg/kg, po, daily, for 8 days; for children ≥6 years, 15 mg/kg/day, po, given in two divided doses, q12h, for 3–8 days
- Surgery, when necessary and possible.

Preventive Measures

- Wash hands before eating.
- Treat all tapeworm infections in pigs and humans.

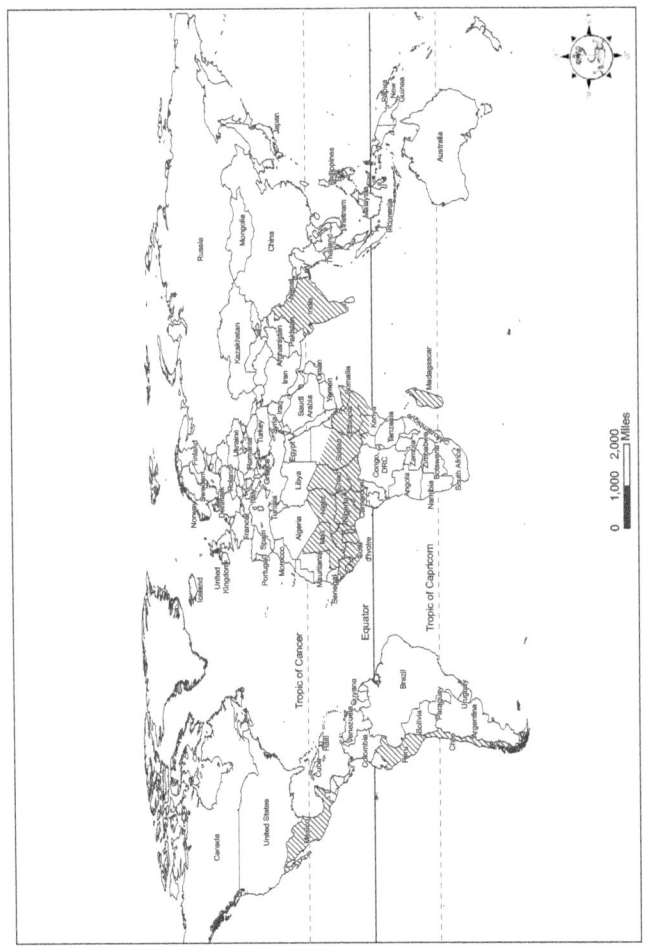

Geographic Distribution of Cysticercosis

///// Endemic_Areas

Gnathostomiasis

Gnathostoma spinigerum

Geographic Distribution

Gnathostomiasis is endemic to Southeast Asia (in particular Thailand) and Japan. It has also been reported from Australia, the Middle East, Mexico, China, and India. Martin S. Wolfe reported the first cases of the disease in East Africa (from the Selous game reserve in southeast Tanzania). Domestic and wild canines and felines are the natural final hosts of the parasite.

Main Symptoms

One to 10 days after eating contaminated raw or marinated freshwater fish (*ceviche* in hispanophone Latin America and *lap* in Vietnam and Cambodia), chicken (or other fowl), frogs, porks, or snakes, the following symptoms may appear: acute gastralgia, pain in the right upper quadrant, nausea, emesis, urticaria, and fever. This phase lasts 24–48 h. Then, larvae of the parasite migrate farther and can be found anywhere in the body.

Under the skin

Sub-cutaneous is the most frequent location. Larvae cause recurrent and erratic edema and form papules and nodules. These symptoms last on average 3 weeks.

In the CNS

The cerebral location is the most serious. Symptoms include radiculitis with intense pain, encephalitis, myelitis, meningitis with involvement of cranial nerves, and meningeal hemorrhage. Thirty percent of patients with CNS symptoms have sequelae, and the mortality rate reaches 25% without treatment.

In the lungs

Larvae trigger dyspnea, cough, hemoptysis, chest pain, and pleuritis.

Other locations

Hemospermia, hematuria, or renal colic may be the first symptoms of the disease. Gastrointestinal symptoms include appendicitis and intestinal occlusion. Ocular symptoms encompass decreased visual acuity, photophobia, and photalgia. Other organs can be involved such as the ears, nose, throat, and liver.

Treatment

- Albendazole or ivermectin can be used.
- Dosing:
    * Albendazole, 400–800 mg/day, po, for adults, for 21 days
    * *or* Ivermectin, 200 µg/kg, twice, 48 h apart, po, for adults and children
- Surgery, when necessary and feasible

Preventive Measures

- Cook all freshwater fish, fowl, frogs, porks, and snakes.

Geographic Distribution of Gnathostomiasis

Endemic Areas
● Isolated Cases

Hydatidosis

Echinococcus granulosus

Geographic Distribution

Hydatidosis is widely spread but only highly endemic in countries where large sheep herds are kept by dogs, which are the natural final host of the parasite, for example, in South America (Argentina, Uruguay), northern and eastern Africa, Australia, New Zealand, Spain, Portugal, and the Middle East.

Main Symptoms

Months to years after contact with an infected dog or eating fruits or vegetables contaminated by the feces of a dog carrying the disease, one or a few hydatid cysts form.

In the liver

The liver is the most frequent location (50–60% of cases). The following symptoms often appear: hepatomegaly, usually well tolerated forming an abdominal mass, with or without pain (spontaneously or under pressure), in the right upper quadrant.

Complications include (1) infection of the cyst(s), creating the clinical picture of a liver abscess; (2) rupture in the biliary tract with hepatic colic, angiocholitis, and icterus (from blockage created by parasitic debris); (3) rupture in the peritoneum, causing peritonitis; and (4) compression of the biliary ducts with icterus and sometimes lithiasis, the portal veins with portal hypertension, and the sus-hepatic veins (Budd-Chiari syndrome).

In the lungs

The lungs are the second most frequent location (30–40% of cases). Pulmonary cysts are asymptomatic. Complications include (1) infection and fissure into a bronchus with abundant hemoptysis and (2) rupture into a bronchus with limpid vomit.

Slowly leaking cysts cause allergic reactions including asthma and urticaria. If a cyst ruptures in a vessel, it causes diffuse hydatidosis and if the the rupture is sudden, allergic shock and death may ensue.

Other locations

Cysts can also grow in the spleen, kidneys, genital tract, thyroid, behind the bladder, left ventricle, and brain (mainly in children, causing seizures). They are seldom found in muscles.

Treatment

- Surgery should be performed, if possible. Sometimes the number of cysts and/or their location precludes an operation.
- Utmost care should be taken by the surgical team to avoid dissemination of parasites.
- Operations should be surrounded with pre- and post-albendazole treatments.
- Dosing:
    * Albendazole, 15 mg/kg/day, po, in two divided doses, q12h, for adults and for children ≥6 years old, 1 month prior to surgery and at least 3 months after.

Preventive Measures

- Always wash hands after patting a dog in endemic areas.
- Avoid contact with unknown dogs.
- Avoid eating fruits that cannot be peeled and uncooked vegetables.

Espen was a 45-year-old Norwegian living in Algeria, where he worked for an oil company. After discovering a lump on his right thigh, he decided to seek medical advice. His parasitological checkup was completely negative. Surgery was performed and revealed a cyst full of blood and serous fluid in which a membrane was found. Microscopic examination revealed a scolex and the membrane of a hydatid cyst. Hydatidosis serology came back positive 30 days after the operation and reverted to negative 30 days later.

DID YOU KNOW THAT:

- Hydatidosis is endemic to northern Africa.
- Muscular hydatid cysts are very rare, usually isolated, and primary.
- Their evolution is slow and they are often asymptomatic.
- Unlike other localizations, muscular hydatidosis serology becomes negative quickly after surgery.
- Surgery is the treatment of choice.
- Prevention in endemic areas is based on (1) avoiding contact with unknown dogs, (2) not eating uncooked vegetables or fruits that cannot be peeled, and (3) always washing hands after petting dogs.

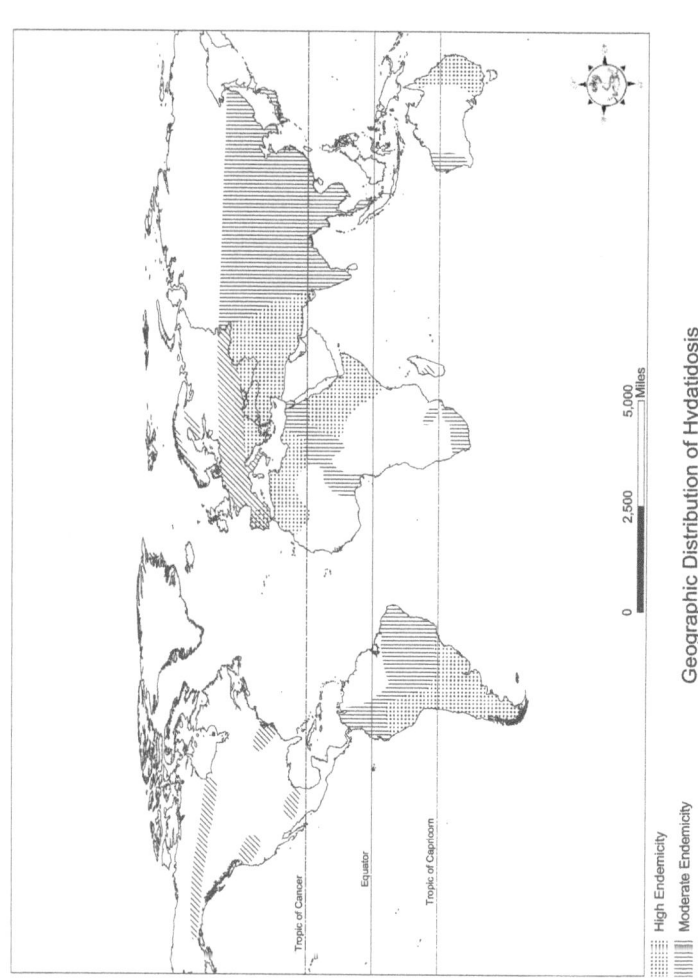

Larva Migrans (Cutaneous, or Creeping Eruption)

Mainly due to *Ancylostoma ceylanicum*

Geographic Distribution

Cutaneous larva migrans is common in the intertropical zone because of the large number of stray dogs. It is found predominantly in sub-Saharan Africa, Madagascar, Southeast Asia, the Caribbean Islands, and South America. The natural final hosts of the parasite are dogs for *Ancylostoma ceylanicum* and other animals (cattle, pigs) for other specific species. Animal larvae can penetrate under the human skin erratically.

Main Symptoms

Two to 3 days after contact with contaminated soil (sand or mud), a small red burrow appears under the skin, progressing several millimeters each day in a serpentine manner on the feet, hands, arms, legs, or torso. It is extremely itchy (especially at night), and symptoms can last from weeks to months. Secondary bacterial infections occur due to scratching.

Treatment

- Ivermectin, po, and thiabendazole cream are both effective.
- Dosing:
  * Ivermectin, 150–200 µg/kg, po, once, for adults and children
  * Thiabendazole cream, apply directly to the affected area, bid, as many days as needed
- Broad-spectrum antibiotics are required to treat secondary bacterial infections.
- Update tetanus immunization.

Preventive Measures

- Avoid beaches where wild dogs roam.
- Wear proper shoes.

Nunzio and Maria were 26- and 24-year-old, respectively, Italian citizens who came to medical consultation complaining of itching all over their bodies, which was worse at night. They had come back from their honeymoon in Guadeloupe and mentioned skinny-dipping and rolling naked in the sand. They said they had red spots on their skins that were moving. Upon clinical examination, both exhibited multiple typical skin lesions of *Ancylostoma ceylanicum*: snake-like tunnels that were erythematous and slightly elevated on the surface of the skin. The couple was successfully treated with ivermectin.

DID YOU KNOW THAT

- In dogs, cattle, and pigs, ancylostomiasis parasites have the same cycle as their equivalent in humans.
- Because they are specific to species and their tissues, animal larvae of ancylostoma cannot complete their cycles and are trapped under human skin.
- Untreated, this creeping disease can last for months.
- In tropical areas some workers are very exposed to the disease, like farmers, especially rice farmers.

Linguatulosis

Linguatula serrata

Geographic Distribution

Linguatulosis is ubiquitous but far more frequent in central Europe, the Middle East, and Brazil. Halzoun is a form of linguatulosis found mainly in Lebanon, Syria, and northern Africa. The natural final host of the parasite is a dog, a fox, or a wolf.

Main Symptoms

Humans are infected by ingesting eggs of the parasite on vegetables or by contact with infested dogs (except for halzoun). Two forms of the disease have been described.

Human larval form

Parasitic cysts are usually stuck in the liver, lungs, or mesenteric lymph nodes and do not provoke symptoms. Rarely, icterus, bronchial or brain compression, or glaucoma may occur.

Halzoun

The disease is contracted by ingesting contaminated raw goat or mutton liver or lymph nodes. Symptoms include pharyngeal tingling, dysphagia, dysphonia, and occasionally dyspnea and epistaxis. It is a mostly benign disease.

Treatment

- Extraction of parasites, when necessary and possible (for halzoun, after gargling with local anesthetics)

Preventive Measures

- Cook vegetables, mutton and goat liver, and lymph nodes.
- Stay away from stray dogs.

Porocephalosis

In Africa: *Armilifer armilatus*, *Armilifer grandis*
In Asia: *Armilifer moniliformis*

Geographic Distribution

Porocephalosis can be found in Asia and Africa. The natural final hosts of the parasite are snakes (e.g., *Pytho seboe* or *Bitis gabonica*).

Main Symptoms

Humans become infected by

- Ingesting parasite eggs from the ground, in food, or on snake skin
- Eating uncooked snake
- Swallowing fragments of an adult worm

In the majority of cases, no symptoms are noticed. The only indirect signs of the disease are unexplained eosinophilia (which can last for years) and/or calcification on chest or abdominal X-rays (1–2 cm in diameter, crescent-shaped, and dense images).

Rare symptoms are caused by compression, for example, of the eye or extrahepatic biliary ducts.

Treatment

- None available

Preventive Measures

- Wash hands before eating.
- Cook snakes well before eating them.

Sparganosis

Sparganum of *Spirometra mansoni*

Geographic Distribution

Sparganosis is endemic to the Far East. Frogs are intermediary hosts of sparganum, the parasite larva of *Spirometra mansoni*, which is an animal bothriocephalus.

Main Symptoms

Various forms of sparganosis exist according to the parasite's location.

Ocular

Infection occurs after the eye touches an infested, skinned frog (used as traditional medicine for various ailments in some Asian countries). The parasite grows on site, causing the eyelids and/or sockets to swell.

Visceral

After ingestion of contaminated water, one may experience abdominal pain.

Other locations

Skin and vaginal lesions have been described.

Treatment

- Surgery is the only treatment available. However, sometimes the parasitic location makes it impossible.

Preventive Measures

- Do not apply skinned frogs to the eyes or other parts of the body.
- Filter/boil water or drink it only from encapsulated bottles.

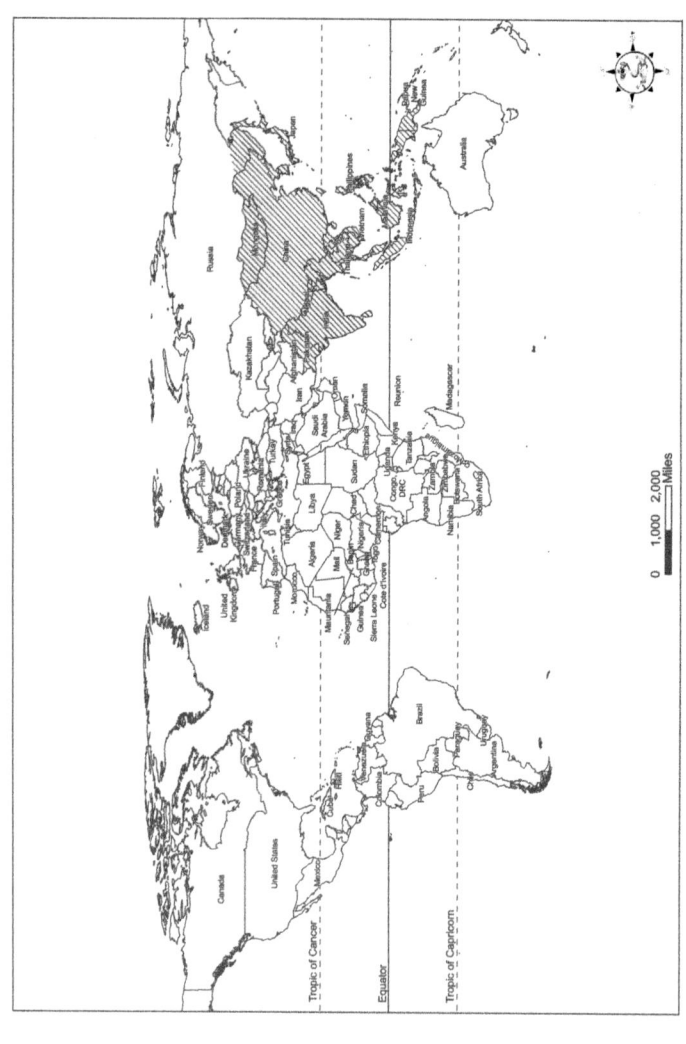

Geographic Distribution of Sparganosis

Endemic Areas

Toxocariasis (Toxocarosis, Visceral Larva Migrans or Roundworm Infection)

Toxocara canis, Toxocara cati

Geographic Distribution

Toxocariasis is a ubiquitous disease. Its prevalence varies, and serologic studies have shown that it is much higher in some tropical areas than in the Western world, with, for example, 63.2% in children and teenagers on Bali, 86% in children under age 15 on Saint Lucia, and 92% in adults on Reunion Island. In mountain aboriginal schoolchildren in Taiwan, the overall seroprevalence of toxocarosis was 77%. By comparison, the frequency of immunoglobulin G antibodies against *Toxocara* in developed countries is 2–5% in urban areas and up to 37% in rural areas.

Main Symptoms

Human infection occurs (1) when embryonated eggs of *Toxocara canis* or *Toxocara cati* are ingested with contaminated soil (by geophagia like with pica or when children play in sand pits) or vegetables or (2) by swallowing raw or poorly cooked meat contaminated with live larvae. Outbreaks sometimes emerge within families or collectivities of children (particularly in low-income neighborhoods).

The symptomatology varies with the level of infection.

After one or very few infestations
Usually no symptoms appear.

After multiple infestations
Symptoms can be divided in three categories.

In children
Systemic form: Anorexia, malaise, fever, cephalgia, myalgia, arthralgia, hepatomegaly (smooth, firm, and painless), mild splenomegaly, upper abdominal discomfort, and adenopathy. Some patients may also experience diarrhea, nausea, emesis, or respiratory signs such as wheezing, coughing, and dyspnea. Pruritic rashes, macular skin eruption, petechiae, chronic urticaria, lymphadenopathy, and angioneurotic edema can also occur. All symptoms usually recede spontaneously, but it may take several weeks.

In teenagers and adults
Benign form: Thwarted clinical pictures.
Ocular form: Retinal granulomas, retinal detachment, uveitis, optic neuritis, keratitis, iritis, endophthalmitis, vitreous abscesses, and hypopyon can occur. The infection is usually unilateral and with a single larva. However, bilateral infections have also been reported. Other symptoms may include leukocoria, decreased visual acuity, strabismus, opththalmalgia, and photopsia. Amaurosis may be progressive or sudden and can be permanent.

At all ages
Neurological form: Dementia, meningoencephalitis, myelitis, cerebral vasculitis, epilepsy, and optic neuritis can occur. Manifestations of the peripheral nervous

system comprise radiculitis, cranial nerves or musculoskeletal involvement. This form is exceptional (fewer than 50 reported cases).

Treatment

- Systemic form:
  - Albendazole, 10–15 mg/kg/day, po, for 2 weeks (75% cure rate)
  - Mebendazole, 20–25 mg/kg/day, po, for 3 weeks (70% cure rate)
  - D.E.C., 3–4 mg/kg/day, po, for 3 weeks (70% cure rate). It must be started progressively (see page 2) and should not be associated with steroids.
- Initial treatment of ocular forms: topical or systemic steroids
- For ocular involvement with retinal detachment, laser treatment may be considered.

Preventive Measures

- Treat cats and dogs.
- Keep cats and dogs away from sand pits.
- Cover sand pits when unused.
- Home gardens should be fenced to prevent fecal contamination by dogs and cats.
- Wash vegetables thoroughly.
- Cook meat sufficiently.
- Personal hygiene: wash hands particularly after handling soil.

Trichinosis (or Trichinellosis)

Trichinella spiralis

Geographic Distribution

Trichinosis is a nematodosis endemic to Germany, North America, India, China, Indonesia, the Middle East, and Africa. All mammals can be natural final hosts of the parasite, but most frequently they are carnivorous or omnivorous.

Main Symptoms

Symptoms appear in four phases, according to the parasite cycle.

Incubation

Asymptomatic, it lasts 1–2 days.

Invasion

Two to 6 days after eating contaminated meat such as ham or sausage, one may experience diarrhea, abdominal cramps, and general malaise.

Acute

Symptoms may only appear at this phase, which occurs 10 days after infection. They include a high and constant fever, face and eye infiltrating edema (hence the name "big head disease" given to trichinosis in Germany), retro-orbital pain, photophobia, myalgia (including when opening the mouth [with pseudotrismus], swallowing, breathing, talking, and walking), tachycardia, and subconjunctival or subungual hemorrhage. Allergic reactions include urticaria and asthma-like dyspnea.

Chronic

Three weeks after infection the fever disappears, but myalgias (due to larval cysts) and allergies persist for months.

Asymptomatic and benign forms have been reported. Complications include toxic shock, encephalitis, myocarditis, pulmonary edema, pneumonia, and acute nephritis.

Treatment

Invasion phase

- Albendazole offers good tolerance but with variable success rates.
- Dosing:
  * Albendazole, 400 mg, po, bid, q12h, for 14 days for adults; for children ≥6 years, 15 mg/kg/day, po, in two divided doses, q12h for 14 days

Acute phase

- *Symptomatic*: Each symptom is treated accordingly with various medications including corticosteroids.
- *Dosing*:
  * Prednisone, 30–60 mg/day, po, for adults, for 10–15 days (for severe symptoms)

Chronic phase

- Medicate the pain with ASA or NSAIDs

Preventive Measures

- Pork meat should be well cooked at a minimum temperature of 63°C (146°F).

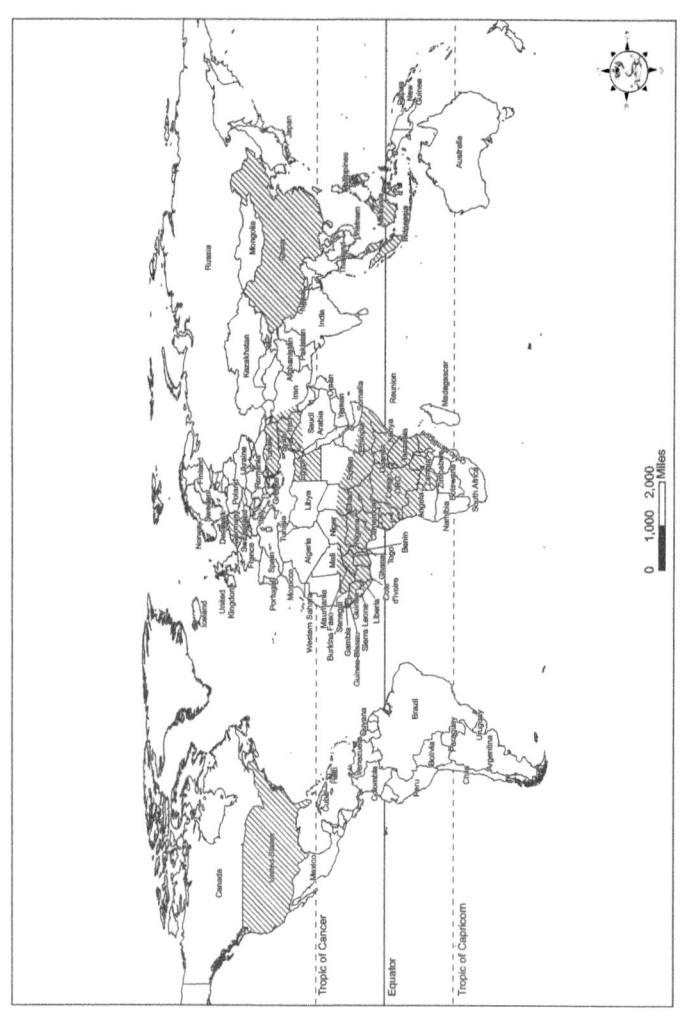

Geographic Distribution of Trichinosis

Endemic Areas

Part 2
Deep Fungal Diseases

Basidiobolomycosis

Basidiobolus ranarum

Geographic Distribution

Basidiobolomycosis is endemic to rural areas of the intertropical zone, particularly in Indonesia, Burma, India, and sub-Saharan Africa.

Main Symptoms

The mode of transmission of the parasite is unclear. Two types of symptoms can be experienced.

Inflammation

A constantly painful inflammation occurs under the skin of the limbs, shoulders, or buttocks. Occasionally, the torso and face may be the sites of bouts of hot swelling.

Edema

The swollen areas are mainly cold and painless, erratically becoming hot and sensitive.

Treatment

- Potassium iodide offers good tolerance but success rates vary. Alternatives are ketoconazole, itraconazole, or fluconazole.
- Dosing:
  * Potassium iodide, 1.5–2 g/day, po, for adults and 30 mg/kg/day, for children, both for many months
  * Ketoconazole, 200–400 mg/kg/day, for adults, for many months
  * Itraconazole, 100–200 mg/kg/day, for adults, for many months
  * Fluconazole, 200 mg/day, for adults, for many months
- Azole antifungals are not used in pregnant women because they are teratogenic.
- With ketoconazole, itraconazole, and fluconazole liver enzymes must be monitored on a monthly basis.
- Associated corticosteroids may help in some cases.
- Surgery, when possible

Preventive Measures

- There is no known prevention.

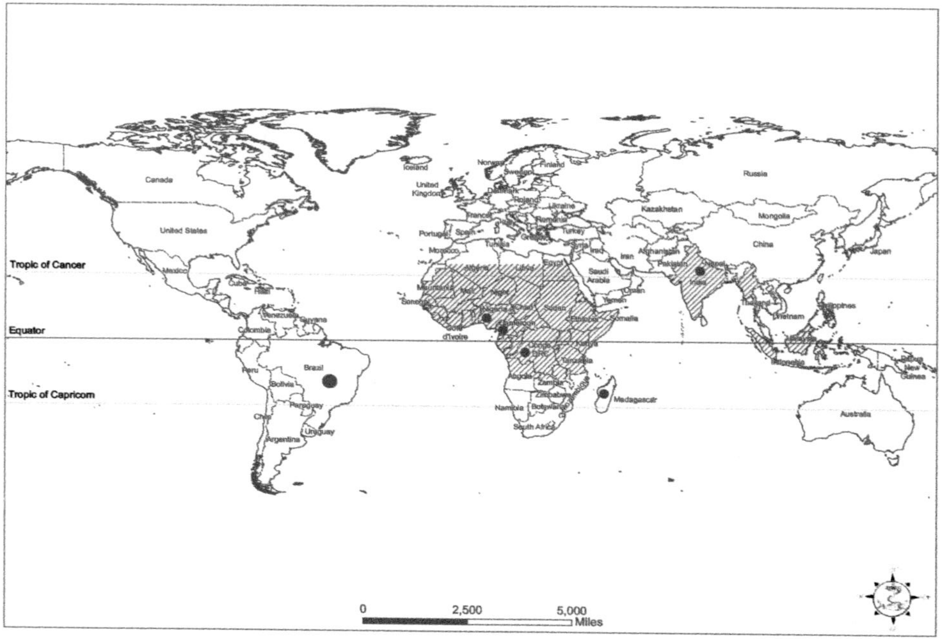

Basidiobolomycosis

Conidiobolomycosis

Geographic Distribution of Tropical Mucormycoses

Blastomycosis (North American or Gilchrist Disease or Chicago Disease)

Blastomyces dermatidis

Geographic Distribution

North American blastomycosis is endemic mainly to the south-central and midwestern United States and Canada but can also be found in Mexico, North Africa, Democratic Republic of Congo, and South Africa. The disease is predominantly rural, with men being more affected than women. It is rare in children.

Main Symptoms

Blastomyces dermatidis can be found in the environment on wet leaves, and it usually enters the human body through the lungs. After a variable incubation period, Gilchrist disease can be divided into five forms. The asymptomatic form is the most frequent. Fulminant forms have been described beside three other ones:

Acute

It affects the lungs. Symptoms include cough, moderate to high fever, dyspnea, hemoptysis, chills, weight loss, and asthenia.

Chronic

It affects bones and skin
Bones: Lesions grow rapidly and multiply, destroying the bones.
Skin: Papules and pustules form, increase in size centrifugally, and begin to bleed. Scar tissue emerges in their center. They are surrounded by a raised edge that enlarges and is occasionally filled with abscesses. Although lesions begin on the skin, they can subsequently penetrate deeply and reach the bones.

Disseminated

The lungs, bones, skin, lymph nodes (in the chest), sometimes kidneys and urogenital tract, ENT, and thyroid can be involved. Complications happen occasionally in the CNS, stomach, and bowel.

Treatment

Form	Treatment of Choice	Remarks
Mild to moderate pulmonary or disseminated disease	200 mg itraconazole, po, once or bid, for 6–12 mo	Osteoarticular disease: treat for 12 mo
Moderately severe to severe pulmonary or disseminated disease, but not in the CNS	0.7–1.0 mg amphotericin B deoxycholate/kg/day, or 3–5 mg lipid amphotericin B/kg/day for 1–2 wk, followed by 200 mg itraconazole, bid, for 6–12 mo (pulmonary) or 12 mo (disseminated)	Amphotericin B deoxycholate given at a total dose of 2 g can be used for the entire course of treatment, but most clinicians prefer to step-down to itraconazole after initial improvement; lipid amphotericin B products have fewer adverse effects than deoxycholate

(continued)

Form	Treatment of Choice	Remarks
CNS disease	5 mg lipid amphotericin B/kg/day for 4–6 wk, followed by an oral azole for at least 1 yr	Azole options for step-down therapy include 200 mg itraconazole, bid or tid, 800 mg fluconazole/day
Immunosuppressed patients	0.7–1.0 mg amphotericin B deoxycholate/kg/day, or 3–5 mg lipid amphotericin B/kg/day for 1–2 wk, followed by 200 mg itraconazole, bid, for 12 mo	Lifelong suppressive therapy may be necessary for patients whose immunocompetence does not improve
Pregnant patients	3–5 mg lipid amphotericin B/kg/day	Systemic azole therapy is contraindicated in pregnancy

- For children with severe blastomycosis, amphotericin B deoxycholate, IV, 0.7–1.0 mg/kg/day, or lipid formulation amphotericin B, IV, 3–5 mg/kg/day, for initial therapy, followed by itraconazole, 10 mg/kg/day (up to 400 mg/day), po, for 12 months. For children with mild to moderate infection, itraconazole, 10 mg/kg/day (to a maximum of 400 mg/day orally), po, for 6–12 months
- Itraconazole and ketoconazole can be hepatotoxic, and liver enzymes must be monitored on a monthly basis.

Preventive Measures

- No preventive measures are known.

Blastomycosis (South American or Lutz-Splendore-Almeida Disease)

Blastomyces brasiliensis

Geographic Distribution

South American blastomycosis or paracoccidioidomycosis is endemic to Central and South America.

Main Symptoms

The disease is contracted from an infected person, and the fungus always enters through the lungs. Two forms have been described.

Acute

In adolescents and young adults symptoms include cervical adenopathy, fever, asthenia, weight loss, and skin lesions (in about 50% of cases with ulcerated or vegetative papules or nodules on the face or limbs). Abdominal symptoms include hepatosplenomegaly and ascites. Bones can be involved. Mucous and pulmonary symptoms are rare. This form can be lethal.

Chronic

After a latent phase of about 30 years, the disease is reactivated from dormant lung lesions. In 90% of cases, this form is the initial presentation of the disease with various symptoms. They can be:

Mucocutaneous
Involving the lips, nostrils, mouth, and occasionally pharynx or larynx. It begins with an ulcerated papule, which grows rapidly. Local lymph nodes become swollen and painful. The lesions can progress toward mutilation or severe stenosis of the digestive and respiratory tracts.

Pulmonary
A mild productive cough (sometimes mimicking tuberculosis) is the prominent feature.

Lymphatic
Lymph nodes are swollen and painful, with very few other symptoms.

Other locations of the disease include the liver, spleen, bowels, adrenal glands, meninges, urogenital tract, and bones.

Treatment

- Itraconazole is the drug of choice as it appears to have the lowest rate of relapse. Ketoconazole can also be used.
- Dosing:
  * Itraconazole, 200–400 mg, daily, po, for adults, and 10 mg/kg/day, for children, both for 6 months
  * A loading dose is recommended in life-threatening situations: 200-mg caps, po, tid, for the first 3 days, followed by usual oral dosage of 200–400 mg/day, for adults
  * Ketoconazole, 400–800 mg, daily, po, for 6 months, for adults
  * For children with severe blastomycosis, amphotericin B deoxycholate, IV, 0.7–1.0 mg/kg/day, or lipid formulation amphotericin B, IV, 3–5 mg/kg/day, for initial therapy, followed by itraconazole, 10 mg/kg/day (up to 400 mg/day), po, for 12 months. For children with mild to moderate infection, itraconazole, 10 mg/kg/day (to a maximum of 400 mg/day orally), po, for 6–12 months
- Azole antifungals are not used in pregnant women because they are teratogenic. Amphotericin B lipid complex, IV, 2.5–5 mg/kg/day for 6–12 months, can be used instead.
- Ketoconazole and itraconazole can be hepatotoxic, and liver enzymes must be monitored on a monthly basis.
- Patients must be monitored for years because relapses are possible.
- Incapacitating sequelae (mainly pulmonary fibrosis) constitute major problems.

Preventive Measures

- No preventive measures are known.

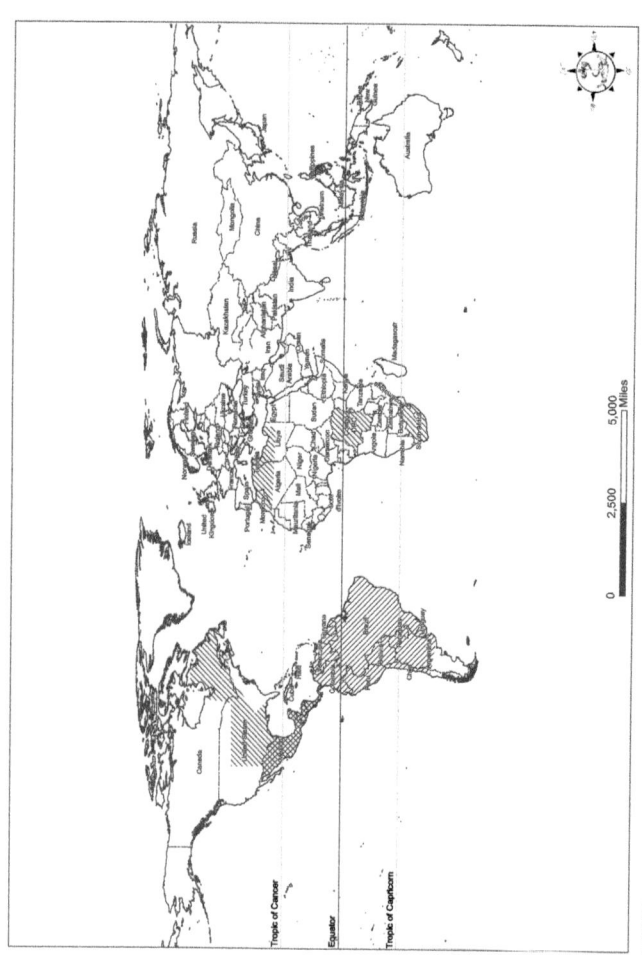

Geographic Distribution of Blastomycoses

Chromomycosis

Due to various fungal genera: Fonsevaea, Phialophora, Wangiella, and Cladosporium

Geographic Distribution
Mainly a rural disease, chromomycosis is frequently found in the intertropical zone but only endemic to Central America, the Greater Antilles, and Madagascar. It has been reported in South America, equatorial Africa, Australia, and Asia and is also known as "chromoblastomycosis."

Main Symptoms
After being pricked by a contaminated thorn, skin lesions slowly appear. First, a nodule or ulcer forms, which can either remain as such or grow into a wart-like lesion with hyperkeratosis over months or years. Several lesions may be seen, and their locations of predilection are the feet and the legs. Secondary bacterial infections are common with lymphatic stasis. Elephantiasis may occur. Complications include cancerization of lesions.

Treatment
- Surgery is performed to remove the lesions. Laser and cryotherapy can also be used.
- Itraconazole in association with flucytosine seems to produce good results, but it requires hospital monitoring. Thiabendazole can be efficient.
- Dosing:
  * Flucytosine, 50–150 mg/kg/day, po, divided, q6hr, for adults, for many months. For children:
    - < 1 month: 25 to 100 mg/kg/day, po, in divided doses, q12–24hr
    - 1 month -18 years: 50 to 150 mg/kg/day, po, in divided doses, q6hr, for many months.
    - Itraconazole, 200mg, po, once a day, for adults, for 6–12 months. For children, 10 mg/kg/day (to a maximum of 400 mg/day), po, for 6–12 months
    - Thiabendazole, 25 mg/kg/day, po, for adults and children, for many months
- Azole antifungals are not used in pregnant women because they are teratogenic.
- Pregnant women should be given flucytosine only if the potential benefits exceed the potential harm to the fetus. Women should not breastfeed during treatment.
- Broad-spectrum antibiotics are used for secondary bacterial infection.
- Tetanus immunization must be updated.

Preventive Measures
- Avoid contact with thorny plants.

Geographic Distribution of Chromomycosis

Coccidioidomycosis (or Posadas-Wernicke, or Posadas-Rixford Disease)

Coccidioides immitis

Geographic Distribution

Coccidioidomycosis is endemic to the United States, Mexico, and South America. Indigenous peoples and African Americans appear to be more susceptible to the disease. It is also known as "San Joaquin Valley fever" or "desert rheumatism."

Main Symptoms

Infection occurs when humans inhale dust contaminated by infested rodents. The period of incubation varies. Most patients are asymptomatic or have limited symptoms. Three stages of the disease have been described.

Primary

The lungs or the skin are affected. In the lungs, the fungus induces a flu-like illness causing asthenia, fever, backache, cephalgia, and cough. In the skin, a nodule, ulcer, or wart-like lesion or a papular nonpruritic rash, erythema nodosum (often pretibial), or erythema migrans may appear. After the primary stage, the disease either heals spontaneously within 1 or 2 weeks or progresses to the secondary or to the residual stage.

Secondary

The fungus reaches another organ, particularly the bones, CNS, or urogenital tract, via the bloodstream or lymphatic vessels. Progression of the disease is severe. This form is seen mostly in pregnant women, newborns, and HIV-positive patients. It is more common among Indians, blacks, and Asians.

Residual

Chronic lesions appear in the lungs, causing bronchiectasis, fibrosis, emphysema, and cavities that can burst into the pleura.

Treatment

- Itraconazole, ketoconazole, and amphotericin B can be used. However, in some severe cases, they can be inefficient.
- Dosing
  - Itraconazole, 200 mg, bid or tid, daily, po
  - Ketoconazole, 400 mg/day, po
  - Amphotericin B deoxycholate, 0.5–1.5 mg/kg/day, IV
  - Lipid formulations of amphotericin B, 2–5 mg/kg/day, IV
  - All for at least 6 months
- Azole antifungals are not used in pregnant women because they are teratogenic. Pregnant women may be treated with amphotericin B.
- Patients with more advanced disease require more aggressive treatment. In particular, patients who exhibit signs of meningitis need either intravenous therapy with amphotericin, unless otherwise contraindicated, or high-dose azole therapy with or without intrathecal amphotericin.

- Ketoconazole and long-term itraconazole can be hepatotoxic, and liver enzymes must be monitored on a monthly basis.
- Surgical management can be of help in the treatment of pulmonary and extrapulmonary lesions
- Patients must be monitored for years because relapses are possible.

Preventive Measures

- Avoid traveling on dirt tracks, when possible.

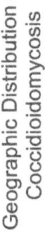

Geographic Distribution of Coccidioidomycosis

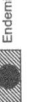 Endemic Areas

Conidiobolomycosis

Coniobolus coronatus

Geographic Distribution
Conidiobolomycosis is found predominantly in Cameroon, Nigeria, Democratic Republic of Congo, Madagascar, India, and Brazil.

Main Symptoms
The mode of transmission is unclear (inhalation or inoculation by contaminated fingers). Infected patients experience a painless, tumor-like mass in the nose, which progressively grows toward the larynx, sinuses, base of the nose, and upper lip, eventually involving the entire face. Other symptoms include rhinorrhea and epistaxis. As lesions progress, the nose loses its original shape and becomes snout-like. Palate and bone invasion may occur.

Treatment
- Potassium iodide offers good tolerance, but success rates vary. Alternatives are ketoconazole, itraconazole, or fluconazole.
- Dosing:
  * Potassium iodide, 1.5–2 g/day, po, for adults and 30 mg/kg/day, for children, for many months
  * Ketoconazole, 200–400 mg/kg/day, for adults, for many months
  * Itraconazole, 100–200 mg/kg/day, for adults, for many months
  * Fluconazole, 200 mg/day, for adults, for many months
- With ketoconazole, itraconazole, and fluconazole liver enzymes must be monitored on a monthly basis.
- Azole antifungals are not used in pregnant women because they are teratogenic.
- Pregnant women should not use potassium iodide.
- Associated corticosteroids may help in some cases.
- Surgery, when possible.

Preventive Measures
- Unknown

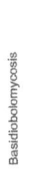

Geographic Distribution of Tropical Mucormycoses

Basidiobolomycosis
Conidiobolomycosis

Histoplasmosis (African)

Histoplasma duboisii

Geographic Distribution

African histoplasmosis is a rare fungal disease, which can be contracted only in Africa.

Main Symptoms

The modes of infection remain unclear. Two forms of the disease have been described.

Localized

Skin

Papules, nodules, and abscesses, sometimes with fistulae appear on the head and torso and last for months or years.

Bones and joints

Vertebral lesions, which mimic Pott disease, are common. Other locations include the wrists, elbows, knees, sternum, and ribs.

Lymph nodes

They can be involved primarily or secondarily with other lesions, and symptoms mimic TB.

Diffuse

Cases are rare but very severe, involving the liver, spleen, peritoneum, and gastrointestinal and urogenital tracts.

Treatment

- Amphotericin B is the drug of choice, requiring hospital monitoring. Success rates vary. Itraconazole and ketoconazole can also be used.
- Dosing:
  * Amphotericin B, 2–4 g/day, IV in courses, for adults, for 6–12 months
  * Itraconazole, 600–800 mg/day, po, for adults, for 6–12 months
  * Ketoconazole, 600–800 mg/day, po, for adults, for 6–12 months
  * Itraconazole, a loading dose is recommended in life-threatening situations, 200 mg caps, tid, for the first 3 days of therapy, followed by usual oral dosage of 200–400 mg/day, po.
- Azole antifungals are not used in pregnant women because they are teratogenic. They can use amphotericin B instead.
- Ketoconazole and long-term itraconazole can be hepatotoxic, and liver enzymes must be monitored.
- Surgery is sometimes necessary depending on the symptoms, the lesion locations, and their severity.

Preventive Measures

- Not enough is known about the transmission of the disease for effective prevention measures to be formulated.

Nuigi was a 64-year-old villager from Senegal who sought medical attention after noticing that he had multiple skin abscesses. Fourteen months earlier, he had seen a growth under his left nipple, which had ulcerated. Three months later, his left shoulder became painful and swollen. He had undergone several traditional treatments (including plasters and scarifications) before his hospitalization. He lost 15 kg (33 lb) over 6 months but experienced no fever. A left shoulder mass felt firm, hot, and tender; and a clear liquid oozed from multiple spots. A second mass was detected under his left armpit and a third one behind his skull. X-rays showed bone decalcification and destruction in various places. The histoplasmosis serology was positive, and amphotericin B was prescribed repeatedly. Surgery was necessary but could not completely restore the bone structure.

DID YOU KNOW THAT:

- The mode of contamination and means of prevention of African histoplasmosis are unknown.
- It can mimic extrapulmonary TB.
- It is endemic to western, central, and equatorial Africa.
- It mainly involves soft tissue, the skeleton, and lymph nodes.
- Skin lesions progress chronically in various forms: maculae, papulae, nodules, or abscesses forming fistulae.
- Treatment is difficult and often not completely successful.

PART 2 **Tropical Diseases**

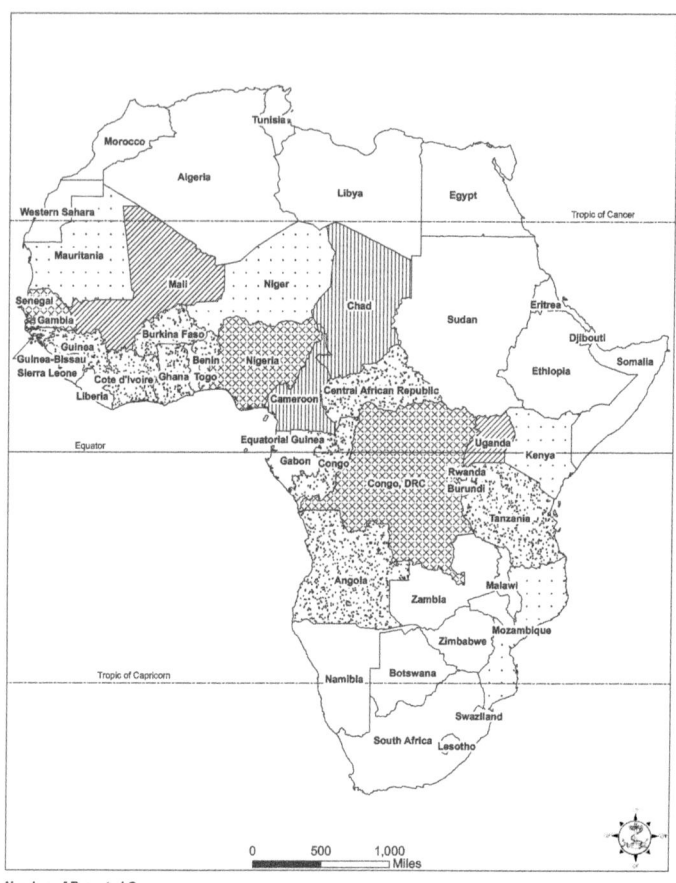

Number of Reported Cases

- 0
- 1
- 2 - 4
- 5 - 9
- 10 - 20
- More than 20

Geographic Distribution of
African Histoplasmosis
(Cases Reported in 1980)

Histoplasmosis (American or Darling Disease)

Histoplasma capsulatum

Geographic Distribution

American histoplasmosis is endemic to North, Central, and South America as well as South Africa. It has also been reported in the Middle East, India, Southeast Asia, Australia, New Zealand, and New Caledonia.

Main Symptoms

The disease is caused by inhaling dust containing the feces of infested birds or bats. Common places of contamination include farms, pigeon houses, caves, and sometimes forests. American histoplasmosis evolves in three phases.

Acute

Symptoms appear 3–14 days after infection with a flu-like syndrome. In case of massive infection, cough, hemoptysis, chest pain, and dyspnea may occur. Joint pain and skin lesions can be seen in 5–6% of patients, mostly in females.

Chronic

Symptoms include cough, fever, weight loss, and malaise. Cavities may form and cause hemoptysis with increasing dyspnea.

Disseminated

This phase appear mostly in immunocompromised people or infants and can be seen years after initial infection. Fever is high and the clinical picture, severe.

Symptoms of American histoplasmosis vary with the duration of the disease. Many systems can be involved.

- GI with diarrhea and abdominal pain
- Cardiac with valvular disease, angina, and cardiac insufficiency
- CNS (in 5–20% of patients) with headache, visual and gait disturbances, confusion, seizures, and altered consciousness
- Mucous membrane lesions are common.

Other forms include ocular syndrome (macular involvement may result in blindness) and mediastinitis with lymph node enlargement.

Treatment

Form	Remarks	Regimen
Acute Pulmonary	Treatment is indicated only with hypoxemia or if the disease lasts for >1 mo	Amphotericin B +/− corticosteroids, followed by itraconazole for a total of 6–12 wk of therapy (see dosing below_
Chronic Pulmonary	Treatment is indicated	Amphotericin B followed by Itraconazole for a total of 12–24 mo (see dosing below)

(continued)

Form	Remarks	Regimen
Disseminated (without AIDS)	Treatment is indicated	Amphotericin B followed by Itraconazole for a total of 12 wk minimum (see dosing below)
Disseminated in AIDS	Treatment is for life	Amphotericin B followed by itraconazole for life (see dosing below)
Fibrotic Mediastinitis	Controversial. Treatment can be considered when ESR is elevated or complement fixation titers are >1:32	Itraconazole for 3 mo (see dosing below)

- With self-limited pulmonary disease, no treatment is necessary.
- In other cases, itraconazole is the drug of choice. Ketoconazole can also be used. Amphotericin B is used initially for CNS and disseminated histoplasmosis.
- Dosing:
  * Itraconazole, 400 mg/day, po, for adults, for months to years (see above). For children: (1) acute pulmonary infection, 5–10 mg/kg/day orally in two divided doses (up to 400 mg/day); (2) progressive disseminated histoplasmosis (following an initial regimen of IV amphotericin B), 5–10 mg/kg/day orally in two divided doses (up to 400 mg/day), for at least 3 months
  * A loading dose is recommended in life-threatening situations: one 200-mg cap, po, three times a day for the first 3 days, followed by usual dosage of 200–400 mg/day, po
  * Ketoconazole, 400–600 mg, daily, po, in courses of 2–4 weeks, for at least 3 months
  * Ketoconazole and long-term itraconazole can be hepatotoxic, and liver enzymes must be monitored.
  * Azole antifungals are not used in pregnant women because they are teratogenic. Amphotericin B can be used instead.
  * Amphotericin B IV, 3–5 mg/kg, daily, over 1–2 h, every 2–3 days, for adults and children, for weeks, or amphotericin B lipid complex, IV, 2.5–5 mg/kg/day for adults and children, both until cure

Preventive Measures

- Stay away from infested farms, pigeon houses, caves, and forests.

Ayako was a 25-year-old Japanese flight attendant who sought medical attention after feeling tired and short of breath. She explained that she had been in Peru 7 weeks earlier, where she visited some caves with local friends. Her symptoms began 4 weeks after her exploration and included fatigue, shortness of breath, dry cough, joint and muscle pain, and headache. One week later, she was running a low-grade fever (38.5°C or 101.3°F). Her clinical exam showed diffuse rhonchi and rales throughout both lungs. The histoplasmosis histology came back positive. She was successfully treated with ketoconazole.

DID YOU KNOW THAT:
- The reservoir of *Histoplasma capsulatum* is the soil.
- Infection occurs through inhalation of contaminated particles.
- American histoplasmosis is endemic to the United States but also found in Latin America and South Africa.
- Serology can be very useful when the yeast cannot be isolated from sputum or by gastric lavage.
- Itraconazole is very efficient and less toxic than amphotericin B, the traditional treatment.
- Prevention consists of avoiding suspicious caves or bird nesting places.

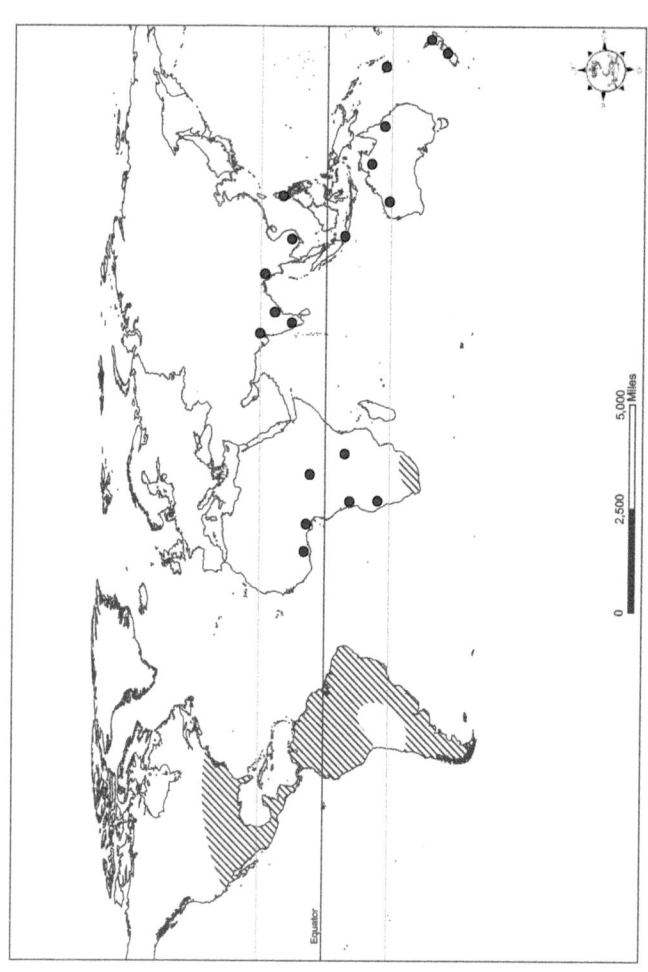

Geographic Distribution of American Histoplasmosis

Lobomycosis (or Jorge Lobo Disease)

Lacazia loboi

Geographic Distribution
Lobomycosis is endemic to the Amazon basin in Brazil, Guiana, and Venezuela.

Main Symptoms
Strictly cutaneous symptoms can be found on the limbs and the ear lobes in the form of cheloid nodules and tumoral or ulcerated plaques. They evolve slowly and generally toward healing.

Treatment
- Surgery but relapses are common

Preventive Measures
- Unknown

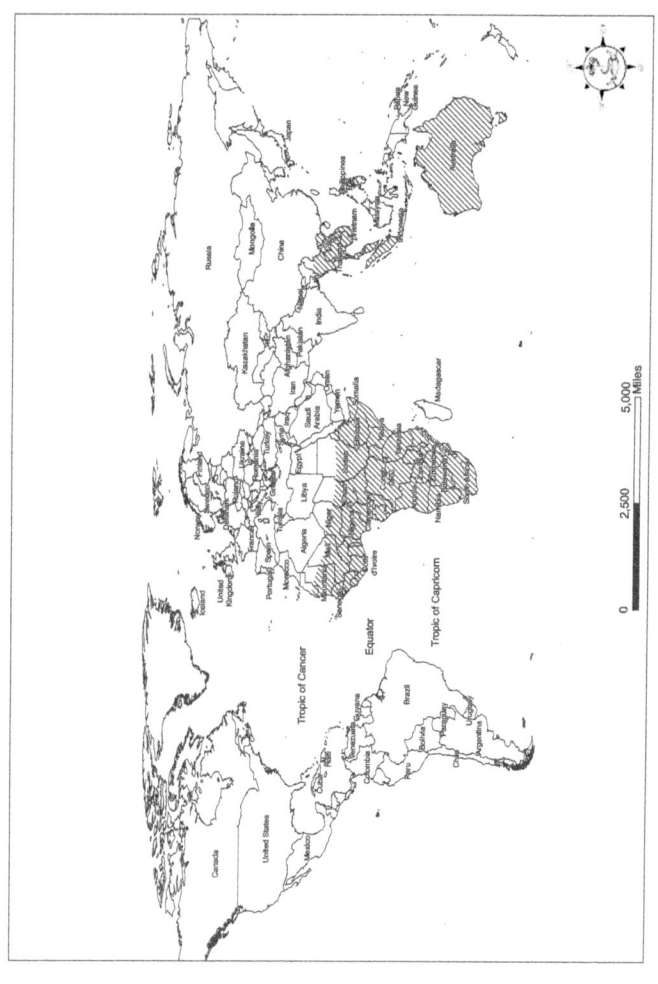

Geographic Distribution of Lobomycosis

////// Endemic Areas

Mycetoma (or Madura Foot)

Maduromycosis is caused by true fungi. Actinomycetoma is due to *Nocardia* and *Actinomadura* sp.

Geographic Distribution

Mycetoma is endemic to areas north and south of the 15th degree of north latitude (for more details please see the map).

Main Symptoms

The disease can be contracted after a scratch or a prick from a contaminated plant. The fungus then penetrates under the skin. It is a rural disease, mainly found among people who walk barefoot. From months to years after contamination, symptoms slowly appear.

African cases

The foot begins to swell without any pain. Black or white grains may ooze from multiple ulcers appearing on the foot. The fungi spread into underlying bones, slowly causing perforations. Although mycetoma predominantly affects the feet, it can sometimes involve the limbs, buttocks, torso, or scalp. Secondary bacterial infections are common.

Central American cases

The disease induces a painful swelling, which is more inflammatory and spreads wider and faster than in the African form. The ulcers are also more numerous. Grains exiting the lesions are very small and white, yellow, or red. The disease can spread to the lymph nodes.

Treatment

Actinomycetomas

- Cotrimoxazole (trimethoprim + sulfamethoxazole) is the treatment of choice.
- Best results are obtained with *Nocardia* spp.
- Dosing:

Table 2.1 Cotrimoxazole adult presentations

Formulation	Trimethoprim	Sulfamethoxazole
Tab (single-strength)	80 mg	400 mg
Tab (double-strength)	160 mg	800 mg
Suspension	80 mg/10 ml	400 mg/10 ml
Parenteral	80 mg/5 ml	400 mg/5 ml

* Adults: 2 single-strength or 1 double-strength tab, po, bid
* Children:

Table 2.2 Cotrimoxazole pediatric doses for the treatment of actinomycetomas

5–8 kg: 120 mg*	9–14 kg: 240 mg*	15–20 kg: 360 mg*	>21 kg: 480 mg*

*Sulfamethoxazole dose (trimethoprim's is automatically proportional)

- All per day and for at least 1 year
- Amikacin can be added to shorten courses
- Dosing:
  * Amikacin, 250 mg, IV or IM, q12h for adults; newborns: 7.5 mg/kg, q12h; other children and older infants: IM inj or IV infusion over 30–60 min, 15 mg/kg/day in two or three divided doses (7.5 mg/kg, q12h, or 5 mg/kg q8h); max 15 mg/kg/day

Fungi mycetomas

- Itraconazole produces good results.
- Dosing:
  * Itraconazole, 400 mg, daily, po, for adults, for months to years; for children, 5–10 mg/kg/day, po, in two divided doses (up to 400 mg/day)
- Azole antifungals are not used in pregnant women because they are teratogenic. Amphotericin B can be used instead.
- Surgery, when necessary and possible.

Always

- Broad-spectrum antibiotics are necessary for secondary bacterial infections.
- Update tetanus immunization.

Preventive Measures

- Disinfect all scratches, cuts, and wounds.
- Wear adequately protective shoes.

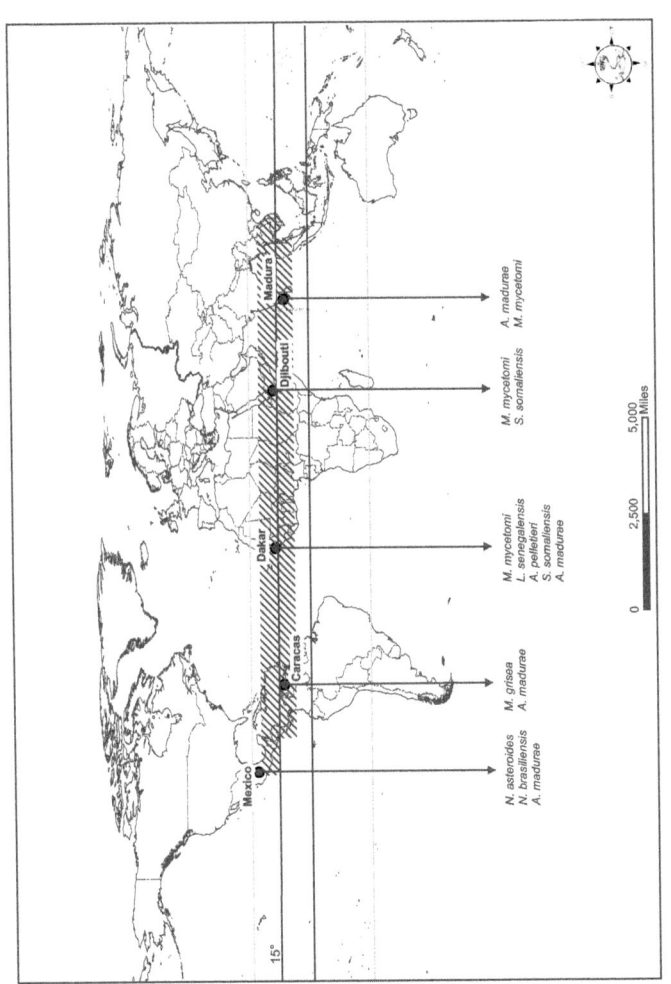

Geographic Distribution of Mycetomas

Pythiosis

Pythium insidiosum

Geographic Distribution

The disease can be found in Thailand and Africa. It affects mainly farmers.

Main Symptoms

Cutaneous or subcutaneous lesions including nodules, sometimes ulcerating, and edema, mainly on the limbs, occur. Ocular forms have been described with keratitis and corneal ulcerations. Other forms include severe vascular lesions, gangrene, and disseminated lesions, which are often lethal. The latter are associated with thalassemia.

Treatment

- Itraconazole can be used.
- Dosing:
  * Itraconazole, 10 mg/kg/day (up to 400 mg/day), po, for adults, for 12 months; for children with mild to moderate infection, itraconazole, 10 mg/kg/day (to a maximum of 400 mg/day, orally); duration is determined on a case-by-case basis
  * Azole antifungals are not used in pregnant women because they are teratogenic. Amphotericin can be used instead (amphotericin B lipid complex, IV, 2.5–5 mg/kg/day for adults and children, both until cure).
  * Long-term itraconazole can be hepatotoxic, and liver enzymes must be monitored.

Preventive Measures

- Unknown

Geographic Distribution of Pythiosis

Endemic Areas
Endemic Areas

Rhinosporidiosis

Rhinosporidium seeberi

Geographic Distribution

Rhinosporidiosis is endemic to the intertropical zone, with a higher prevalence in India, Sri Lanka, and Brazil.

Main Symptoms

The disease can be contracted from contact with infested fish, birds, or mammals or by swimming in infested water. Symptoms include granulomas, papillomas, polyps, or tumor-like masses appearing inside the eyelids, nose, external auditory canal, vagina, and rectum.

Treatment

- Surgery

Preventive Measures

- Avoid contact with disease-carrying animals in endemic areas.
- Do not swim in unknown bodies of water in endemic areas.

Geographic Distribution of Rhinosporidiosis

- Endemic Areas
- Areas of Higher Prevalence

Scytalidiosis

Nattrasia mangiferae and Neosytalidium

Geographic Distribution

Scytalidiosis can be found in the West Indies, Brazil, Guiana, Cameroon, Gabon, Mali, Senegal, and Thailand.

Main Symptoms

The fungus is contracted by walking barefoot or by contact with an infected plant. Symptoms mimic dermatophytosis with onyxis, intertrigo, interdigital skin eruption, and palmo-plantar hyperkeratosis.

Treatment

- Cut damaged nails
- Terbinafine can be used.
- Dosing (Terbinafine)
  - For adults: 250 mg, once daily, po, for 6 weeks (treatment of fingernails) or 12 weeks (treatment of toenails)
  - For children 4 years of age and older and weighing over 35 kg (77 lb): usually 250 mg, once a day, po, for 6 or 12 weeks
  - For children 4 years of age and older and weighing 25 kg (55 lb) to 35 kg (77 lb): usually 187.5 mg, once a day, po, for 6 or 12 weeks
  - For children 4 years of age and older and weighing less than 25 kg (55 lb): usually 125 mg, once a day, po, for 6 or 12 weeks

Preventive Measures

- Wear adequate shoes.

Geographic Distribution of Scytalidiosis

Part 3

Bacterial, Chlamydial, and Prion Diseases

Bacterial Diseases

Anthrax

Bacillus anthracis

Geographic Distribution

Anthrax can be found in many countries but is more common in Asia (Iran), Africa (Senegal, Mauritania, Mali, Niger, Burkina Faso, Ivory Coast, Guinea, Benin, Togo, Chad), South America, and the West Indies. It affects mainly breeders in contact with sick sheep and more rarely caprines and bovines. Internal anthrax is more frequent in Asia and Africa. Other names for anthrax include "black bane," "malignant pustule," "wool sorter's disease," and "tanner's disease."

Main Symptoms

There are four forms of the disease.

External

Spores of *Bacillus anthracis* penetrate humans through skin lacerations, abrasions, or fly bites. After 2–3 days of incubation, a malignant pustule appears at the inoculation site. It is a typical black eschar surrounded with blisters and accompanied with extensive inflammatory edema. Local adenopathy and lymphangitis occur. The lesions chronify and ooze pus. Hematogenous dissemination occurs in 5–10% of untreated cases.

Intestinal

Two to 5 days following ingestion of contaminated meat, abdominal pain and fever appear, followed by nausea, emesis, malaise, anorexia, intestinal edema, ascites, hematemesis, hematochezia, and, rarely, watery diarrhea. Hypovolemic shock may occur from interstitial and intraperitoneal volume losses. The anthrax toxin causes intrinsic renal failure independent of prerenal azotemia. The mortality rate is 50% without treatment.

Thoracic

One to 60 days after inhalation of anthrax spores, symptoms appear, with low-grade fever and a non-productive cough. After initial improvement, the clinical picture deteriorates rapidly with hemorrhagic mediastinitis, high fever, severe dyspnea, tachypnea, cyanosis, profuse diaphoresis, and hematemesis. Chest pain may mimic acute myocardial infarction.

Septicemic

This form results from massive infection by anthrax bacilli. The very large quantity of toxin causes shock and death.

Treatment

Table 3.1 Drug regimens for the treatment of anthrax		
Adults	Ciprofloxacin, 500 mg, po, bid, q12h or Doxycycline, 100 mg, po, bid, q12h	60 days
Children	Ciprofloxacin, 10–15 mg/kg, po, bid, q12h (max 1 g/day) or Doxycycline: >8 yr and >45 kg: same as adult >8 yr and ≤45 kg: 2.2 mg/kg, po, bid, q12h	60 days

Preventive Measures

- Wear masks and gloves.
- During epidemics health-care personnel must use splash protection, gloves, and a full-face respirator with high-efficiency particulate air filters or a self-contained breathing apparatus.
- Seroprevention, either by (1) anthrax immune globulin antitoxin derived from the plasma of individuals previously immunized with the anthrax vaccine or (2) human monoclonal protective antigen-targeted antibodies against toxins, when antibiotics might not be effective.
- A three-dose postexposure anthrax vaccine regimen (at 0 weeks, 2 weeks, and 4 weeks) is recommended by the CDC, in conjunction with antibiotics.
- The standard treatment of anthrax consists of a 60-day antibiotic regimen. Ciprofloxacin or doxycycline can be used. Initial therapy should be IV for internal anthrax and po for external anthrax. Treatment is more effective when started early in the disease.
- Advanced inhalation anthrax may not repond to antibiotics (by the later stages of the disease, the bacteria have often produced more toxins than drugs can eliminate.)
- Dosing:
  * *Ciprofloxacin*
    * Adults: 1 tab of 500 mg, po, bid, q12h.
    * Children 15 mg/kg (maximum 500 mg per dose), po, bid, q12h

Take the drug 2 hours before or after a meal with one large glass of water. If an upset stomach occurs, take it with food. Avoid dairy products such as milk and yogurt for at least 3 hours before and after taking the medicine.

- *Doxycycline*
  * Adults: 1 tab of 100 mg, po, bid, q12h
  * Children: 2 to 4 mg/kg/day (up to 200 mg/day), po, divided, bid, q12h
- Doxycycline is not indicated for use in children < 8 years old, due to staining of teeth and inhibition of bone growth associated with tetracyclines
- Chemoprophylaxis for people who have been exposed: tetracycline (including doxycycline) penicillin, or amoxicillin at their usual dosages, for 60 days. For example, amoxicillin, postexposure inhalational prophylaxis: 500 mg, po, q8hr
- Immunize animals.

Bartonellosis (or Carrion Disease)

Bartonella bacilliformis

Geographic Distribution

Bartonellosis is endemic to the western part of tropical South America. This mainly rural disease is found in the Andes at altitudes ranging from 600 to 3,000 m (approximately 1,970–9,850 feet).

Main Symptoms

Approximately 3 weeks after being bitten at night by an infected *Phlebotomus* sand fly, symptoms appear in two phases.

Acute or Oroya fever

After an incubation period lasting 1–14 weeks, symptoms include irregular fever, anemia, mild icterus, hepatosplenomegaly, and adenopathy. The fever lasts 7–28 days.

Chronic or Peruvian verruga

After the acute phase or as first symptoms, skin lesions appear. Three types can be seen: (1) numerous and small lepromatous-like papules, (2) rare nodules at least 3 mm in diameter, and (3) deep subcutaneous nodules. Low-grade fever, arthralgia, malaise, and cephalgia often occur concomitantly. Symptoms evolve toward spontaneous healing in 4–6 months. A second bout is possible in 5% of cases.

Treatment

- Chloramphenicol is very active when bacilli are in the blood.
- Dosing:
  * Chloramphenicol, 50 mg/kg, daily, IV, in four divided doses, q6h, (maximum 4,000 mg/day), for children and adults, until 10 days after apyrexia is reached. Repeated CBC controls are needed.

Preventive Measures

- Use insecticides to kill vectors.
- Use repellents containing DEET (15–30%). Be aware that they can only provide transitory protection.
- Treat clothes with insecticides containing permethrin.
- Be aware that usual mosquito nets are not efficient because sand flies can fly through their holes.
- Use air conditioning in the bedroom (low temperature makes mosquitoes less active).

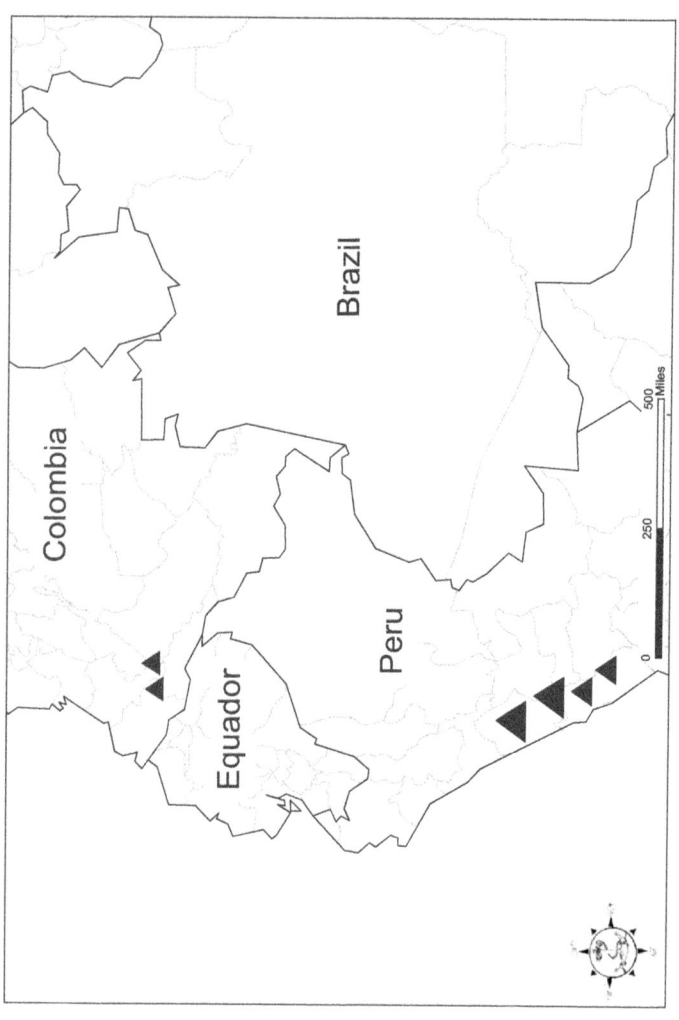

Geographic Distribution of Bartonellosis

Foci of Bartonellosis

Bejel (or Endemic Syphilis)

Treponema pallidum var. endemicum

Geographic Distribution

Bejel is endemic to the Sahel area in Africa, the Middle East, Southeast Asia, and the western Pacific.

Main Symptoms

Transmission is made directly from humans to humans through skin or mucosal contact. Symptoms appear chronologically in two phases.

Early

Buccal plaques
Round or oval soft ulcerations, which bleed easily and become covered with a gray coating. They can hypertrophy into papillomatous or vegetative lesions. Their most common locations are inside the lips or cheeks, on the tongue, and at the corner of the mouth.

Anogenital plaques
Between the buttocks, in the perineum, on the foreskin, or on the penis.

Cutaneous lesions
Papillomatous, circinate, or more rarely serpiginous lesions in the folds of the axillae or elbows

Bone lesions
Identical to those of yaws, involving the legs and forearms

Late

After years, gummas develop. When they affect the nose, they can cause severe mutilations. Polymorphous skin lesions (pseudotuberculous or pseudopsoriatic) are common.

Treatment

- Penicillin is the drug of choice.
- Erythromycin or doxycycline can be used for patients allergic to penicillin.
- Dosing
  * Benzathine penicillin, 1.2–2.4 M IU, IM, for adults and 600,000–1.2 M IU, IM, for children depending on the duration of symptoms, both once
  * Erythromycin, 250–500 mg (base, estolate, stearate) or 400–800 mg (ethylsuccinate), po, q6h for adults, for 2–3 weeks; for children, 40–50 mg/kg/day, po, divided, q6h, for 2–3 weeks; max 2 g/day (not for infants <1 month of age)
  * Doxycycline, 100 mg, po, bid, q12h, for 2–3 weeks. Not for children <8 years old.

Preventive Measures

- Avoid contact with sick people.
- Avoid endemic areas.

Buruli Ulcers (or Bairnsdale, Daintree, Mossman, or Searls Ulcer or Mycoburuli Ulcers)

Mycobacterium ulcerans

Geographic Distribution

Buruli ulcers endemic to black Africa, Australia, Southeast Asia, and Guiana. They were named after a county in Uganda.

Main Symptoms

The disease starts with a cold and painless papule, nodule, plaque, or skin edema on a lower (60% of cases) or upper (30% of cases) limb, rarely on the face or on the body trunk. The nodules and papules ulcerate. Ulcers have elevated edges, usually chronify, and can be numerous. Local adenopathies result mainly from secondary bacterial infections. Spontaneous healing may occur with sequelae such as cheloid scars, retraction, and ankylosis. Relapses on the same site are frequent. Complications include destruction of tendons, muscles, nerves, bones, and other organs. Arthritis and osteomyelitis may occur. Bone deformities remain as sequelae.

Treatment

- *Mycobacterium ulcerans* is resistant to numerous antibiotics.
- The best approach is to choose an efficient antibiotic according to antibiogram results.
- Surgery and resection of infected and necrotic tissue are often necessary.
- Amputation may be required.

Preventive Measures

- Unknown

Geographic Distribution of Buruli Ulcers

Chancroid (or Soft Chancre or Ulcus Molle)

Haemophilus ducreyi

Geographic Distribution and New Problems

Chancroid is endemic to Asia and Africa, where it is a public health concern particularly since it has become resistant to sulfas and macrolides.

Main Symptoms

One to 5 days after sexual contact with an infected individual, a small bump appears on the genitalia or around the anus. It becomes an ulcer within 24 h, with the following features.

- Its size varies between 3.2 and 50.8 mm (0.13 and 2 in).
- It is painful.
- It has sharply defined, eroded, irregular, or ragged borders.
- Its base is covered with a gray or yellowish-gray material.
- It bleeds easily when traumatized.

In women, who are often asymptomatic carriers of the disease, the main symptom may be dysuria or dyspareunia with lesions of the vulva, vagina, or cervix. Painful inguinal lymphadenopathy, usually unilateral, develops in approximately 50% of patients within 1–2 weeks. Lymph nodes can become soft with fistulae.

Treatment

- Erythromycin is efficient and has few side effects. Ceftriaxone and azithromycin are alternatives.
- Dosing:
    * Erythromycin, 2g (2 × 500 mg, bid), po, for 7 days
    * Azithromycin, 1 g, po, once
    * Ceftriaxone, 250 mg, IM, once
- Local adenopathies should not be incised and drained.
- Treat partner(s).
- Check for other STDs.

Preventive Measures

- Wear condoms when having sex with casual partners.
- Use only water-based lubricants.
- Practice strict body hygiene.
- Avoid sharing towels or underclothing.
- Wash before and after intercourse.
- Urinate after intercourse.
- Know the health of your sexual partner(s).

Cholera

Toxigenic Vibrio cholerae O-group 1 or O-group 139

Historical Background

The historical epicenter of cholera is the Ganges delta in India and Bangladesh. From there, six worldwide epidemics have started.

Due to the panic surrounding cholera, an international conference was held in Paris in 1851, making it the first globalized public health problem. Robert Koch discovered the causal agent of the disease, *Vibrio cholerae* in 1883.

The seventh cholera pandemic started in 1961 and can be traced from the Celebes to other islands of Indonesia and India, Afghanistan, Iran, Iraq (August 1966), the Suez Canal, Israel, Jordan, Turkey, Russia, Czechoslovakia, Egypt, Libya, Tunisia, Morocco, Algeria, Somalia, Ethiopia, Sudan, Kenya, Uganda, Rwanda, Tanzania, Guinea (August 1970), Mali (November 1970), Cameroon (March 1971), Burkina Faso, Niger, Nigeria, Chad, Central African Republic (June 1971), Mauritania and East Senegal (summer 1971).

In 1972, the epidemic spread to other continents: Europe (Spain, Portugal, Italy, France, Great Britain), Oceania (Australia), North America (United States), and South America (Brazil). In 1978, the great lakes area of East Africa was hit, as well as some islands in the Indian Ocean.

In 1979, the disease infiltrated South Africa. In 2006, there were outbreaks reported from Yemen, the Philippines, Thailand, Myanmar, Malaysia, Indonesia, India, Bangladesh, Zimbabwe, Zambia, Uganda, Tanzania, Sudan, South Africa, Sierra Leone, Sao Tome and Principe, Rwanda, Nigeria, Mozambique, Malawi, Liberia, Kenya, Guinea Bissau, Guinea, Ghana, Democratic Republic of Congo, Cameroon, Burundi, and Angola. There was a high-mortality outbreak in Zimbabwe in 2008, which subsequently spread to South Africa, Botswana, Mozambique, and Zambia. A cholera epidemic started in the UN camp of Mirabalais in Haiti, which was established after the earthquake in late 2010. More than 7,500 people had died from it as of November 16, 2012 (more than twice as many as on the whole African continent in the same period of time).

New Problems

The late 1990s saw a resurgence of cholera with many outbreaks. The most notorious have been in East Africa, coinciding with the flow of people uprooted from their country by civil conflict. In 1994, an epidemic killed at least 30,000 refugees within weeks, after over 1 million Hutus fled from Rwanda to then eastern Zaire in fear of genocide by the Tutsis. The Hutus were gathered in camps that were quickly organized without sufficient time for hygienic structures to be built. Moreover, the turmoil of the environment made medical screenings and checkups impossible until adequate support arrived. As a result of the high concentration of people and lack of basic hygienic conditions, cholera broke out rampantly. Cholera epidemics continue to be a public health threat in Africa where *V. cholerae* has become resistant to sulfas.

Geographic Distribution

Cholera has been reported from many countries in Africa, Central and South America, and Asia. In 2009, 45 countries reported 221,226 cholera cases

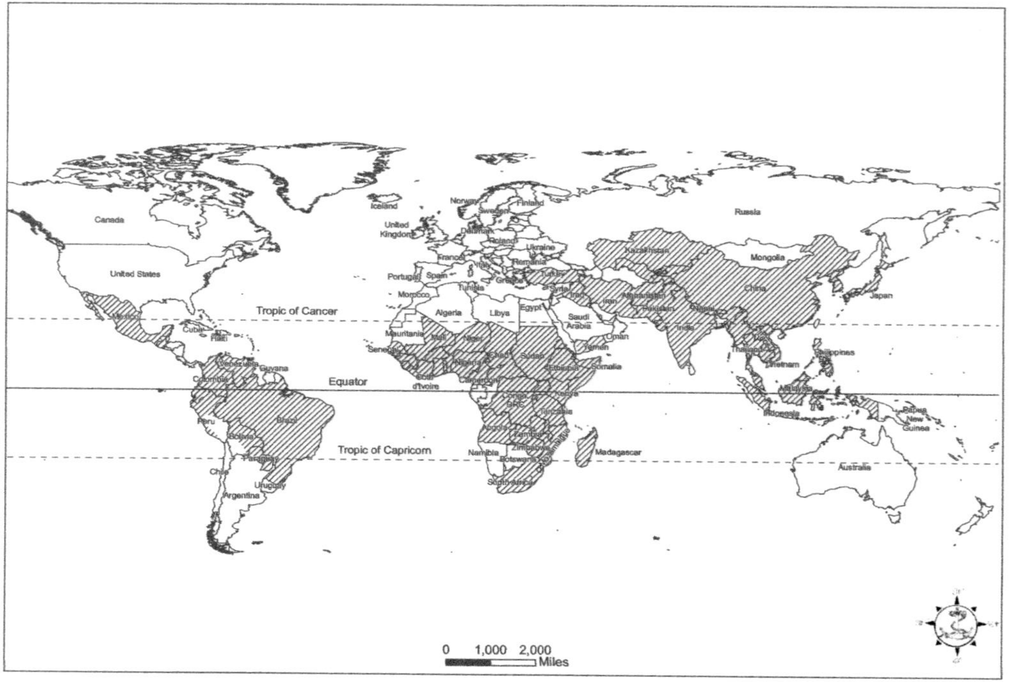

Reported Cases

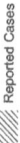

Geographic Distribution of Cholera

including 4,946 deaths to the WHO (case-fatality rate 2.24%). 99% of cases were from Africa, continuing a trend.

Main Symptoms

Four forms of the disease have been described.

Classic

Two to 3 days after ingesting contaminated food or water or becoming infected by direct human contact, gastralgia, anxiety, moderate diarrhea, and emesis appear abruptly. Within 2 h, the patient experiences numerous bowel movements, without abdominal cramps but with some tension in the stomach. Stools are very watery, colorless, odorless, and bloodless (rice water stool). Vomit has the same characteristics. The patient rapidly becomes weak and dehydrated, getting a hoarse and weak voice, a gaunt face, and circles around the eyes, which sink into the sockets. The skin becomes cyanotic and is covered with cold sweat. Death occurs usually within 48–72 h.

Dysenteric

This form represents about 5% of all cases. Diarrhea can become bloody, and emesis is less intense.

Fulminant

"Dry" cholera kills by hypovolemic shock before diarrhea can be seen. It occurs mainly in children.

Benign

This form may be misleading by its milder onset.

Severe forms of cholera rarely heal spontaneously.

Treatment

- Large amounts of IV fluids and electrolytes are essential. Rehydration is accomplished in two phases: (1) replenishing and (2) maintenance. Antibiotics are useful.
- Dosing
  * (1) Lactated Ringer, IV, over up to 4 h, 50–100 ml/kg/h
  * (2) Oral rehydrating solution: 500–1,000 ml/h
- Sulfadoxine, one IM injection of 1.5–2 g for adults and 0.5–1 g for children

Preventive Measures

- During epidemics, sulfadoxine 1.5–2 g, daily, po, for adults, and 250 mg–1 g, daily, po, for children
- Practice personal hygiene and systematically wash hands before meals.
- Immunization is possible and 4 vaccines are available. The inactivated WC/rBS oral vaccine is given in 2 doses, 1 week apart. No significant adverse reactions have been described and protection rates range from 85–90% after 6 months to about 60% after 2 years.

Progression of the Cholera Pandemic in West Africa (1970-1979)

Cholera Pandemic (1961-1991)

Diphtheria

Corynebacterium diphtheriae

Geographic Distribution

Because of partial immunization coverage of populations, diphtheria is still common in some developing countries; but it is rare in black Africa. There were 4,887 cases reported in the world in 2011.

Main Symptoms

Infection is direct from humans to humans. Several forms of the disease have been described.

Pseudomembranous tonsillitis

It is the most common form. After a 2- to 5-day incubation period, pharyngitis appears, usually in the absence of systemic complaints (fever is rare and mild, and malaise, dysphagia, and cephalgia are not prominent features). Membranes start to develop and involve the pharyngeal walls, tonsils, uvula, and soft palate. They may extend to the larynx and trachea, causing airway obstruction and eventual suffocation. Lymphadenopathy and edema of the neck may lead to a bull-neck appearance. Complications include myocarditis and neurological symptoms causing rapid death.

Laryngeal

It is the most common form in infants, with hoarseness leading to aphonia and severe respiratory tract obstruction. A foul smell may appear. Croup is a serious complication.

Cutaneous

It is relatively frequent in central and eastern Africa, with painful and erythematous lesions progressing to impetiginous or eczematiform ulcers with sharply defined borders and a brownish gray membrane. Symptoms can last for months.

Paralytic

Paralytic symptoms appear late in the disease.

Other forms

External ear, palpebral conjunctivae, and the genital mucosa can be involved. Endocarditis cases have been reported. Septicemia is rare but always fatal.

Treatment

- Strict isolation until at least two subsequent cultures taken 24 h apart after cessation of therapy come back negative.
- Specific antitoxin is the mainstay of therapy.
- Dosing:
    * Mild or moderate severity: 4,000–30,000 U, IM, after a test dose to eliminate hypersensitivity
    * Severe: 40,000–100,000 U, IV, over 30–60 min
- Antibiotics help kill bacteria in the body and reduce the length of the contagious period.

- Amoxicillin, penicillin, and erythromycin are the treatments of choice.
- Dosing:
  * Amoxicillin, for adults, 1 g, tid, po; for children, see Table 3.2.

Table 3.2 Amoxicillin pediatric doses for the treatment of diphtheria

5–9 kg: 62.5 mg*	10–19 kg: 125 mg*	20–39 kg: 250 mg*	>40 kg: 250–500 mg*

* tid, po.

  * Benzathine penicillin, for adults and children >27 kg (60 lb), 1.2 M units, IM, daily; for children <27 kg (60 lb), 600,000 units, IM, daily, for a few days
  * Erythromycin, for adults, 400 mg, po, divided in two doses, q12h; for children with mild to moderate infection, 30–50 mg/kg/day, po, divided in 4 doses, q6h; for children with severe infection, 60–100 mg/kg/day, po, divided in four doses, q6h; for neonates <1.2 kg, 20 mg/kg/day, po, divided in two doses, q12h; for neonates ≥1.2 kg, 7 days or older, 30 mg/kg/day, po, divided in three doses, q8h
- All for 14 days. Two negative cultures, taken at least 24 h apart, indicate successful treatment. If either culture is positive, a further treatment with erythromycin or penicillin must be initiated, for 10 days.
- Croup: urgent intubation or tracheotomy
- For severe cases: ICU

Preventive Measures

- Immunization. The vaccine is made of an inactivated diphtheria toxin. In the United States, 5 IM injections are given at 2, 4, 6 and between 15-18 months old with a booster between 4-6 years of age. Thereafter, the Tdap vaccine, which protects adolescents and adults against diphtheria as well as tetanus and pertussis is given only once from 11-64 years of age. In other countries the immunization schedule may differ.
- Strict isolation and treatment of healthy carriers (antibiotics for 7–10 days + age-appropriate diphtheria toxoid if the patient has not received a booster injection within 1 year)

Gonorrhea (or Clap)

Neisseria gonorrhoeae

Historical Background

Until the middle of the 19th century, every STD was thought to be caused by the same bacterial agent. In 1838, Philippe Ricord, a French surgeon born in Baltimore, proved that gonorrhea and syphilis were two different entities.

In 1879, Albert Neisser provided the first details of the bacteria that became known as *Neisseria gonorrhoeae*. The disease is also known as "blenorrhea."

New Problems

The second part of the 20th century saw the emergence of N. gonorrhoeae strains that are increasingly resistant to many antibiotics. The wave of resistance began in Southeast Asia (Thailand in particular), then spread to Brazil, Africa, and the rest of the world. Strains of N. gonorrhoeae resistant to penicillin and tetracyclines can now be found in most major cities. In 2012, 35% of strains in sub-Saharan Africa and >90% in Asia were resistant to penicillin. Up to 70% were resistant to azythromycin in South America. N. gonorrhoeae resistance to fluoroquinolones is higher in Asia than in Africa and South America.

Geographic Distribution

Gonorrhea is present everywhere in the world but is more prevalent in the intertropical zone because of poor local hygienic and socioeconomic conditions.

Estimated new cases of gonorrhea infections (in millions) in adults, 1995 and 1999 (from WHO)

Region	1995			1999		
	Female	Male	Total	Female	Male	Total
North America	0.92	0.83	1.75	0.84	0.72	1.56
Western Europe	0.63	0.60	1.23	0.63	0.49	1.11
North America and Middle East	0.77	0.77	1.54	0.68	0.79	1.47
Eastern Europe and Central Asia	1.16	1.17	2.32	1.81	1.50	3.31
Sub-Saharan Africa	8.38	7.30	15.67	8.84	8.19	17.03
South and Southeast Asia	14.55	14.56	29.11	15.09	12.12	27.20
East Asia and Pacific	1.47	1.80	3.27	1.68	1.59	3.27
Australia and New Zealand	0.07	0.06	0.13	0.06	0.06	0.12
Latin America and Caribbean	3.67	3.45	7.12	4.01	3.26	7.27
Total	31.61	30.54	62.15	33.65	28.70	62.35

Main Symptoms

Men

Five to 6 days after direct infection from sexual contact with an infected person, dysuria and a milky discharge from the urethra often appear. One to 3 days later, pain increases and the discharge becomes yellow. Complications include epididymitis, which can lead to sterility.

Women

The disease often remains asymptomatic. When present, symptoms include dysuria, polyuria, urgency, and vaginal discharge with pus. Complications encompass vaginitis, cervicitis, bartholinitis, metritis, salpingitis, and pelvic inflammatory disease. Symptoms of pelvic inflammatory disease include lower abdominal pain, cervical motion tenderness, adnexal tenderness (usually bilateral) or adnexal mass, intermenstrual bleeding, fever, chills, nausea, and sometimes emesis. PID can damage the fallopian tubes and lead to infertility. It also increases the risk of ectopic pregnancy.

Men and women
Pharyngitis, conjunctivitis, and rectitis. Systemic complications (disseminated gonococcal infection) include fever, tenosynovitis, arthritis (mainly knees, ankles, wrists), and skin eruption with the following characteristics:

- Small papules that turn into pustules on broad erythematous bases with a necrotic center
- Located on the trunk, limbs, palms, and soles (usually it spares the face, scalp, and mouth)

Other skin lesions include purpura, erythema nodosum, urticaria, and erythema multiforme. They occur less frequently.

In rare cases, pericarditis, endocarditis, or meningitis can develop. Gonorrhea increases the risk of HIV transmission.

Newborns
Bilateral conjunctivitis (ophthalmia neonatorum) with ophthalmalgia, hyperemia, and a purulent discharge. Neonates may also acquire a pharyngeal, respiratory, rectal, or disseminated gonococcal infection.

Treatment

- The antibiotic of choice depends on the region of origin of the bacteria:
  - Asia: Cefuroxime, 1,000 mg, po, in a single dose
  - United States: Ceftriaxone, 250 mg, IM, single dose + azithromycin, 1 g, po, single dose, or doxycycline, 100 mg, bid, q12h, po, for 7 days
  - Other areas: Choose efficient antibiotics, recommended by local colleagues, based on their daily practice (foci of drug resistance are often not published in the international literature).
- The antibiogram result will enable treatment adjustment, if needed.
- Check for other STDs (in particular HIV, syphilis, and chlamydia).
- Any sexual partner(s) must be treated concomitantly.

Preventive Measures

- Use condoms with new sexual partner(s).
- Use only water-based lubricants.
- Practice strict body hygiene.
- Avoid sharing towels or underclothing.
- Wash before and after intercourse.
- Urinate after intercourse.
- Postcoital minocycline, po, is effective on sensitive strains.
- Prophylactic antibiotic combinations are effective against both gonorrhea and syphilis and vary geographically.
- Know the health of your sexual partner(s).

Granuloma Inguinale (or Donovan Disease)

Klebsiella granulomatis

Geographic Distribution

Granuloma inguinale is found only in the intertropical zone, where it is endemic to the West Indies, South America, India, Papua New Guinea, and some Pacific islands.

Main Symptoms

Eight to 12 days after infection, mainly (but not only) by sexual contact with an infected partner, symptoms begin on the skin or mucous membranes of the genital or anal area. The lesion(s) spreads progressively to the lower abdomen and thighs. Five types of symptoms have been described.

Ulcerovegetative lesions

Most common. Large, usually painless, expanding, suppurative ulcers develop from nodules. They have clean, friable bases with distinct, raised, rolled margins and bleed easily. They slowly expand centrifugally in the skinfolds. Smelly secondary bacterial infections are usual.

Nodular lesions

A papule or a soft, often pruritic, and erythematous nodule arises at the site of inoculation. The latter eventually ulcerates.

Hypertrophic or verrucous lesions

Relatively rare. Proliferative reaction, with large vegetating masses, which may resemble genital warts.

Cicatricial lesions

Cicatricial plaques, which may be associated with lymphedema.

Complications

Autoinoculation may lead to involvement of the lips, oral/gastrointestinal mucosa, scalp, abdomen, arms, legs, and bones. Elephantiasis-like swelling of the external genitalia is a frequent complication in females in the late stage of the disease. Disseminated lesions to the spleen, lungs, liver, bones, and orbits associated with systemic symptoms can be observed. They occasionally result in death. Squamous cell carcinoma and less often basal cell carcinoma can develop from long-standing lesions or scars.

Treatment

- Trimethoprim + sulfamethoxazole or doxycycline. Alternatives include ciprofloxacin, erythromycin, and azithromycin. Tetracycline resistance has been reported from various countries.
- Dosing:
  * Trimethoprim 80 mg + sulfamethoxazole, 400 mg, po, bid, q12h
  * or doxycycline, 100–200 mg, po, bid, q12h
  * or erythromycin, 2 g/day
  * or azithromycin, 1 g/week
  * Regimens vary but courses should last at least 3 weeks, alternating antibiotics until all lesions have healed.
- Treat partner(s).
- Check for other STDs.

Preventive Measures

- Use condoms during sexual intercourse with new partners.
- Use only water-based lubricants.
- Avoid sharing towels or underclothing.
- Wash before and after intercourse.
- Urinate after intercourse.
- Practice strict personal hygiene.
- Know the health of your sexual partner(s).

Geographic Distribution of Donovan Disease

///// Endemic Areas

Leprosy (or Hansen Disease)

Mycobacterium leprae

Geographic Distribution

Pockets of high endemicity of leprosy can be found in Indonesia, the Philippines, Democratic Republic of Congo, India, Madagascar, Mozambique, Nepal, Tanzania, and some areas of Brazil. According to the WHO, there were approximately 219,000 new cases reported worldwide in 2011, mainly from Asia and Africa

Main Symptoms

The mode of transmission is unclear. Classically, infection occurs after close and long contact with an infected person presenting a multibacillary form. Clinically, leprosy is a spectrum disease with thresholds. With time, in the same patient it may evolve between two poles or forms. On one end stands the tuberculoid form (TT) and on the other the lepromatous form (LL). In between other forms have been described as borderline, interpolar, and indeterminate (I) (Table 3.3).

Table 3.3

Tuberculoid end ←				→ Lepromatous end
Few bacilli				Many bacilli
TT	BT	BB	BL	LL

TT = tuberculoid form; BT = borderline tuberculoid form; BB = borderline form; BL = borderline lepromatous form; LL = lepromatous form.
From the Ridley Jopling classification.

Nevertheless for therapeutic reasons, the WHO has adopted a classification based on bacteriological criteria: (1) pauci and (2) multibacillary leprosy.

Paucibacillary I form

This form is mainly seen in children. It represents about 50% of all cases of leprosy.

Skin lesions are hypochromic or slightly red, flat maculae with well-defined borders. Sometimes repigmentation occurs at their center. The lesions are few. Hypoesthesia, anhidrosis, and alopecia occur.

Paucibacillary T form

Skin lesions are erythematous on light skin, or hypopigmented or copper-colored on dark skin, plaque (5–20 cm [2–7.8 in] diameter); typically salient and concave with an elevated edge; round or oval in shape. The central area is often atrophic. Alternatively, it can be a large erythematous macule (>5 cm [2 in]) with occasional central healing and repigmentation. Hypoesthesia or anesthesia (no response to touch, heat, or pain stimuli) of these lesions is typical with anhidrosis and alopecia. In children below 3 years of age, the only skin lesion can be a purple nodule, which will heal spontaneously in 6–24 months. The lesions are well defined, few, and asymmetrical.

Neurological lesions are usually located close to the skin lesions. Peripheral hypertrophic neuropathy with mono- or polyneuritis, which is erratic but severe occurs with hyper- or anesthetic nerves. Lesions evolve toward sclerosis, mutilation, and aseptic abscesses. In decreasing order of frequency the following nerves are affected: cubital, external popliteal sciatic, facial, radial, median, and the superficial cervical plexus.

Sensitivity is altered with hypo- or anesthesia, paresthesia, and neuralgia. Anhidrosis, amyotrophy, cubital claw, facial palsy with lagophthalmos, neurotrophic disorders (whitlow, plantar ulcers, osteoporosis, osteolysis, and mutilation of toes, fingers, and feet) can occur.

Ocular lesions include keratitis and corneal ulcers.

Multibacillary LL form

Skin lesions are erythematous or hypopigmented (on dark skin) macules or infiltrated papulonodules called "lepromas," which are salient and convex. They are small (up to 2 cm [0.8 in] in diameter) and appear most often on the face. Eyebrows and eyelashes can be destroyed, but hair is intact. The lesions are numerous (50–100), ill-defined, symmetrical, and bilateral. Neurological lesions are the same as in the paucibacillary T form, but many more nerves are involved. The evolution of lesions is slow.

ENT symptoms include ear lobes infiltrated with lesions. In 80% of cases, rhinitis occurs, producing pus and blood. Perforation and destruction of nasal cartilage, glossitis, pharyngitis, and laryngitis are less common.

Visceral manifestations include polyadenopathy, gynecomastia, and infiltration of the testicles, liver, bones, and kidneys (which causes 13–38% of deaths).

The main complication is Lucio phenomenon which consists of blue hemorrhagic plaques and necrotic ulcerations, followed by necrotic epidermis and vasculitis with thrombus formation and endothelial proliferation.

BT form

Skin lesions differ from the TT form by the following characteristics: more numerous (2–10), possible satellite small lesions, with less anesthesia. The lesions are round or oval, erythematous, infiltrated, and somewhat well defined. Their edge is papular, elevated, with an abrupt slope outward and a gentle slope inward. The central area is typically hypopigmented and occasionnaly atrophic. Nerve involvement is common and early. Mutilation is asymmetrical, affecting one or several nerves.

BB form

This form is rare. Skin lesions are ill defined and consist of infiltrated papules of annular shape with broad edges. There is no or little hypoesthesia. Hair or mucosal involvement is rare. Neurological lesions become more bilateral and symmetrical toward the LL pole.

BL form

Skin lesions are more numerous (10–50), bilateral, symmetrical without hypoesthesia, but with partial or total peripheral infiltration (lepromas). Hair and mucosal involvement is more frequent toward the LL pole. Neurological lesions are grossly bilateral and symmetrical.

Treatment
- The regimens are shown in Table 3.4.
- Leprous reactions can occur at any time during treatment. Three types are possible: (1) reversion from borderline toward tuberculoid, (2) degradation from borderline toward lepromatous, and (3) erythema nodosum leprosum (ENL)
- ASA, NSAIDs, thalidomide, corticosteroids, or clofazimine (only as an adjunct to corticosteroids) can be used for ENL.
- Dosing
  * Mild ENL reactions
    - ASA, 600–1,200 mg/day, po, divided in four to six doses, for adults; for children, initially 60–90 mg/kg/day in divided doses, q6–8h, and maintenance 80–100 mg/kg/day, in divided doses q6–8h, po, monitoring serum concentrations
    - Thalidomide, initial dose 100–300 mg, po, once a day with water, preferably at bedtime and at least 1 h after the evening meal; patients <50 kg should be started at the low end of the dose range; for adults and children >12 yr. It is contraindicated in pregnant women (please see Contraindications for Drugs page 314).
  * Severe ENL reactions
    - Prednisone, 60–80 mg/day, po, slowly tapering by reducing by 5–10 mg every 2–4 weeks, for adults; for children, 0.14–2 mg/kg/day in three or four divided doses, po (4–60 mg/m^2/day)
    - Thalidomide, initial dose up to 400 mg/day, po, once a day at bedtime or in divided doses with water, at least 1 h after meals. In general, dosing should continue until active reaction subsides (usually at least 2 weeks), then tapered in 50-mg decrements every 2–4 weeks. Patients with a history of requiring prolonged maintenance to prevent recurrence or who flare during tapering should be maintained on the minimum dose necessary to control the reaction. Tapering off medication should be attempted every 3–6 months, in decrements of 50 mg every 2–4 weeks, for adults and children >12 yr. It is contraindicated in pregnant women (please see Contraindications for Drugs page 314).

Table 3.4 Treatment regimens for leprosy

	Daily (self-administered)	Monthly (under supervision)	Treatment duration
Paucibacillary	Dapsone 100 mg, po	Rifampicin 600 mg, po	6–12 months
Multibacillary	Dapsone 100 mg, po Clofazimine 50 mg, po	Rifampicin 600 mg, po Clofazimine 300 mg, po	24 months
Pediatric	Dapsone 2 mg/kg, po Clofazimine 1 mg/kg, po	Rifampicin 10 mg/kg, po Clofazimine 6 mg/kg, po	Same as in adults

- Clofazimine, 200–300 mg, po, daily, for adults and children, for up to 3 months. Dosage should be tapered to 100 mg daily as quickly as possible after the reactive episode is controlled.
- Decompressive surgery for the relief of mechanical compression in cases of severe neuritis or in patients with neuritis not responding to medical therapy
- Amputation is sometimes necessary.
- Physiotherapy accelerates functional recovery.
- Patient should be monitored for 5–10 years post-treatment.

Preventive Measures

- A vaccine should be soon available to prevent lepromatous leprosy.
- The BCG vaccine produces a protection against leprosy in about 50% of recipients and is more effective in paucibacillary forms. It is recommended for household contacts of patients with leprosy.

Leptospirosis (or Weil Disease or Nanukayami Fever)

Serovars of *Leptospira interrogans*

Geographic Distribution

Leptospirosis is prevalent in Japan, Vietnam, Malaysia, Indonesia, and Australia. The disease can also be found in Africa (Democratic Republic of Congo, Senegal, and Morocco), Reunion Island, New Caledonia, and Central and South America. Isolated cases have been reported from Europe and California. Other names for leptospirosis include "canicola fever," "canefield fever," and "7-day fever."

Main Symptoms

Means of contamination include

1. Ingesting food or drink contaminated by the urine of an infested animal (rat, dog, cat, cow, sheep, or pig)
2. Being bitten by an infested rat
3. Direct contact with a sick animal
4. Swimming in water contaminated by the urine of an infested animal

Symptoms occur on average 10 days after infection and include sudden high fever, cephalgia, arthralgia and myalgia (involving particularly the calf muscles), neck stiffness, icterus, oliguria, and exanthem. After 7–10 days of evolution, improvement can be seen: temperature returns to normal and jaundice subsides. A possible relapse without jaundice begins on the fifteenth day. Twenty days after contamination, the healing process begins. Recuperation from the disease may take weeks, with complete recovery in most cases.

Milder forms of leptospirosis exist, particularly without jaundice. Complications include myocarditis, aseptic meningitis, hepatic failure with or without renal failure, pulmonary hemorrhage, iridocyclitis, seizures, ARD, and coma. Poor prognostic signs are oliguria, lung involvement, hypotension, and hypokalemia.

Treatment

- For mild leptospirosis, doxycycline is the drug of choice. Alternative drugs include amoxicillin and azithromycin dihydrate.
- For moderate and severe leptospirosis, penicillin G remains the drug of choice.
- Doses should be increased progressively over 3–4 days at the start until reaching the optimal dosage, to avoid a Jarisch-Herxheimer reaction.
- Dosing:
  * Penicillin, 1.5 M units, IV or IM, q6–8h, for 10 days
  * Doxycycline, 100 mg, po, bid, q12h, for 10 days

Preventive Measures

- Immunize people who are exposed to leptospirosis in their profession (the vaccine protects for a short period of time, and none covers all serogroups. In France, a vaccine is available against serovar *icterohaemorrhagiae*.
- Doxycycline on a weekly basis can be prescribed for short stays in high-risk areas.
- Wear protective clothing (gloves, boots, overalls) in high-risk areas.
- Avoid swimming in suspicious bodies of freshwater (including swimming pools).

Melioidosis (or Whitmore Disease)

Burkholderia pseudomallei

Historical Background

Melioidosis was first identified in 1911 by Alfred Whitmore and his assistant C. S. Krishnaswami in Yangon, Burma. During the Second Indochina War, many cases of melioidosis were treated in the United States.

New Problems

Progressive worldwide drug addiction has created new human reservoirs of Whitmore's bacillus. The disease has dispersed widely and is no longer restricted to rural areas of Asia. *Burkholderia pseudomallei* is now challenging major city hospitals. In some regions of Southeast Asia, each year melioidosis kills as many people as tuberculosis.

Geographic Distribution

Traditionally, melioidosis has been endemic to Burma, Malaysia, Thailand, Vietnam, Indonesia, Northern Australia and the Philippines. Rare cases have been identified in the Middle East, Africa, and South America. For example, from 1989 to 1996, there were 372 cases in Singapore, resulting in 147 deaths. Melioidosis is a major cause of death in Thailand. In 2012, the paucity of information about the disease created an incomplete map of global risk with vast regions of the world completely unchartered, including India, Africa, and most of South America.

Main Symptoms

The incubation period of the disease is unknown. Human contamination occurs from contact with contaminated water or mud in ponds, rice paddies, or rivers. *Burkholderia pseudomallei* enters the human body through a wound or a break in the skin (e.g., from dirty needles). Four forms of the disease have been described.

Inconspicuous
It is very common. No symptoms appear, and only serology can show previous contact with *Burkholderia pseudomallei*.

Localized
The skin (ulcers), lymph nodes (chronically oozing pus), muscles, or bones can be involved.

Pulmonary
It is the form most frequently seen by physicians. Symptoms often include fever, weight loss, and a cough producing mucus, pus, and blood. It can evolve in an acute or chronic mode which mimics TB. The mortality rate is about 10%.

Septicemic
Five to 10 days after infection, fever, chills, diarrhea, and respiratory symptoms appear suddenly. Usually, the port of entry can be seen as a wound with local adenopathy. Symptoms gradually deteriorate to stupor, coma, or shock within a few days. Before death, the disease appears in the lungs, skin, bones, joints, meninges, liver, spleen, or kidneys. In drug addicts, the incubation period is 2–3 days and the mortality rate about 50%.

Risk factors include diabetes, liver or kidney disease, thalassemia, immunosuppression (not related to HIV), chronic lung disease, and bronchiectasis.

Treatment

- Sulfamethoxazole + trimethoprim are the drugs of choice. In case of allergy to sulfa, chloramphenicol and doxycycline can be prescribed. Both drugs offer very high success rates.
- Usually treatment is started by the IV route with ceftazidime.
- A complete blood count should be checked periodically with chloramphenicol.
- Dosing:
  * Sulfamethoxazole + trimethoprim, 6 tabs, daily, po, in two divided doses, for adults, for at least 1 month and up to 4 months
  * Chloramphenicol, 4 g, daily, po, for adults, for at least 1 month and up to 4 months
  * Doxycycline, 100 mg, po, bid, q12h, for at least 1 month and up to 4 months
  * Ceftazidime, 50 mg/kg (up to 2 g), IV, q6h, daily, for adults
- In the septicemic form, a combination of drugs is needed, usually doxycycline + chloramphenicol + sulfamethoxazole/trimethoprim

Preventive Measures

- Practice good skin hygiene and promptly clean scrapes, burns, and wounds.
- Avoid contact with infested water or mud.
- Use sterile needles and do not share needles.

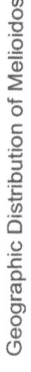

Geographic Distribution of Melioidosis

▨ Main Focus
● Reported Autochthonous Cases
– – – Limits of Main Focus

Meningococcal Meningitis

Neisseria meningitidis

Historical Background

Meningococcal meningitis was first recognized by Gaspard Vieusseux in Geneva in 1805 and by Lothario Danielson and Elias Mann in Massachusetts in 1806. In 1887, *Neisseria meningitidis* was found to be the bacterium responsible for the disease. In 1944, John Turner, John Russell Reynolds, and Roy Richard Grinkler discovered the mode of transmission. Two years earlier, Henry Stanley-Banks and James McCartney had distinguished two complications: cerebral and adrenal (the latter is called "Waterhouse-Friderichsen syndrome"). The main groups of meningococcus are A, B, C, Y, and W-135.

New Problems

Historically, sporadic meningitis infections have been seen in all areas of the world. Major epidemics have traditionally been caused by group A organisms and were thought to occur in approximately 20-year cycles. World War I and World War II triggered massive outbreaks. Other major epidemics due to A-group meningococcus include Detroit in 1929, Santiago (Chile) in 1941 and 1942, Brazil in 1974, and Africa (recurring epidemics). However, in the second part of the 20th century, this pattern seemed to have changed. Group C bacteria have been responsible for outbreaks in the United States and for lethal waves of disease in Africa: Nigeria in 1975, Chad in 1976, and Chad and Ethiopia in 1977. From January 1 to April 17, 2012, outbreaks of meningococcal disease were reported in 42 districts in 10 of the 14 countries of the African meningitis belt. Benin, Burkina Faso, Chad, Central African Republic, Ivory Coast, Gambia, Ghana, Mali, Nigeria, and Sudan reported a total of 11,647 cases including 960 deaths (case/fatality ratio of 8.2%). The outbreaks were mainly caused by the W-135 serogroup of *N. meningitidis*.

Geographic Distribution

Meningococcal meningitis is endemic to intertropical Africa, where a meningitis belt was first described by Leon Lapeyssonie. It is in sub-Saharan Africa, stretching from Senegal in the west to Ethiopia in the east and it has the highest rates of the disease.

Group A meningococcus accounts for an estimated 80–85% of all cases in the meningitis belt, with epidemics occurring at intervals of 7–14 years. In the 2009 epidemic season, 14 African countries reported 88,199 suspected cases, including 5,352 deaths, the largest number since a 1996 epidemic. Elsewhere, meningococcal meningitis appears in sporadic outbreaks.

Main Symptoms

Infection occurs by inhaling contaminated microscopic air particles. Occasionally, the disease begins with a flu-like syndrome. Two to 10 days after contamination, high fever, chills, cephalgia, pain (in the back, abdomen, hands, and feet), tachycardia, tachypnea, hypotension, nausea, and emesis follow. These symptoms are often primary. Neck and back rigidity are present, and a skin eruption occurs in most cases, ranging from pinhead-size macules to gangrene. Seizures are seen in about 20% of patients at presentation and in an additional 10% within 72 h (40% in children in the first few days). The patient can go into shock. Other complications include the following:

- Arthritis, cranial nerve damage (particularly to the VIII, which can cause deafness), hydrocephalus, myocarditis, nephritis, and DIC
- Chronic meningococcemia can last from 1 week to several months. The fever tends to be intermittent, with afebrile periods lasting 2–10 days. As the disease progresses, the febrile bouts become more frequent.
- Cutaneous manifestations appear later, consisting of pink-colored macules and papules, indurated nodules, petechiae, purpura, or large hemorrhagic areas.

A physically demonstrable sign of meningitis is Brudzinski's sign: severe neck stiffness causes a patient's hips and knees to bend when the neck is flexed. Another one is Kernig's sign: the maneuver is usually performed with the patient supine and hips and knees in flexion. Extension of the knees is attempted and the inability to perform beyond 135 degrees without causing pain constitutes a positive Kernig's sign. Both reactions to the maneuvers show evidence of the meningeal irritation present in meningitis. In young children the diagnosis of meningococcal meningitis may be difficult because headache and nuchal rigidity are often absent.

Treatment

- Ampicillin IV is the drug of choice and, in epidemic conditions, ceftriaxone
- Dosing:
  * Ampicillin, 12 g daily, IV (six injections of 2 g), for adults, and 200 mg/kg/day for children, for 10 days
  * Ceftriaxone, 2 g IM, for adults, and 50 mg/kg, IM, for children, both once

Preventive Measures

- Vaccines are available for groups A, C, Y, and W-135. 2 types of vaccines are on the market: (1) meningococcal conjugate vaccine is preferred for people 9 months to 55 years of age (in particular, MCV4—MenACWY-D) and (2) meningococcal polysaccharide vaccine (MPSV4) is for people older than 55. Immunization should be provided as early as possible in endemic countries, to children at risk in others and to people traveling to some endemic countries (for example, Saudi Arabia during the Hajj). A single dose is given IM for MCV4 and S/C for MPSV4. If risk persists a second dose is necessary at least five years after the first one. For both types of vaccine protection reaches about 93%.
- People who are in contact with patients infected with meningitis should take rifampicin or spiramycin, po.
- Dosing: Rifampin, 600 mg, bid, q12h, for 2 days; for children 1 month old or older, 10 mg/kg, po, bid, q12h; and 5 mg/kg, bid, q12h, po, for infants <1 month of age; both for 2 days

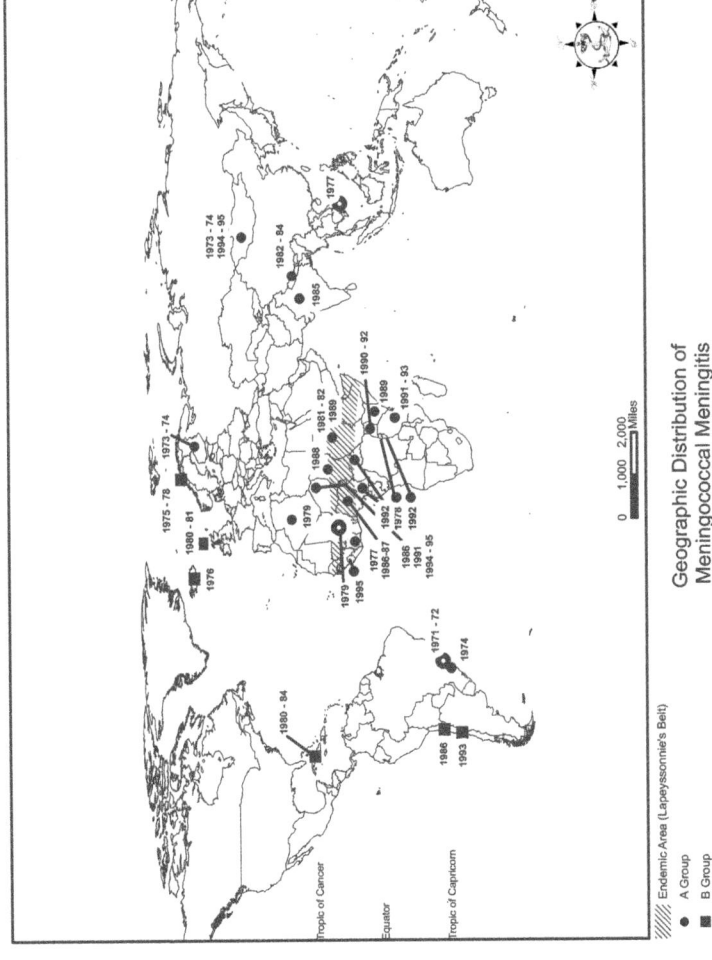

Geographic Distribution of Meningococcal Meningitis

Pertussis (or Whooping Cough)

Bordetella pertussis, Bordetella parapertussis

Geographic Distribution

Because of partial immunization coverage of populations, pertussis is more frequent in developing countries, where it is also more severe because of frequent complications.

Main Symptoms

Infection is interhuman by inhalation of air droplets coming from a coughing sick person. After an incubation period of 3–12 days, the disease lasts about 6 weeks. In children, three stages have been described. In older patients, symptoms are milder and centered on cough. Each stage lasts 1–2 weeks. Estimates from WHO suggest that in 2008 about 16 million cases of pertussis occurred worldwide, 95% of which were in developing countries. About 195,000 children died from the disease that year. The three different forms are:

Catarrhal

Upper respiratory tract infection with nasal congestion, rhinorrhea, sneezing, and sometimes low-grade fever, lacrimation, and conjunctival hyperemia. Pertussis is most infectious at this stage.

Paroxysmal

Intense coughing (lasting up to several minutes) occasionally followed by a loud whoop in younger patients. Infants may experience apneic spells. Pertussis remains communicable 3 weeks or more after the cough onset.

Convalescent

Chronic cough, which may last for weeks is the main symptom.

Complications include asphyxiating cough, emesis, malnutrition, seizures in the second or third week, otitis media, hernias, intestinal infections, pneumonia, hypoxic encephalopathy, tuberculosis activation, epistaxis, hemoptysis, cerebral hemorrhage, coma, and death (in about 15% of inpatients).

Treatment

- Supportive: oxygenation, breathing treatments, mechanical ventilation, prn
- Hospitalization for at-risk patients
- Observation of infants for apnea, cyanosis, and/or hypoxia
- Antitussive medications
- Antibiotics given early reduce the infectious period to 5 days but do not alter the duration of cough. (see Table 3.5)
- Treat with antibiotics in case of (1) persons older than 1 year within 3 weeks of cough onset and (2) infants younger than 1 year and pregnant women (especially near term) within 6 weeks of cough onset.

Table 3.5 Treatment regimens for pertussis

Type	Adult doses	Child doses
Azithromycin	500 mg, po, on day 1, then 250 mg, po, for 4 days	<6 months: 10 mg/kg/day, po, for 5 days >6 months: 10 g/kg (up to 500 mg), po, on day 1, then 5 mg/kg/day (up to 250mg), po, for 4 days
Clarithromycin	500 mg, q12h, po, for 7 days	>1 month: 7.5 mg/kg, q12h (up to 500 mg), po, for 7 days
Erythromycin	250 mg, q6h, po, for 7 days	>1 month: 10 mg/kg, q6h (up to 250 mg), po, for 7 days
Erythromycin (ethyl succinate formulation)	400 mg, q6h, po, for 7 days	>1 month: 10 mg/kg, q6h (up to 400 mg), po, for 7 days
Trimethoprim+sulfamethoxazole	160+800 mg, q12h, po, for 7 days	>2 months: 4+20 mg/kg, q12h (up to 160+800 mg), po, for 7 days

Preventive Measures

- Isolation of patients (not always feasible)
- Immunization. In the United States, 5 IM injections are given at 2, 4, 6 and between 15–18 months old with a booster between 4-6 years of age. Thereafter, the Tdap vaccine, which protects adolescents and adults against pertussis as well as tetanus and diphtheria is given only once from 11-64 years of age. In other countries the immunization schedule may differ.
- The same antibiotics can be used for 10–14 days for post-exposure prophylaxis.

Pinta (or Carate)

Treponema carateum

Geographic Distribution

Pinta is endemic to warm valleys crossed by water streams in Mexico, northern South America (mainly Colombia), and the Caribbean. *Treponema carateum* thrives in warmth and humidity. Other names of pinta include "azul," "empeines," "lota," "mal del pinto," and "tina."

Main Symptoms

The disease can be transmitted by direct human contact or by *Simulium* fly bites. It is a purely cutaneous disease, which evolves in three stages.

Primary

A chancre appears on uncovered skin areas (face, limbs), which starts as a small papule and turns into an erythematous squamous plaque in a few weeks ("empeine"). It is circinate and depressed in the middle and disappears within a few months, leaving a dyschromic scar.

Secondary

Diffusion of dyschromic lesions with the appearance of bluish, pinkish, or white macules, which form a benign leucomelanous dermitis.

Tertiary

Vitiligoid maculae appear. They are symmetrical, more frequent on extremities, and will last for the rest of the patient's life.

Notably absent are osseous and visceral lesions.

Treatment

- Treatment will completely but slowly heal hyperchromic and pinkish lesions but will have no influence on white lesions.
- Penicillin is the drug of choice.
- Erythromycin or doxycycline can be used for patients allergic to penicillin.
- Dosing
  * Benzathine penicillin, 1.2–2.4 M IU, IM, for adults, and 600,000–1.2 M IU, IM, for children depending on the duration of symptoms, both once
  * Erythromycin, 250–500 mg (base, estolate, stearate) or 400–800 mg (ethylsuccinate), po, q6h for adults, for 2–3 weeks; for children, 40–50 mg/kg/day, po, divided q6h, for 2–3 weeks; max 2 g/day (not for infants <1 month of age)
  * Doxycycline, 100 mg, po, bid, q12h, for 2–3 weeks, for adults and children > 8 years old

Preventive Measures

- Avoid contact with sick people.
- Avoid endemic areas.
- Use insecticides to kill vectors.
- Use repellents containing DEET (15–30%). Be aware that they can only provide transitory protection.
- Treat clothes with insecticides containing permethrin.
- Use repellents.
- Usual mosquito nets are not useful because *Simulium* flies can fly through their holes.

Geographic Distribution of Pinta

Endemic Areas

Plague (or Black Death)

Yersinia pestis

Historical Background

Since the beginning of Christianity, plague has been responsible for three main pandemics.

In the 6th century
Justinian's plague occurred in the Mediterranean basin.

In the 16th century
The black plague originated in India, devastated Europe, and killed more than 2 million people.

In the 19th century
The third pandemic started in Yunnan, China, in 1855 and spread around the world by ships. In 1894, Alexandre Yersin identified the bacteria causing the disease, and in 1897 he and Pierre Roux defined the role of rats in its transmission.

In 2011 and 2012, Madagascar and the Democratic Republic of Congo reported the majority of cases to the WHO. Other countries where the plague is endemic include Tanzania, Peru, the United States, China, Mongolia, and Vietnam.

New Problems

Since the third pandemic, the plague bacteria have spread, infesting rats all over the world. This large animal reservoir presents a potentially serious threat. In the late 20th century, outbreaks of the disease occurred in many countries, including the United States. Therefore, the specter of a pandemic remains constant.

Geographic Distribution

Plague currently exists in North America, South America, Africa, the Middle East, and the Far East. Between 1,000 and 2,000 cases each year are reported to the WHO, though the true number is probably much higher. It is hard to assess the mortality rate of plague in developing countries, as relatively few cases are reliably diagnosed and reported to health authorities. The WHO cites mortality rates of 8–10%; however, studies suggest that the figure may be much higher in some plague endemic areas.

Main Symptoms

Three forms can be found.

Bubonic

One to 2 days after being bitten by a flea from an infested rat, malaise, diffuse pain, cephalgia, chills, and fever appear. Sometimes a blister can be seen at the bite site. Later, a painful adenopathy (bubo) emerges in the groin, armpit, neck or under the jaw. The patient's condition worsens with prostration, delirium, diarrhea, emesis, and dehydration. On days 8–10, the lymph node bursts and oozes with pus. Oozing will persist for weeks to months. Complications include ulceration of the boil, involvement of the eyes and meninges, and occasionally pneumonia.

Pneumonic

A few hours after inhalation of contaminated microscopic air particles, the disease begins abruptly with fever, chills, prostration, chest pain, dyspnea, tachypnea, cyanosis, and a cough producing bloody, foamy phlegm. Complications include acute pulmonary edema and death.

Septicemic

No localization can be found. The patient usually dies within 24 h.

Treatment

Streptomycin is the drug of choice, particularly for the pneumonic form. Sulfonamides and cyclines can also be used with high success rates. Gentamicin is the drug of choice for pregnant women.

- Dosing:
  * Streptomycin, 30 mg/kg/day (max 2 g/day) in divided doses, IM, for adults and 30 mg/kg/day, in two divided doses, q12h, for children, for 10 days, or 3 days after the temperature has returned to normal
  * Tetracycline, 2 g, daily, po, for 14 days, for adults and children >8 yr
  * Sulfadiazine, 4–6 g, daily, po, for at least 10 days, for adults
  * Sulfadoxin, 0.5–1 g, IM (single injection), for children
  * Gentamicin, 3 mg/kg/day, IM or IV, in three divided doses, q8h, for adults; 6.0–7.5 mg/kg/day, IM or IV, in three divided doses, q8h, for children; 7.5 mg/kg/day, IM or IV, in three divided doses, q8h, for infants/neonates for at least 10 days

Preventive Measures

- Rodent-proof home.
- Flea treatment for pets.
- Use repellents containing DEET (15–30%). Be aware that they can only provide transitory protection.
- Doxycycline (100 mg, po, bid)
- Strict isolation of patients with plague pneumonia is imperative.
- Immunization is recommended for people who reside in rural areas with enzootic or epidemic plague where avoidance of rodents and fleas is impossible, and persons in regular contact with wild rodents or rabbits in these areas.
  - *Adults and children ≥ 11 years old*: 3 doses of vaccine are given IM. The second dose of 0.2 ml follows the first one of 0.1 ml, 1 month later. The third one of 0.2 ml, is administered 5 months after the second one. If an accelerated schedule is essential, 3 doses of 0.5 ml each, administered at least 1 week apart, may be given. The efficacy of this schedule has not been determined.
  - *Children <11 years old*: The primary series is also 3 doses of vaccine, but the doses are smaller. The intervals between injections are the same as for adults.
  - *Booster Doses*: When needed because of continuing exposure, 3 booster doses should be given at approximately 6-month intervals. Thereafter, antibody levels decline slowly and booster doses at 1- to 2-year intervals, depending on the degree of continuing exposure, should provide good protection.
  - The recommended booster dosages for children and adults are the same as the second and third doses. If serious side effects to the vaccine occur, their severity may be reduced by using half the usual dose.

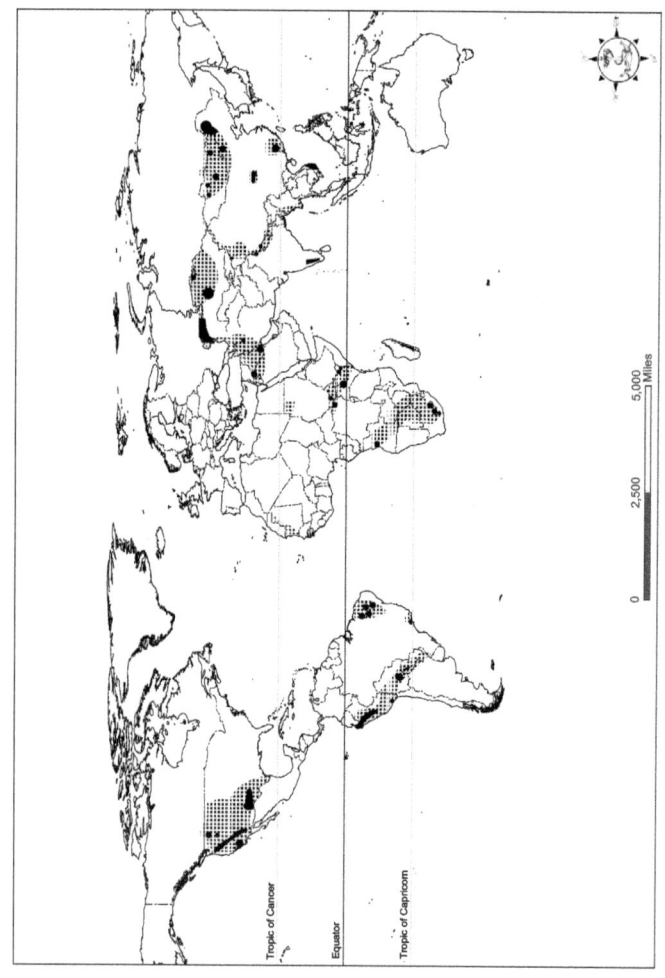

Geographic Distribution of Plague

Pneumococcal Disease

Streptococcus pneumoniae or pneumococcus

Geographic Distribution

Streptococcus pneumoniae is ubiquitous. According to the WHO, 1.6 million people die each year from pneumococcal infection including 800,000 children under 5 years old. This lethality strikes mainly poor tropical countries. The primary cause of death is pneumococcal pneumonia but pneumococcal meningitis also kills or disables 40–70% of the children it infects. Children under 2 years old and the elderly are at highest risk for pneumococcal disease. Children with HIV/AIDS are 20-40 times more likely to develop a pneumococcal infection than healthy chidren. Underweight children are 4 times more likely to die of pneumonia than normal weight children. Children who are not breastfed are twice more likely to die of pneumonia before age 18 months than those who are breastfed. Additional risk factors include: immune deficit caused by malignancy, diabetes mellitus, conditions associated with decreased pulmonary clearance functions (eg, asthma, chronic bronchitis, or chronic obstructive pulmonary disease), and the inability to distinguish *S pneumoniae* pneumonia from other pneumonias.

Main Symptoms

Steptococcus pneumoniae can cause a wide range of infections from conjunctivitis, otitis media, osteomyelitis, septic arthritis, endocarditis, pericarditis, peritonitis, myositis, periorbital cellulitis, skin abscess, pneumonia, meningitis, and brain abscess to sepsis. Symptoms vary accordingly, for example:

Meningitis

Please see meningococcal meningitis, page 167

Acute Otitis media

In adults

- Sharp, sudden, or dull, continuous pain in the ear
- Warm discharge from the external ear canal
- A feeling of fullness in the ear
- Nausea
- Decreased hearing acuity

In children

- Pulling at the ear
- Insomnia
- Irritability, restlessness
- Fever
- External ear canal discharge
- Anorexia
- Crying when lying down

These symptoms are accompanied by abnormal otoscopic findings of the tympanic membrane, which may include the following: opacity, bulging, erythema, middle ear effusion, decreased mobility with pneumatic otoscopy.

Pulling the ear lobe upward usually triggers pain.

Complications of otitis media occur (1) intracranially, by spreading of infection from the ear and temporal bone through 3 routes: direct extension, thrombophlebitis, and hematogenous dissemination and (2) extracranially, being usually direct sequelae of localized acute or chronic inflammation. They include the following: chronic suppurative otitis media, postauricular abscess, facial nerve paresis, labyrinthitis, labyrinthine fistula, mastoiditis, temporal abscess, petrositis, intracranial abscess, meningitis, otitic hydrocephalus, sigmoid sinus thrombosis, encephalocele, and CSF leak.

Pneumonia

- Cough, often productive of rusty, green, or tinged with blood mucus
- Fever (less common in older adults)
- Chills
- Tachypnea
- Shortness of breath
- Chest pain often worsened by coughing or deep inspiration
- Tachycardia
- Asthenia
- Nausea and emesis
- Diarrhea

If consolidation occurs, the signs are (1) on palpation, increased fremitus where the consolidation is located, (2) on percussion, dullness in the same area, and (3) on auscultation, a variety of crackles with lobar and occasional rhonchi, bronchial breath sounds, egophony, bronchophony and whispered pectoriloquy.

Complications of pneumonia can be (1) local: lung abscess, pleurisy, pleural effusion, emphysema, dyspnea, ARDS, respiratory failure, or (2) distant: bacteremia, septicemia, meningitis, septic arthritis, endocarditis, or pericarditis.

Sepsis

The diagnosed of sepsis, is based on the presence of at least two of the following signs and symptoms:

- Fever > 101.3 F (38.5 C) or < 95 F (35 C)
- Heart rate > 90 beats/min
- Respiratory rate > 20 breaths/min
- Probable or confirmed infection

It is classified as severe if at least one of the following signs and symptoms are also present (they indicate that an organ may be failing):

- Significantly decreased urine output
- Abrupt change in mental status
- Difficulty breathing
- Abnormal heart pumping function
- Abdominal pain
- Thrombocytopenia

It is classified as septic shock if severe sepsis is accompanied by extremely low blood pressure that doesn't adequately respond to simple fluid replacement.

Treatment

The key to successful antibiotic therapy of pneumococcal disease is achieving good drug concentrations in the affected area of the body. For all treatments adjust the antibiotic(s) best choice to the sensitivity results of the antibiogram, when available.

- Amoxicillin

Acute Otitis Media

- It is the drug of choice for acute otitis media in high doses

Children

- >3 months old and <40kg: 80-90 mg/kg/day, po, divided q8-12hr, for 10–14 days
- >40 kg: 500 mg, po, q12hr, or 250 mg, po, q8hr, for 10-14 days

Adults

- 250 to 500 mg, po, tid, for 10 to 14 days; alternatively, 500 to 875 mg, po, tid, for 10–14 days

Mild Pneumonia

- It is the drug of choice for the outpatient treatment of mild pneumonia only.

Children

- 90 mg/kg/day in 2 doses or 45 mg/kg/day in 3 doses, for 7 to 10 days

Adults

- 500 mg, po, tid, or 875 mg, po, bid, for 7 to 10 days

- Ceftriaxone

Children

Meningitis

<12 years old: 100 mg/kg (not to exceed 4 g) IV/IM; may be administered q24h or divided q12hr for 7–14 days
>12 years old: As in adults

Serious Infections Other Than Meningitis

<12 years old: 50–75 mg/kg IV/IM divided q12hr for 4–14 days
>12 years old: As in adults

Adults

Meningitis and Pneumonia

- 1-2 g IV/IM q24h or divided, bid, for 4–14 days depending on type and severity of infection

- Cefotaxime

Children

Meningitis and Pneumonia

- <12 years old or < 50 kg: 200 mg/kg/day, IV/IM, divided q6hr
- >12 years old or >50 kg: As in adults

Adults

Moderate to Severe Infections
- 1 to 2 g IV/IM, q8hr

More Severe Infections
- 2 g IV, q6-8hr

Life-Threatening Infections
- 2 g IV, q4hr, up to 12 g/day
- **Vancomycin**

Children
- Vancomycin is frequently the preferred drug for the treatment of severe penicillin-resistant pneumococcal infections outside the CNS and for patients with an IgE-type allergy to penicillin. Only IV administration is effective.
- Dosing
- < 7 days, < 1,200 g: 15 mg/kg IV, q24 h
- < 7 days, 1,200 to 2,000 g: 10 to 15 mg/kg IV, q12-18 h
- < 7 days, > 2,000 g: 10 to 15 mg/kg IV, q8-12 h
- 7 days-1 month, < 1,200 g: 15 mg/kg IV, q24 h
- 7 days-1 month, 1,200-2,000 g: 10 to 15 mg/kg IV, q8-12 h
- 7 days-1 month, > 2,000 g: 10 to 15 mg/kg IV, q6-8 h
- 1 month-18 years: 10 to 20 mg/kg IV, q6-8 h (total 40 to 60 mg/kg/day)

The manufacturer recommends an initial dose of 15 mg/kg in neonates, followed by 10 mg/kg, q12 h for neonates in the first week of life and q8 h thereafter up to 1 month of age. They recommend 10 mg/kg IV, q6 h for pediatric patients.

Adults
For pneumonia: 5 to 20 mg/kg IV, q8-12hr, for 7 to 21 days, depending on the nature and severity of the infection. For meningitis: 10 to 14 days or at least 1 week after the patient becomes afebrile and cerebrospinal fluid normalizes.

Preventive Measures
- Adequate nutrition to ensure a well-functioning immune system (including exclusive breastfeeding during the first six months of life)
- Immunization
  - There are currently 2 types of pneumococcal vaccines: PCV13 and PPSV23.
  - PCV13 is recommended for all children younger than 5 years old and for adults with certain risk factors.
  - Children 2 years or older who are at high risk of pneumococcal disease should also receive the PPSV23.
  - All adults 65 or older (and those 19 or older with risk factors) should receive PPSV23.
  - Vaccination Schedule

1) Children

Children < 2 years of age

- PCV13 is routinely given to infants as a series of 4 doses, one dose at each of these ages: 2, 4, 6, months and 12-15 months.
- Children who miss their shots or start the series later should still get the vaccine.
- The number of doses recommended and the intervals between doses will depend on the child's age when vaccination begins.

Children 2–5 years of age

- Healthy children 24 months-4 years of age who are unvaccinated or have not completed the PCV13 series should get 1 dose.
- Children 24 months-5 years of age not having completed the 4-dose series should get 1 or 2 doses of PCV13, if they have the following medical conditions: Sickle cell disease, a damaged spleen or no spleen, cochlear implant(s), cerebrospinal fluid leak(s), HIV/AIDS or other diseases that affect the immune system (such as diabetes, cancer, or liver disease), chronic heart or lung disease, undergoing chemotherapy or taking steroids.

Children 6–18 years of age

- A single dose of PCV13 may be given to children 6–18 years of age with certain medical conditions (i.e., sickle cell disease, HIV-infection, or other immunocompromising condition, cochlear implant(s), or cerebrospinal fluid leaks), regardless of whether they have previously received a pneumococcal vaccine.
- Children with a damaged spleen or no spleen should complete the PCV13 recommended series before getting meningococcal conjugate vaccine.
- PCV13 may be given at the same time as other vaccines, except for meningococcal conjugate vaccine.

2) Adults

- All adults 65 years of age and older.

3) Specific Cases

- Anyone 2–64 years of age who has a long-term health problem such as: heart disease, lung disease, sickle cell disease, diabetes, alcoholism, cirrhosis, leaks of cerebrospinal fluid or cochlear implant(s).
- Anyone 2–64 years of age who has a disease or condition that lowers the body's resistance to infection, such as: Hodgkin's disease, lymphoma or leukemia, kidney failure, multiple myeloma, nephrotic syndrome, HIV infection or AIDS, damaged or no spleen, organ transplant.
- Anyone 2-64 years of age who is taking a drug or treatment that lowers the body's resistance to infection, such as: long-term steroids, certain cancer drugs, radiation therapy.
- Any adult 19-64 years of age who is a smoker or has asthma.
- Residents of nursing homes or long-term care facilities.

The CDC conducted studies with PCV7 and found that the vaccine was 96% effective against pneumococcal disease in healthy children who received one dose or more and 81% effective in children with medical conditions that put them at risk of pneumococcal disease. The vaccine was also highly effective at preventing pneumococcal disease caused by antibiotic-resistant serotypes. Since routine vaccine introduction in the US, rates of invasive pneumococcal disease caused by the seven serotypes included in the vaccine have declined by 99%. PPSV may be less effective for people with lower resistance to infection. However, they should still be vaccinated, because they are more likely to have serious complications from pneumococcal disease.

Salmonellosis (Typhoid Fever or Enteric Fever) and Paratyphoid Fever

Salmonella typhi, *Salmonella paratyphi* A, *Salmonella paratyphi* B, *Salmonella paratyphi* C

Historical Background, Geographic Distribution, and New Problems

Typhoid and paratyphoid fevers are caused by different bacteria with various origins. *Salmonella typhi* is present virtually everywhere. However, tropical countries are endemic areas for *S. paratyphi* A, which is encountered mainly in Africa, and *S. paratyphi* C, which is found in Asia. Typhoid fever is common in the intertropical zone due to local climatic, hygienic, and socioeconomic conditions. Humans are the only reservoir of the disease.

The resistance of *S. typhi* to chloramphenicol and other antibiotics has been known for many years and poses a therapeutic challenge for its treatment. It first appeared sporadically in various countries: Greece, Israel, and Kuwait (1967); Spain (1969); France and Romania (1972); Algeria (1974); and Chile and Indonesia (1975). Epidemics of resistant strains occurred in Vietnam (1971–1975), Mexico (1972–1975), India (1972–1978), Taiwan (1973–1974), Thailand (1973–1975), Cambodia (1974), and Peru (1974–1976). Multidrug-resistant (including to nalidixic acid and ciprofloxacin) strains of *S. typhi* also emerged as the cause of typhoid fever epidemics in various Asian countries, first in India (1990–1993), then in other countries (late 1990s). In Asia *S. paratyphi* A is resistant to quinolones. In Africa, multiresistant strains have been found in foci in Kenya and Egypt. An outbreak of typhoid fever in the Democratic Republic of Congo in 2004 and 2005 involved more than 42,000 cases and caused 214 deaths. In 2011, there were 20 million new cases and 200,000 deaths due to typhoid fever worldwide. A big challenge are the chronic and healthy carriers of the disease (2–5% of all cases), threatening starts of outbreaks. In the United States most cases (up to 75%) are acquired while traveling internationally. Typhoid fever is still common in the developing world, where it affects about 21.5 million persons each year.

Main Symptoms

Seven to 14 days after ingesting contaminated food or water, or after oro-anal sex with an infected partner the disease begins. Its course can be divided into four phases, each lasting approximately 1 week.

First phase

Cephalgia, dizziness, sleeplessness, epistaxis, anorexia, constipation, undulating fever, asthenia, and myalgia can occur.

Second phase

Fever with paradoxical bradycardia (Faget's sign), diarrhea or constipation, pharyngitis, and a skin eruption consisting of rose spots (truncal maculopapules, 4 cm [1.6 in] in diameter and fewer than five in number) can appear. They generally disappear within 2–5 days.

Third phase

General signs and symptoms

The patient becomes more toxic and anorexic with significant weight loss. Conjunctivitis and tachypnea occur, and a weak pulse and crackles over the lung bases can be found.

GI signs and symptoms

Abdominal distension becomes severe. Foul, green-yellow, liquid diarrhea (pea-soup diarrhea) occasionally occurs. Intestinal perforation and resulting peritonitis may appear.

Neurological signs and symptoms

Typhoid state is characterized by apathy, confusion, and psychosis. The stupor has been described as "muttering delirium" or "coma vigil". Picking at the bedclothes and at imaginary objects (carphology and floccillation) are characteristic, as is muscular twitching (subsultus tendinum).

Complications

They include toxemia, myocarditis, GI hemorrhage, liver or pancreas abscess, cholecystitis, encephalitis, meningitis, phlebitis, enteritis, and lung involvement. Muscle and/or joint lesions can also occur.

Fourth phase

The fever, mental state, and abdominal distension slowly improve over a few days. Intestinal and neurologic complications may still occur. Weight loss and severe asthenia last for months. Among survivors a few become healthy carriers.

Atypical forms are common and can have the following features: sudden onset of high fever, major stomach and bowel disturbances, respiratory and joint symptoms.

Treatment

- Antibiotic treatment should best be based on antibiogram results. Doses must be increased progressively. If not, encephalitis may ensue. Monitoring during the treatment includes stomach palpation, level of consciousness, blood pressure, pulse, temperature, appearance of the stool, and antibiogram.
- Resistance patterns have led to a shift toward the third-generation cephalosporins, azithromycin, and fluoroquinolones as empiric therapy for typhoid fever while awaiting the results of antimicrobial susceptibilities.
- Doses must be increased progressively over 3–4 days until reaching optimal dosage.

Table 3.6 Typhoid fever treatment: antibiotics of choice by disease origin and severity

Origin	Severity	First line	Second line
South or East Asia	Mild/moderate	Cefixime, po	Azithromycin, po
	Severe	Ceftriaxone, IV, or cefotaxime, IV	Aztreonam, IV, or imipenem, IV
Eastern Europe, Middle East, sub-Saharan Africa, South America	Mild/moderate	Ciprofloxacin, po	Cefixime, po; amoxicillin, po; trimethoprim + sulfamethoxazole, po; or azithromycin, po
	Severe	Ciprofloxacin, IV	Ceftriaxone, IV; cefotaxime, IV; ampicillin, IV; or trimethoprim + sulfamethoxazole, IV
Unknown or Southeast Asia	Mild/moderate	Cefixime, po, + ciprofloxacin, po	Azithromycin, po
	Severe	Ceftriaxone, IV, or cefotaxime + ciprofloxacin, IV	Aztreonam, IV, or imipenem + ciprofloxacin, IV

Precaution: The combination of azithromycin and fluoroquinolones is not recommended.

- Abundant bed rest is needed.
- Dosing (for empirical treatment)
  * Ceftriaxone, (1) severe disease, 4 g, IV, once a day, for adults and 75 mg/kg of body weight for children for 3–5 days or 1–2 g, IV, once a day for 7–14 days, (2) mild/moderate disease, 1–2 g/day, IV. It is the drug of choice for children.
  * Cefotaxime, for mild/moderate disease 1–2 g, IV, q8h, for adults; for children 100–150 mg/kg/day, IV, in four divided doses, q6h, both until the patient is afebrile for 7 days.
  * Ciprofloxacin, 500 mg, po, bid, q12h, for 7–14 days, for adults; 10 mg/kg/day, IV over 10 min, in two divided doses, q12h, for children. When patients are able to take substances orally, switch to ciprofloxacin po at the same dosage regimen. Continue for 7 days after the patient becomes afebrile.
  * Cefixime, 400 mg, po, bid, q12h, for adults; 5–10 mg/kg, po, bid, q12h, for children, both for 7–10 days.
- Chronic carriers
  - Ciprofloxacin, 500–750 mg, po, bid, q12h, for adults, for 28 days.
  - Ofloxacin, 400 mg, po, bid, q12h, for adults, for 28 days.

Preventive Measures

- Immunization. The oral vaccine is given in 3 or 4 doses, 2 days apart. The capsules are not adequate for children under 5 years old. The IM vaccine is given once. It is inefficient under 2 years old. For both, protection ranges from 60–70% and is achieved only against *S. typhi*. It lasts about 3 years and immunization should take place 1–2 weeks prior to travel.
- Boil or filter water or drink only from encapsulated water bottles.

- Eat only fruits that need to be peeled.
- Avoid salads and uncooked vegetables or wash them with water sterilized with potassium permanganate.
- Avoid ice cream and ice cubes.
- Always wash hands before meals.
- Know the health of your sexual partner(s)

Geographic Distribution of Typhoid Fever

////// Highly Endemic Areas

Salmonellosis (*Salmonella* gastroenteritis)

Numerous *Salmonella* species

Geographic Distribution and New Problems

Salmonella gastroenteritis is common in the intertropical zone. In contrast to enteric fever, animals can be a reservoir of bacteria, particularly cattle, birds, and reptiles. In Africa, Asia, and South America, *Salmonella enteritidis* and *Salmonella typhimurium* are resistant to ampicillin, cotrimoxazole, chloramphenicol, and fluoroquinolones.

Main Symptoms

Six to 72 h after ingesting contaminated food (meat, milk, eggs, fruit, vegetables) or water or after direct contact with a sick person (including oro-anal sex with a contaminated partner) or a carrier animal, symptoms occur. They include chills, fever, nausea, emesis, abdominal cramps, and diarrhea (sometimes with blood). In severe cases, cholera-like diarrhea may be associated with tenesmus. They usually subside spontaneously within 2–5 days.

Complications include dehydration, septicemia, septic arthritis, osteomyelitis, meningitis, pyelonephritis, cholecystitis, acute appendicitis, and pleuropneumopathy (especially in infants and patients with sickle cell disease, cancer, therapeutic immunosuppression, or AIDS).

Treatment

- For uncomplicated forms, symptomatic treatment is sufficient.
- Severe cases and sickle cell and AIDS patients warrant the use of antibiotics: trimethoprim+sulfamethoxazole, ampicillin, or ciprofloxacin.
- Dosing:
  * Two tabs of 80-mg trimethoprim + 400 mg sulfamethoxazole, po, bid, q12h, for 3–7 days for adults; for children, 40 mg of sulfamethoxazole + 8 mg of trimethoprim/kg body weight, po, in two divided doses, q12h, continued for 3–7 days.
  * Ampicillin, 100 mg/kg/day, in four doses, q6h, po or IM, for adults; for children, 50–100 mg/kg, daily, po or IM, for 3–7 days.
- Trimethoprim+sulfamethoxazole should not be given to children <2 yr.
- IV fluid replacement is necessary in severe cases.

Preventive Measures

- Boil or filter water or drink only from encapsulated water bottles.
- Only eat fruits that need to be peeled.
- Avoid salads and uncooked vegetables, or wash them with water sterilized with potassium permanganate.
- Avoid ice cream and ice cubes.
- Always wash hands before meals.
- Know the health of you sexual partner(s)

Shigellosis

Shigella dysenteriae, Shigella flexneri, Shigella boydii, Shigella sonnei

Geographic Distribution and New Problems

Shigellosis is endemic to the intertropical zone because of local climatic, hygienic, and socioeconomic conditions. The disease is held annually responsible for approximately 120 million cases of severe dysentery. The overwhelming majority occurs in developing countries and involves children less than 5 years of age. About 1.1 million people are estimated to die from *Shigella* infection each year, with 60% of the deaths occurring in children under 5 years of age. In developing countries *Shigella flexneri* and *Shigella sonnei* present high levels of resistance to chloramphenicol, ampicillin, tetracyclines, and fluoroquinolones.

Main Symptoms

One to 7 days after ingestion of contaminated food or water or after oro-anal sex with an infected partner, the following symptoms may appear in severe cases: abdominal cramps, tenesmus, diarrhea (up to 100 BMs/day with mucus, pus, and blood), emesis, high fever, dehydration, asthenia, myalgia, arthralgia, and tachycardia. Complications include shock, renal failure, hemorrhage, gangrene, intestinal perforation, and peritonitis. In tropical countries the mortality rate can reach 20%. Mild forms of the disease are common and cause moderate diarrhea and low-grade fever.

Treatment

- Ampicillin or sulfamethoxazole+trimethoprime is the historical treatment of choice, but it is no longer used because of the spread of bacterial resistance.
- Cetriaxone is the recommended treatment in tropical countries.
- Dosing:
  * Ceftriaxone, 1 g for adults and 50 mg/kg for children, IM for both, once a day, for 2–5 days

Preventive Measures

- Boil or filter water or drink it from encapsulated water bottles.
- Only eat fruits that need to be peeled.
- Avoid salads and uncooked vegetables, or wash them with water sterilized with potassium permanganate.
- Avoid ice cream and ice cubes.
- Always wash hands before meals.
- Know the health of your sexual partner(s)

Geographic Distribution of Shigellosis

////// Highly Endemic Areas

Syphilis (or Hard Chancre)

Treponema pallidum, subsp. pallidum

Historical Background

The first appearance of syphilis dates back to the 15th century in Europe, but the initial syphilitic focus was in the West Indies.

In 1905, Fritz Gerard Schaudinn and Erich Hoffmann identified the causal agent of the disease and a year later, August Paul Von Wassermann created the first serological test. The first treatment, based on arsenic derivatives, was proposed by Paul Ehrlich in 1909. The prognosis of the disease became much more favorable when penicillin became available after 1928.

Estimated new cases of syphilis (in millions) among adults, 1995 and 1999 (from WHO)

Region	1995			1999		
	Male	Female	Total	Male	Female	Total
North America	0.07	0.07	0.14	0.054	0.053	0.107
Western Europe	0.10	0.10	0.20	0.069	0.066	0.136
North Africa and Middle East	0.28	0.33	0.62	0.167	0.197	0.364
Eastern Europe and Central Asia	0.05	0.05	0.10	0.053	0.052	0.105
Sub-Saharan Africa	1.56	1.97	3.53	1.683	2.144	3.828
South and Southeast Asia	2.66	3.13	5.79	1.851	2.187	4.038
East Asia and Pacific	0.26	0.30	0.56	0.112	0.132	0.244
Australia and New Zealand	0.01	0.01	0.01	0.004	0.004	0.008
Latin America and Caribbean	0.56	0.70	1.26	1.294	1.634	2.928
Total	5.55	6.67	12.22	5.29	6.47	11.76

New Problems

The latter part of the 20th century saw the appearance of *Treponema pallidum* strains resistant to penicillin, causing a public health concern in many countries. Later, *T. pallidum* became resistant to other antibiotics (macrolides, clindamycin, and rifampicin, in particular).

Since the 1970s, the incidence of syphilis has been on the rise. Homosexual men with multiple partners and the spread of drug addiction (crack cocaine in particular), which promotes exchange of sex for drugs, are two factors influencing progression of the disease. More than 90% of all the cases of syphilis are in the developing world.

Hindering the fight against syphilis includes (1) limited access to health care due to economic and/or cultural reasons and (2) sexual promiscuity, which makes tracking contacts difficult. In certain places like Southeast Asia, the illegal trafficking of women and children for sex to several countries creates additional problems. The WHO estimated in 1999 that out of 12 million adults with syphilis worldwide, 11 million were living in sub-Saharan Africa, Latin America, and southern and southeastern Asia.

Main Symptoms

The evolution of syphilis is divided into three stages, which are separated by symptom-free periods.

Primary (early stage)
Approximately 3 weeks after contracting the disease through sexual contact with an infected partner, an isolated chancre (superficial ulcer with clear-cut edges on a firm base), frequently located on the genitalia, rectum, or inside the cheek, appears with painless local adenopathy.

Secondary
Lesions usually appear a few weeks (and sometimes up to 6 months) after the chancre. Skin lesions include a non-itching eruption (roseola). Syphilis must be particularly suspected when skin lesions appear on the palms of the hands and/or the soles of the feet.

Mucous membrane lesions (ranging from ulcers to nodules) can be seen on the lips, mouth, throat, genitalia, and anus. Both skin and mucous membrane lesions are highly contagious at this stage. Alopecia may occur.

Complications include involvement of the meninges, liver, kidneys, bones, joints, eyes, and heart.

Tertiary (late stage)
The following symptoms can be found in about one-third of untreated patients: infiltrative tumors of the skin, bones, and liver (gummas) and lesions of the aorta (including aneurysms) and heart valves (mainly aortic regurgitation). The eyes, respiratory system, and GI tract can also be affected.

Neurosyphilis can be seen in 15–20% of patients who have tertiary syphilis. It includes meningovascular lesions, which produce cephalgia and irritability, cranial nerve palsy, unequal reflexes, stroke, and tabes dorsalis. The latter produces impairment of vibration and of sensation and poor reaction of pupils to light (Argyll Robertson pupil), muscular weakness, slow reflexes, ataxia, and inability to walk in the dark. Shooting or lightning pain in the muscles accompanied with numbness is also common. Abdominal pain with nausea and emesis, severe attacks of cough, dyspnea, painful bladder spasms, and tenesmus can also be experienced. All these symptoms begin suddenly and last from hours to days.

Joint damage (Charcot joint) and ulcers on the heels are not rare. General paresis is a symptom of neurosyphilis, which appears at the final stage of the disease. At this point, the patient's cortex becomes affected, and the following symptoms gradually emerge: decreased ability to focus, memory loss, dysarthria, tremor of the fingers and lips, irritability, mild cephalgia, and change in personality (gradually becoming lazy, careless, and irresponsible). It leads to a confused and eventually psychotic state.

The causes of death are multiple, such as encephalitis; lesions of the liver (cirrhosis, gummas), meninges, spinal cord, kidneys, larynx, lungs, esophagus, and rectum; and exostoses of the cranium and vertebrae. Death can also occur by progressive cachexia.

Treatment

- In early syphilis, benzathine penicillin is the drug of choice. In case of allergy, erythromycin is used.

- Secondary syphilis is treated with benzathine penicillin.
- At the late stage of syphilis, penicillin does not produce good results.
- Dosing:
  * For the primary stage, benzathine penicillin, 2,400,000 IU, IM, once or twice
  * For the secondary stage, benzathine penicillin, 2,400,000 IU, IM, two or three times with 1-week intervals. To avoid serious side effects, treatment should be started at a low dose and increased progressively until the recommended posology is reached.
- Check other STDs (in particular HIV and chlamydia).
- Any sexual partner(s) must be treated concomitantly.

Preventive Measures

- Wear a condom during sexual activities with new partners.
- Use only water-based lubricants.
- Avoid sharing towels or underclothing.
- Wash before and after intercourse.
- Urinate after intercourse.
- Practice strict personal hygiene.
- Know the health of your sexual partner(s).

Tuberculosis

Mycobacterium tuberculosis

Historical Background

In the 19th century TB assumed epidemic proportions as a result of rapid urbanization and industrialization in Europe. About one-fourth of the adult population had died from TB on the continent by the middle of the century, hence its label "the great white plague."

In 1809, Rene Laennec discovered the pathological process of TB, and Jean Antoine Villemin reproduced the human disease in animals in 1865. In 1882, Robert Koch isolated and cultivated the bacteria causing TB, *Mycobacterium tuberculosis*, also called "Koch's bacillus."

Streptomycin was the first effective anti-TB drug in 1945. In 1951, isoniazid was found to be more efficient than streptomycin. Consequently, the disease became curable in most cases.

TB started to recede progressively from the developed world in the late 20th century through a combination of improved housing, better hygiene, enhanced nutrition, and mass campaigns of detection, treatment, and immunization. In the developing world, the accelerated urbanization of cities in Africa, Asia, Central America, and South America has created de novo conditions conducive to the rapid spread of the disease. In most tropical countries, TB remains a deadly threat and serious public health concern. In 2004, drug-resistant TB cases were mostly found in Kazakhstan (4,828/100,000 people), Russia (3,500/100,000), South Africa (3,060/100,000), Peru (1,911/100,000), and Romania (459/100,000). In 2011, nearly 9 million people worldwide were newly infected with TB (2.3 million in India alone, including 100,000 with resistant strains). There are

490,000 new cases of multiresistant TB worldwide each year, including 100,000 deaths.

New Problems

In the latter part of the 20th century, the appearance of M. tuberculosis strains resistant to one or multiple anti-TB drugs created a new obstacle to the treatment and control of TB. Despite the constant shortening of therapeutic courses (down to 6 months), the first factor in the emergence of resistant strains stems from patients not following their regimen properly, interrupting and restarting it several times. Also, tracking patients is not easy in developing countries. Treatment cost is a major hindrance to eradication campaigns. Furthermore, TB is one of the frequent opportunistic infections associated with HIV/AIDS. The forms of TB in AIDS patients are often more serious, not only because of the deficient immune terrain but also because of the unusually high levels of multiple drug-resistant bacilli. One-third of patients with AIDS die from TB.

This new reservoir of resistant TB presents a real epidemiological threat. The spreading of multidrug-resistant forms of TB is a concern, particularly in countries like India, Brazil, Mexico, Egypt, Nigeria, Thailand, South Africa, and Indonesia. They are present in more than 40 countries. In developing countries there is particular concern for transmission due to health-care personnel and in hospitals because of (1) patient promiscuity, (2) the use of ventilators, and (3) the absence of mask wear.

Geographic Distribution

TB is endemic to many developing countries and more prevalent in slums of large cities. According to the WHO in 2011, there were an estimated 8.7 million new cases of TB worldwide (13% co-infected with HIV) and 1.43 million people died from TB, including almost 1 million deaths among HIV-negative and 430,000 among HIV-positive individuals. TB was one of the top killers of women, with 300,000 deaths among HIV-negative and 200,000 deaths among HIV-positive females.

Main Symptoms

Contamination is interhuman by aerosols containing M. tuberculosis and sent by sneezing, coughing, or loudly speaking sick persons. Symptoms include the following.

In adults

Lung cavities are the most common characteristic associated with the suggestive symptoms of anorexia, weight loss, asthenia, low-grade fever, night sweats, and cough, initially dry but later producing bloody phlegm. This is the most contagious form of the disease.

In children

Primary TB is the form most frequent in children. No symptoms can be observed. In most cases, M. tuberculosis remains dormant in the body and can be reactivated later in life. Other forms are similar to those in adults.

Extrapulmonary TB

This form of TB is especially common in patients with HIV infection. In Africa, it represents 10–20% of all cases, but they play only a minor role in the transmission of the disease. Lymph nodes, spleen, liver, lungs, skin, meninges, bones (usually in the spine, known as Pott disease), and skin TB can occur.

Treatment

- Rifampicin (RIF), isoniazid (INH), pyrazinamide (PZA), streptomycin, sometimes ethionamide (ETA), and ethambutol (EMB) are used in different combinations (triple or quadruple therapy) in regimens lasting 6–12 months (Table 3.7).
- Tablets with fixed dose combinations of INH+RIF or INH+RIF+PZA are available and increase compliance.
- Dosing (immunocompetent patients/susceptible bacillus)

INH

- Presentation: Tabs (50 mg, 100 mg, 300 mg), elixir (50 mg/5 ml), aqueous solution (100 mg/ml) for IV or IM injection
- Adults: 5 mg/kg, po, IM, or IV, q 24 hrs (max 300 mg)
- Children: 10-15 mg/kg, po, IM, or IV, q 24 hrs (max 300 mg)

RIF

- Presentation: (1) Caps (150 mg, 300 mg), or (2) Powder that may be suspended for oral administration, or (3) Ready-to-use aqueous solution for intravenous injection
- Adults: 10 mg/kg/day po, or IV (max 600 mg)
- Children: 10–20 mg/kg/day po, or IV (max 600 mg)

PZA

- Presentation: Tablet (500 mg, scored)
- Adults:
- 40–55 kg, daily, 1,000 mg/kg; thrice weekly, 1,500 mg/kg; twice weekly, 2,000 mg/kg
- 56–75 kg, daily, 1,500 mg/kg; thrice weekly, 2,500 mg/kg; twice weekly, 3,000 mg/kg
- 76–90 kg, daily, 2,000 mg/kg; thrice weekly 3,000 mg/kg; twice weekly, 4,000 mg/kg
- Children: 15–30 mg/kg/day (max 2 g)
- All po

Table 3.7 TB treatment basic regimens

Preferred	Alternative 1	Alternative 2
Initial phase	*Initial phase*	*Initial phase*
Daily INH, RIF, PZA, and EMB for 56 doses (8 weeks)	Daily INH, RIF, PZA, and EMB for 14 doses (2 weeks), then twice weekly for 12 doses (6 weeks)	Thrice-weekly INH, RIF, PZA, and EMB for 24 doses (8 weeks)
Continuation phase	*Continuation phase*	*Continuation phase*
Daily INH and RIF for 126 doses (18 weeks) or twice-weekly INH and RIF for 36 doses (18 weeks)	Twice-weekly INH and RIF for 36 doses (18 weeks)	Thrice-weekly INH and RIF for 54 doses (18 weeks)

EMB
- Presentation: Tablet (100 mg, 400 mg)
- Adults:
- 40–55 kg, daily, 800 mg/kg; thrice weekly, 1,200 mg/kg; twice weekly, 2,000 mg/kg
- 56–75 kg, daily, 1,200 mg/kg; thrice weekly, 2,000 mg/kg; twice weekly, 2,800 mg/kg
- 76–90 kg, daily, 1,600 mg/kg; thrice weekly, 2,400 mg/kg; twice weekly, 4,000 mg/kg
- Children: 15–20 mg/kg (max 1g), daily
- All po
- Periodic checkups help in detecting clinical and biological side effects of drugs.
- Hospitalization is not necessary for most patients.
- First-line drugs include INH, RIF, rifabutin, rifapentine, PZA, and EMB
- Second-line drugs include streptomycin, cycloserine, p-aminosalicylic acid, ethionamide, amikacin, kanamycin, capreomycin, levofloxacin, moxifloxacin, and gatifloxacin
- New drugs and combinations have proven successful. In particular, the 3-in-1 combination, PaMZ (PA 824—novel TB candidate—+moxifloxacin+PZA). It is active on resistant bacilli and could shorten the treatment course to 4 months.

Preventive Measures

- BCG immunization for extended stays in highly endemic countries or when in contact with TB patients. BCG is a live vaccine. In some endemic countries like India, it is given from birth to 15 days of age at the same time as the oral polio vaccine, and over the left arm. A swelling of 6 mm is raised above the skin surface. No alcohol or antibiotic should be applied over the site before injection. Clean locally only with soap and water. BCG can be given up to 5 years of age. Beyond 6 months and in adults a Mantoux test is recommended prior to immunization. If it is positive no immunization is necessary. Some countries like in the Arabian Gulf recommend 1 or more boosters thereafter.
- Proper housing, hygiene, and nutrition.

Yaws (Pian, Parangi, Paru, or Frambesia Tropica)

Treponema pertenue

Geographic Distribution

Yaws is endemic to warm, humid, and tropical forest areas of Africa, Asia (particularly Indonesia and Papua New Guinea), Latin America, and the Pacific. According to the WHO, 2.5 million people were affected by the disease in 2012. Other names for yaws include "granuloma tropicum," "polypapilloma tropicum," and "thymiosis."

Main Symptoms

The mode of transmission is direct from person to person. *Treponema pertenue* penetrates through mucous or cutaneous effractions. The disease is more common in children 4–14 yr old. After an incubation period of 9–90 days, symptoms appear in three phases separated by asymptomatic periods.

Primary

Pruriginous piannic chancre (95% on the lower limbs), squamous macules, maculopapules, nodules, and plaques with lymphadenopathy

Secondary

Six to 16 weeks after the primary stage, disseminated macules, papules, nodules, hyperkeratotic skin and bone lesions, and constitutional symptoms may appear. They are painful like osteoperiostitis and edema of the hands (with hypertrophy or polydactylitis) and feet. Periosteal thickening is often palpable. Hypertrophy of the nasal bone ("ngoudou") can only be seen in Africa. Piannic onychia can occur. These lesions usually heal. About 10% of cases will progress to the the tertiary phase within 5 to 15 years

Tertiary

Painful and crippling periostitis, osteitis, ulcerating rhinophryngitis (gangosa), hyperkeratosis of the palms and soles, nodules, papilloma (serpiginous or ulcerated), chronic ulcers, and dyskeratosis.

Remarkably absent are cardiovascular involement, neurological symptoms, and congenital transmission.

Treatment

- Penicillin is the drug of choice.
- Erythromycin or doxycycline can be used for patients allergic to penicillin.
- Dosing
  * Benzathine penicillin, 1.2–2.4 M IU, IM, for adults and 600,000–1.2 M IU, IM for children depending on the duration of symptoms, both once
  * Erythromycin 250–500 mg (base, estolate, stearate) or 400–800 mg (ethylsuccinate), po, q6h for adults, for 2–3 weeks; for children, 40–50 mg/kg/day, po, divided q6h, for 2–3 weeks; max 2 g/day (not for infants <1 month of age)
  * Doxycycline, 100 mg, po, bid, q12h, for 2–3 weeks, for adults

Preventive Measures

- Avoid contact with sick people.
- Avoid endemic areas.

Chlamydial Diseases

Lymphogranuloma Venereum (or Nicholas-Favre-Durand Disease)

L1, L2, L3 serovars of *Chlamydia trachomatis*

Geographic Distribution

Lymphogranuloma venereum is endemic to the intertropical zone, particularly to India and sub-Saharan Africa. In the developed world, the disease mainly affects male homosexuals.

Main Symptoms

One to 3 weeks after infection by sexual contact with an infected partner, the following symptoms appear in three stages.

Primary

A small, painless papule or pustule appears on the coronal sulcus, prepuce, glans, or scrotum in men. In women, the same type of lesions appears on the posterior vaginal wall or cervix (where they often go unnoticed), fourchette, and vulva.

Secondary

It begins 2–6 weeks after the primary lesion, with painful lymphadenopathy, usually in the inguinal and/or femoral area in men and deep iliac or perirectal area in women. Swollen lymph nodes coalesce to form buboes, which may rupture. Fever, chills, myalgias, and malaise also occur. Complications include arthritis, ocular inflammatory disease, cardiac and/or pulmonary involvement, aseptic meningitis, and hepatitis or perihepatitis.

Tertiary

Bloody purulent discharge, rectal pain, tenesmus, and strictures can be experienced.

Treatment

- Doxycycline and erythromycin offer good results.
- Dosing:
  * Doxycycline, 100 mg, po, bid, q12h, for 21 days
  * Erythromycin base, 500 mg, po, qid, q6h, for 21 days (for pregnant and lactating women, in particular)
- Treat partner(s).
- Check for other STDs.
- In some cases, surgery is necessary.

Preventive Measures

- Always use condoms during sexual activity with new partners.
- Use only water-based lubricants.
- Avoid sharing towels or underclothing.
- Wash before and after intercourse.
- Urinate after intercourse.
- Practice strict personal hygiene.
- Know the health of your sexual partner(s).

Geographic Distribution of
Nicholas-Favre-Durand Disease

Endemic Areas

Trachoma (or Granular Conjunctivitis or Egyptian Ophthalmia)

Chlamydia trachomatis

Geographic Distribution

Trachoma is the first of cause of blindness by infectious diseases in the world. In 2003 according to the WHO, 40 million people carried an active disease, 8 million had a trichiasis entropion, and 7 million suffered from visual deficit or blindness due to corneal scarring. Trachoma is mainly found in rural settings in poor developing countries because of lack of hygiene, nonaccess or difficult access to clean water, and deficient health education.

Main Symptoms

Transmission is direct and interhuman, primarily between children and the women who care for them. Flies can play a role as passive vectors. The disease evolves in two phases.

Active (inflammatory)

Most patients are relatively asymptomatic. Signs and symptoms are linked to conjunctivitis and include red eyes with burning sensation, lacrimation, and the presence of an exudate. Eyelids are thickened and inflamed inside. At the upper side of the cornea, a vascularized grayish veil can develop. It is called *pannus*.

Scarring (cicatricial)

After many years of evolution, scars appear. The lid retraction provokes an inner deformation of the upper tarsus called "entropion." Consequently, some eyelashes can grow inward, causing trichiasis, which triggers an intensely irritating foreign body sensation as well as blepharospasm. These eyelashes sting the cornea, which vascularizes and/or ulcerates. Many patient self-epilate. Simultaneously, the destruction of conjunctival glands stops the production of protective tears. Ultimately, it leads to corneal scarring. Corneal opacities or scars that cover any part of the pupil impair the patient's vision.

The WHO has developed a simplified grading system for trachoma as follows:

- T0: Normal conjunctiva
- TF: Trachomatous inflammation, follicular; five or more follicles >0.5 mm on the upper tarsal conjunctiva
- TI: Trachomatous inflammation, intense; papillary hypertrophy and inflammatory thickening of the upper tarsal conjunctiva obscuring more than half the deep tarsal vessels
- TS: Trachomatous scarring; presence of scarring in tarsal conjunctiva
- TT: Trachomatous trichiasis; at least one ingrown eyelash touching the globe or evidence of epilation (eyelash removal)
- CO: Corneal opacity; corneal opacity blurring part of the pupil margin

Treatment

- Antibiotic therapy
  - Azithromycin. It is better than tetracycline but more expensive. It is easy to administer as a single oral dose of 20 mg/kg, po, once a year in endemic areas. It is safe for pregnant women, and its administration can be directly observed. It has high efficacy and a low incidence of adverse effects. Moreover, infection with *Chlamydia trachomatis* occurs in the nasopharynx; therefore, patients may reinfect themselves if only topical antibiotics are used. Beneficial secondary effects of azithromycin include its treatment of genital, respiratory, and skin infections.
  - 1% Tetracycline ointment. It should be applied daily for 6 weeks. It is the treatment of choice for children under 6 weeks of age. It can be used by pregnant women. However, compliance is worse than with azithromycin, and the ointment causes transitory visual impairment.

Development of significant resistance to either azithromycin or tetracycline has not yet been demonstrated.

- Surgery
  - Eyelid rotation limits the progression of corneal scarring. In some cases, it can result in a slight improvement in visual acuity, probably due to restoration of the visual surface and reductions in ocular infectious secretions and blepharospasm. The WHO has produced a training manual on the bilamellar tarsal rotation procedure:
- It involves a full-thickness incision of the scarred lid and external rotation of the distal margin by using three sutures.
- Results of randomized clinical trials have confirmed the superiority of this method over other techniques.
- Even after successful surgery, patients remain at risk for recurrence. Therefore, long-term follow-up care and intermittent screening are important after surgery.
- Recurrence rates vary greatly between surgeons.
- Prognosis is dependent upon (1) the level of corneal scarring and (2) surgical success.

Preventive Measures

- Facial cleanliness. Epidemiologic studies and community-randomized trials have shown that facial cleanliness in children reduces both the risk and the severity of active trachoma.
- Hygiene. General improvements in personal and community hygiene are almost universally associated with a reduction in the prevalence (and eventually the disappearance) of trachoma. It has been observed not only in Europe, the Americas, and Australia but also in Africa and Asia.
- Environmental improvement. Environmental improvement activities are the promotion of improved water supplies and better household sanitation, particularly methods for safe disposal of human feces (to avoid fly infestation).

Urethritis and Cervicitis

Chlamydia trachomatis

Geographic Distribution

Chlamydial urethritis and cervicitis are found all over the world and are common in tropical countries.

Estimated new cases of chlamydia infections (in millions) among adults, 1995 and 1999 (from WHO)

Region	1995			1999		
	Male	Female	Total	Male	Female	Total
North America	1.64	2.34	3.99	1.77	2.16	3.93
Western Europe	2.30	3.20	5.50	2.28	2.94	5.22
North Africa and Middle Europe	1.67	1.28	2.95	1.71	1.44	3.15
Eastern Europe and Central Asia	2.15	2.92	5.07	2.72	3.25	5.97
Sub-Saharan Africa	6.96	8.44	15.40	7.65	8.24	15.89
South and Southeast Asia	20.20	20.28	40.48	18.93	23.96	42.89
East Asia and Pacific	2.70	2.63	5.33	2.56	2.74	5.30
Australia and New Zealand	0.12	0.17	0.30	0.14	0.17	0.30
Latin America and Caribbean	5.01	5.12	10.13	4.19	5.12	9.31
Total	42.77	46.38	89.15	41.95	50.03	91.98

Main Symptoms

Chlamydial urethritis and cervicitis are STDs. Their symptoms are as follows:

In men

Urethral or rectal discharge, dysuria, proctitis, unilateral pain and swelling of the scrotum, fever, or no symptoms (in 50% of cases).

In women

Vaginal discharge, abnormal vaginal bleeding, dyspareunia, proctitis, rectal discharge, slow onset and progressive lower abdominal pain, fever, or no symptoms (in 80% of cases). If untreated, the disease can spread to the cervix and fallopian tubes and cause infertility.

In newborns

Conjunctivitis with eye discharge and/or swelling developing at 1–2 weeks of age or pneumonia with cough and fever beginning at 1–3 months of age

Treatment

- Doxycycline is the treatment of choice for adults. Azythromycin is the alternative for pregnant women and erythromycin for neonates.
- Dosing (see Table 3.8)
- Treat partner(s).
- Check for other STDs.

Table 3.8 Treatment regimens for chlamydial urethritis and cervicitis

Azithromycin*: 1 g, in a single dose, po
Doxycycline: 100 mg, bid, po
Alternatives
Erythromycin base: 500 mg, qid, po
Erythromycin ethylsuccinate: 800 mg, qid, po
Ofloxacin: 300 mg, bid, po
Levofloxacin: 500 mg once a day, po
All for 7 days, except for *.

Preventive Measures

- Patients should abstain from sexual intercourse for 7 days after single-dose therapy or until the end of a longer regimen.
- Use condoms during sexual activity with unknown partners.
- Avoid sharing towels or underclothing.
- Wash before and after intercourse.
- Urinate after intercourse.
- Practice strict personal hygiene.
- Know the health of your sexual partner(s).

Prion Disease

Variant Creutzfeldt-Jakob Disease

Prion

Historical Background

Creutzfeldt-Jakob disease (CJD) is a rare and incurable degenerative neurological disorder. This spongiform encephalopathy was first described in the Fore tribe of the Eastern Highlands Province of New Guinea. It was named "kuru" and was transmitted by cannibalism. At the end of the 20th century, it was thought to have disappeared.

New Problems

In 1996, scientists found that 10 Britons had been infected with "mad cow disease," which is a variant of CJD (vCJD). Eight of them died. The suspicion was that contamination occurred after eating beef from cattle infected with BSE.

Roughly 160,000 cases of BSE were reported in Great Britain from 1985 to 1996. Cows get this disease by eating the remains of sheep (a practice which was commonly used in cattle breeding in the United Kingdom) infected with scrapie, a brain disease similar to BSE. A law was passed to prevent cattle from feeding on sheep in that country. As a result, the incidence of BSE declined dramatically. Nonetheless, since 1998, 143 cases of vCJD have been reported in the United Kingdom. The disease can also be transmitted via blood transfusion.

Geographic Distribution

The last cases of CJD were reported from New Guinea. None were recorded in people born after 1959. vCJD emerged in Great Britain many years later, as well as in France, Canada, Ireland, Italy, and the United States. The presence or prevalence of vCJD in tropical countries is unknown.

Main Symptoms

For CJD, months to years after eating contaminated human brains (or eyes) or contaminated beef, tremors, somnolence, dysarthria, emotional instability, ataxia, and dementia appear progressively. The disease gradually worsens, resulting in death. Compared to CJD, vCJD affects younger patients (average age 29 vs. 65 years), lasts longer (median 14 vs. 4.5 months), and is strongly linked to food through BSE.

Treatment

- Specific treatment is unknown.
- Symptomatic and supportive.

Preventive Measures

- Avoid eating beef from countries where contamination can occur.
- Control blood donations.

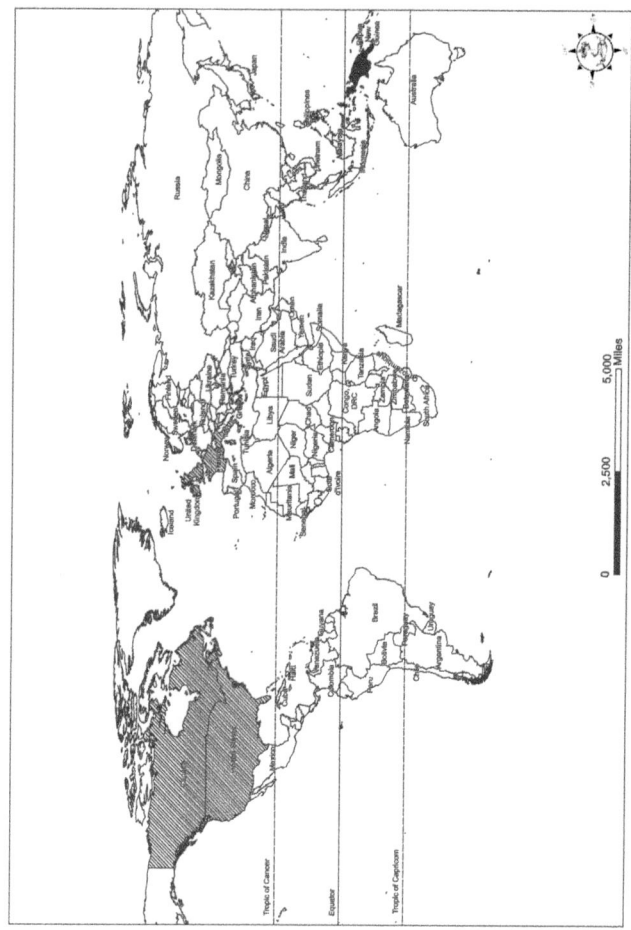

Geographic Distribution of Creutzfeldt-Jacob Disease and Variant

Part 4

Viral Diseases

Viral diseases are divided into two categories, those that are (1) common and familiar to medical practitioners and/or have a high incidence and (2) rare and uncommon to most of them and/or have a low incidence, particularly in tropical countries.

Common Diseases

Dengue Fever (or Breakbone Fever)

Flavivirus types DEN1, DEN 2, DEN3, and DEN4

Historical Background

The first cases of dengue fever were described in Australia in 1897. It was first reported in the United States in 1922, in South Africa in 1927, in Greece in 1928, and in Taiwan in 1931. In Thailand, the first cases were registered at the end of World War II. The disease surfaced in India with an epidemic in 1966, which started in the Philippines in 1953 and spread throughout the main cities of Southeast Asia. In 1964, 4,000 cases were identified in Bangkok. An epidemic struck Ivory Coast, Burkina Faso, and Senegal in 1980–1981. Another outbreak occurred simultaneously in the West Indies, mainly targeting Cuba.

New Caledonia was hit by outbreaks of dengue fever in 1989 and 1995. In both cases, the type 3 virus was predominant. Epidemics of dengue fever occurred in Costa Rica in 1993, Laos in 1994, Venezuela in 1995, and India in 1996.

In 1996, there were 3,128 cases of dengue fever in Singapore (three deaths), 8,000 cases in Vietnam (34 deaths), 14,244 cases in Malaysia (31 deaths), and 3,024 cases in Jakarta, Indonesia (34 deaths). Malaysia experienced another outbreak in 1997. Since then, there has been an increase in dengue epidemics worldwide. In early 2007, Paraguay declared a 60-day state of emergency with tens of thousands of cases and at least 10 deaths. There was also an epidemic in Brazil. Southeast Asia was hit to record levels in the same year. In October 2011, the Republic of the Marshall Islands declared a state of emergency due to a large dengue outbreak. In 2011, 1,034,064 cases were reported to the Pan American Health Organization including 716 deaths with outbreaks in Paraguay, Panama, Aruba, the Bahamas, and Saint Lucia. It is estimated that 37 million cases occur in India annually, resulting in 227,500 hospitalizations. Typically, epidemics occur in 3- to 5-year cycles. Other names for the disease are "dandy fever" and "devil's crunch."

New Problems

Two factors are particularly worrisome:

1. The increase in outbreaks in recent years, which have become more numerous and more frequent
2. The presence of hemorrhagic forms in previously immune areas

A number of reasons have been suggested to explain these phenomena:

- Global warming (which expands the areas where the vector can live) and rapid urbanization in developing countries (which increases the size of populations potentially targeted by the vector)
- Mutation of the virus, making it resistant and/or more virulent
- Successful mass control plans that result in low immunity in populations, which therefore became more susceptible to the virus

Geographic Distribution

Dengue fever is endemic to the intertropical zone, including Central and South America, Africa, Asia, and Oceania. According to the WHO in 2013, over 2.5 billion people – > 40% of the world's population – are now at risk for dengue fever. There may be 50–100 million infections due to the disease worldwide every year.

Main Symptoms

The incubation period lasts 5–8 days after being bitten by an infected *Aedes* mosquito. Symptoms can be classified in various forms.

Classic

Cephalgia, face flushing, back pain followed by chills, high fever, severe arthralgia, myalgia, spinal pain, GI disturbances, photophobia, retro-orbital pain, and adenopathy occur. Three to 4 days later, fever and pain disappear but on the fifth or sixth day, they reappear with a skin eruption (macular or maculopapular exanthem). Hepatomegaly and polyadenopathy can be found. All symptoms subside progressively, but asthenia and arthralgia may persist for weeks.

Mild

This form is common and causes a moderate fever only. It represents more than 60% of all cases.

Hemorrhagic

The onset is the same as in the classic form, but on the third to fifth day, the patient's condition suddenly deteriorates with skin, mucous membrane, and GI tract hemorrhage. Shock may occur. Cardiac, pulmonary, and neurological symptoms (mental confusion, agitation, convulsions, and coma) may also appear. The hemorrhagic form develops more frequently during a second infection by a virus type different from the original infection. Women, children, and Caucasians are more susceptible. The mortality rate is about 5%.

The severity can be graded as shown in Table 4.1.

Table 4.1 Severity Grading for Dengue Fever

Grade 1 Fever accompanied with nonspecific constitutional symptoms Only hemorrhagic manifestation: a positive tourniquet test
Grade 2 Skin and/or other hemorrhages
Grade 3 Circulatory failure: rapid and weak pulse, cold and clammy skin, and restlessness or Narrowing of pulse pressure (20 mm Hg or less) or Hypotension
Grade 4 Profound shock with undetectable blood pressure and pulse

Other severe forms

Cases of meningitis and fulminant hepatitis due to dengue fever have been reported.

Treatment

- Symptomatic and supportive (IV fluid and electrolyte replacement, BP monitoring, transfusion to replace blood loss).
- Avoid NSAIDs and ASA because of increased risk of hemorrhage.
- ICU for hemorrhagic and severe forms.

Preventive Measures

- Use insecticides to kill vectors.
- Use repellents containing DEET (15–30%). Be aware that they can only provide transitory protection.
- Treat clothes with insecticides containing permethrin.
- Use air conditioning.
- Get rid of water reservoirs around houses.

Anders was a 60-year-old Swiss surgeon who experienced a fever after coming back from central Africa, where he had been hunting 2 weeks earlier. Symptoms began 2 days after his return home, including joint and muscle pain, fever, and fatigue. Simultaneously, he noticed swelling of both wrists, which lasted 1 week. In the meantime, both hands had turned purple for a couple of days. The patient also mentioned feeling short of breath on and off and having a low urine output. The blood tests showed slightly elevated alkaline phosphatases, and the arbovirus serology came back positive (without yellow fever vaccination cross-reaction).

DID YOU KNOW THAT:
- Clinical features of dengue fever vary with the type of virus, without any difference in outcome.
- Splenomegaly never occurs in dengue fever.
- Joint pain can last weeks to months after initial symptoms.
- Photophobia and neck stiffness are frequent (they can falsely evoke meningitis).
- Two blood tests at least 2 weeks apart are indispensable for the serology.
- Status of the yellow fever immunization must be known because of possible serologic cross-reactions.

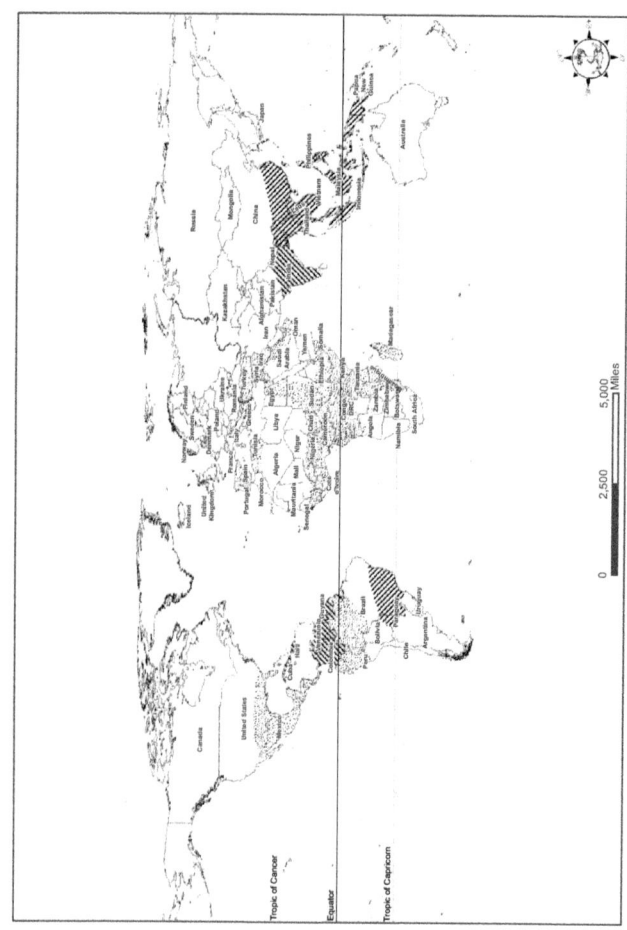

Geographic Distribution of Dengue Fever

Hepatitis

Hepatitis viruses A, B, C, D, E, and G

Geographic Distribution and Etiology
Viral hepatitis can be caused by different viruses.

Hepatitis A
Hepatitis A virus
The A virus is usually transmitted indirectly by food or water contaminated by feces or directly by infected people (oro-anal sex). The incubation period lasts 2–6 weeks. Because of poor local hygiene and socioeconomic conditions, hepatitis A is more common in the intertropical zone. According to the WHO, globally, there are an estimated 1.4 million cases of hepatitis A every year.

Hepatitis B
Hepatitis B virus
Usually transmitted by inoculations (needles) or transfusion of infected blood or blood products (such as plasma or platelets transfusion), hepatitis B can also be spread by sexual contact, including oral sex; but its most common route of transmission worldwide is perinatal. The incubation period is 1–4 months. The disease is more frequent in some parts of the intertropical zone. According to the WHO in 2012, 2 billion people worldwide were infected with the virus and about 600,000 people die every year due to the consequences of hepatitis B.

Hepatitis C
Hepatitis C virus
The C virus is responsible for approximately 80% of hepatitis cases after blood transfusion. The incubation period lasts 15–150 days for the acute phase, but only 15% of patients will present the latter. Chronic symptoms appear 20–40 years after contamination. According to the WHO, about 150 million people are chronically infected with hepatitis C virus, and more than 350,000 people die every year from hepatitis C-related liver diseases.

Hepatitis D
Delta agent
The delta agent has only been identified in association with hepatitis B infection. It increases the severity of the disease.

Hepatitis E
Hepatitis E virus
The mode of transmission of the hepatitis E virus is similar to that of hepatitis A. Hepatitis E is usually mild (except in pregnant women, particularly during the third trimester, and in malnourished and immunodepressed people).

Hepatitis G
Hepatitis GB virus C
The hepatitis G virus is transmitted through blood transfusion, but it does not appear to cause cirrhosis. GB virus C, formerly known as hepatitis

G virus, is a virus in the *Flaviviridae* family and a member of the *Pegivirus* genus.

Other viruses

Other viral agents can cause hepatitis, including Epstein-Barr, yellow fever, Lassa fever, Marburg and Ebola viruses, and CMV.

Main Symptoms

Viral hepatitis symptoms can be divided into three phases, with complications.

Initial Symptoms

Progressive or abrupt appearance of malaise, myalgia, arthralgia, asthenia, rhinorrhea, pharyngitis, anorexia, nausea, emesis, diarrhea or constipation, fever, chills, distaste for cigarette smoke, abdominal pain (right upper quadrant or right flank) aggravated by jarring or exercising, skin eruption, dark urine and pale clay-colored stools

Icterus

With the onset of icterus, initial-phase symptoms usually get worse before slowly improving. Some patients never become icteric.

Recovery

Appetite increases; jaundice, abdominal pain, tenderness, and asthenia disappear progressively.

Evolution

The acute illness frequently subsides within 2–3 weeks with recovery occurring within 9 weeks (hepatitis A) or 16 weeks (hepatitis B and C). Residual asthenia may be pronounced in some cases.

Complications

From 5% to 10% of hepatitis B cases and up to 70–80% of cases of hepatitis C chronify and last longer than 6 months. Rarely, complete liver failure and death occur within a few days, but 75–90% of hepatitis fulminans cases are fatal, without transplant. Chronic hepatitis may lead to cirrhosis (in 20% of cases for hepatitis C), and cirrhosis may lead to hepatoma (in 1–5% of cases for hepatitis C). The symptoms of cirrhosis include weakness, anorexia, weight loss, gynecomastia in men, a skin eruption on the palms, blood-clotting disorders, and telangiectasia.

Treatment

- *Hepatitis A and E*: There is no specific treatment for hepatitis A and E. Rest, avoiding fatty foods and alcohol, staying hydrated, and supportive mesures are recommended.
- *Hepatitis B*: No drug can clear the infection. For chronic disease, antivirals can stop the virus from replicating and therefore minimize liver damage. Lamivudine, adefovir, tenofovir, telbivudine, entecavir, and long-acting pegylated interferon can be used.
  - Check for other STDs.
  - Screen sexual partner(s).

- *Hepatitis C*: For chronic disease, depending on the hepatitis C virus genotype, a combination of pegylated interferon-alpha-2a or pegylated interferon-alpha-2b with ribavirin can be used for 24 or 48 weeks.
- *Co-infection hepatitis B + hepatitis C*: A trial with high doses of interferon is strongly recommended. Interferon-alpha/ribavirin combination therapy has been effective for hepatitis B+C–co-infected patients. However, no standard recommendations exist for the treatment of B+C co-infection. Therefore, it must be individualized based on variables such as hepatitis blood test results, DNA or RNA levels, prior exposure to antiviral treatment, and the presence of other similarly transmitted viruses such as hepatitis D virus and HIV.
  - Supportive measures include bed rest, diet (no fat, no alcohol), and not taking medications metabolized by the liver.
  - Drugs are administered according to symptoms and to the level of liver metabolism.
  - Because treatment regimens for hepatitis are being actively researched and new drugs discovered and medication recommendations, indications, and dosages are constantly evolving, consultations with a gastroenterologist, hepatologist, and/or general surgeon are the best approach.
  - Liver transplant is sometimes the only treatment available to terminally ill patients.

Preventive Measures
- Immunization for hepatitis A and B. Against hepatitis A: 2 IM injections 6 to 12 months apart, after 1 year old. Protection lasts many years. Hepatitis B: 2 IM injections, 2 months apart and a booster 6 months later. Protection reaches high levels.
- Screen blood for transfusions for hepatitis B and C.
- Screen pregnant women for chronic hepatitis B infection and immunize their infants with hepatitis B immunoglobulin as well as hepatitis B vaccine.
- Boil tap water or drink only from encapsulated water bottles; avoid salads and uncooked vegetables; eat only fruits which need to be peeled, and wash hands before meals for hepatitis A and E.
- Practice safe sex for hepatitis A, B, and E.
- Know the health of your sexual partner(s).

Francois, a 50-year-old Caucasian man, presents with the sole complaint of asthenia. For the past week, he has been feeling weak and somnolent and is waking up tired in the morning despite sleeping more than usual. Notably absent symptoms are nausea (in particular provoked by tobacco smoke), vomiting, fever, and joint and muscle pain. The urine and stool colors are unremarkable. His medical history reveals asthma during childhood and no immunization against hepatitis A or B or typhoid fever. The patient has smoked about one pack of cigarettes per day for about 14 years but has not touched a cigarette in 2 months. He travels very frequently throughout Asia. His last trip was to Cambodia 3 weeks earlier. One week prior to consultation he experienced a URTI, which was treated with antibiotics. The clinical examination is noncontributory. Pertinent negatives: no scleral icterus, no hepatomegaly, no upper right quadrant or liver-area tenderness or pain on percussion.

Laboratory tests reveal white blood cell count 10,000, polymorphs 20.9%, lymphocytes 63.8%, monocytes 11.9%, erythrocyte sedimentation rate 11 mm/h, triglycerides 167 mg/dl, total cholesterol/high-density lipoprotein cholesterol 5.26, alkaline phosphatase 150 U/l, serum glutamic pyruvic transaminase 402 U/l, gamma glutamyl transpeptidase 289 U/l, hepatitis B surface antigen negative, hepatitis B surface antibody negative, and hepatitis A immunoglobulin G antibody negative. The provisional diagnosis is viral hepatitis. A few days later, laboratory tests show the following: hepatitis A immunoglobulin M antibody negative; anti–hepatitis E virus immunoglobulin G positive; anti–hepatitis E virus immunoglobulin M positive. The diagnosis is acute hepatitis E. Treatment includes rest and a nonalcoholic/nonfat diet, with advice given regarding drugs metabolized by the liver such as certain antibiotics. The asthenia regresses gradually toward complete disappearance within 3 weeks.

DID YOU KNOW THAT:
- In general, hepatitis E is a self-limited viral infection with full and spontaneous recovery.
- Occasionally, a fulminant form occurs.
- Fulminant hepatitis is found more frequently in pregnant women, inducing a mortality rate of about 20% in the third trimester.
- Hepatitis E virus has been described as a cause of sporadic hepatitis cases in Southeast and central Asia, including China.
- The incubation period varies greatly, with a minimum of 2 weeks, an average of 6 weeks, and a maximum of 10 weeks.
- Prophylactic measures include (1) drinking only mineral water from sealed bottles and (2) if this is not possible, boil the drinking/cooking water for 10 min before use; sterilize it at least 1 h before consumption with additives such as iodine tincture (10 drops/l), potassium permanganate, toluene sodium chloramines, or 1,3 dichloro-striazine 2,4,6 trione; or sieve it through resin or microceramic filters.

Geographic Distribution of Hepatitis A

///// High Risk Areas

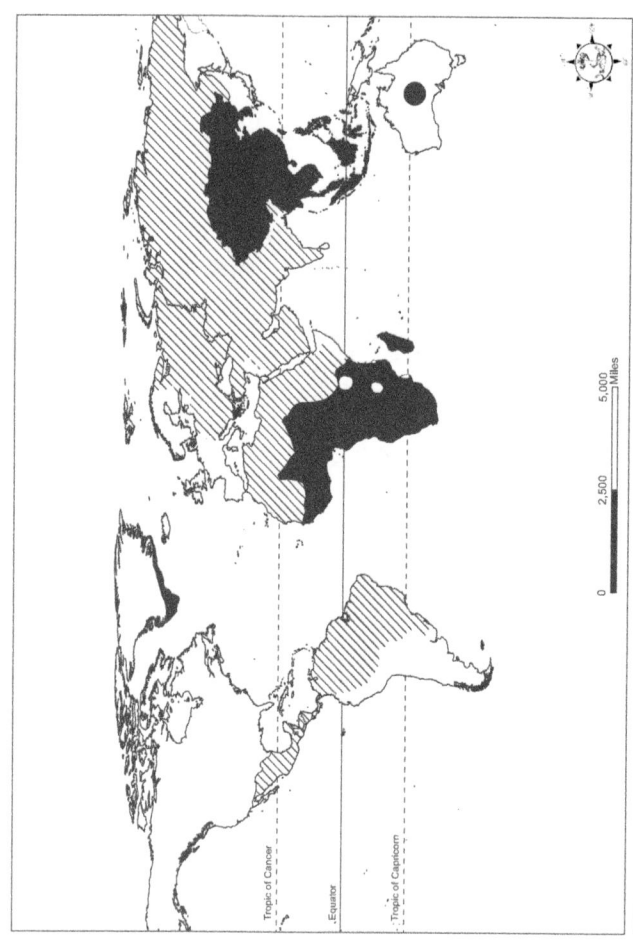

Herpes Simplex (or Cold or Fever Sore)

Herpes simplex virus types 1 and 2 (HSV-1 and HSV-2)

Geographic Distribution
Cold or fever sore is frequently found in the intertropical zone as it can be triggered by sun exposure.

Main Symptoms
Transmission is interhuman. Traditionally, HSV-1 involved the lips and mouth and HSV-2, the genitalia. This distinction is gradually disappearing as both viruses are increasingly being isolated from any of the three areas.

After being acquired from a contaminated person, the virus remains dormant in lymph nodes from months to years. Then, prodromal symptoms of itching and tingling may emerge. However, about 40% of people with these prodromal sensations, which give up to 2 days of warning before further symptoms, do not develop any herpetic lesions later.

When the virus surfaces, small blisters often appear (mostly on the lips, genital area, buttocks, or thighs or around the anus). They are accompanied with a burning sensation. In more severe cases, the skin of the chin, nose, cheeks, and ears may be affected. Genital symptoms also include vaginal or urethral discharge and cervicitis with intermittent bleeding. Local lymph nodes become swollen and tender. General symptoms include fever, malaise, and myalgia. Triggering factors include influenza, malaria, pneumococcal pneumonia, bacterial meningitis, stomach and bowel disturbances, trauma, physical exertion, stress, fatigue, pregnancy, menstruation, and sun exposure.

All symptoms subside spontaneously in 2–7 days but will recur erratically. In severe cases, pharyngitis, aseptic meningitis, encephalitis, transverse myelitis, sacral neuropathy, and erythema multiforme may occur. Other organs may be involved, like the cornea and conjuctiva (keratoconjuctivitis), skin (eczema herpeticum is a serious form of the disease in children), meninges, brain, and viscera (visceral herpes simplex is a fatal disease in newborns who became infected during delivery). In AIDS patients, the herpes virus may cause painful perianal ulcerations.

Treatment
- Acyclovir, valacyclovir, or famciclovir
- Dosing:

First episode
  * Acyclovir, 400 mg, tid, po, or 200 mg, po, five times a day
  * Famciclovir, 250 mg, tid, po
  * Valacyclovir, 1 g, bid, po
  * All for 7–10 days. Treatment can extend if healing is incomplete after 10 days.

Recurrent episodes

- Acyclovir, 400 mg, tid, po, for 5 days; 800 mg, bid, po, for 5 days; or 800 mg, bid, for 2 days
- Famciclovir, 125 mg, bid, po, for 5 days; 1,000 mg, bid for 1 day; or 500 mg once, then 250 mg, bid, po, for 2 days
- Valacyclovir, 500 mg, bid, po, for 3 days or 1 g, once a day, po, for 5 days
  - *Treatment must be started latest on the first day of symptoms.*
  - *Acyclovir topically, five times a day, until clearance of the lesions*
- Life-threatening HSV infections in immunocompromised patients, disseminated herpes, and HSV encephalitis require high-dose IV acyclovir, often started empirically.
- Some viral strains have become drug-resistant.
- Treat partner(s).
- Check for other STDs.

Preventive Measures

- Suppressive long-term regimen for recurrent disease
  - Acyclovir, 400 mg, bid, po
  - Famciclovir, 250 mg, bid, po
  - Valacyclovir, 1 g/day, po
- Refrain from contact during outbreaks.
- Practice safe sex with unknown partners.
- Know the health of your sexual partner(s).

HIV/AIDS

Human Immunodeficiency Virus 1 (HIV-1) and Human Immunodeficiency Virus 2 (HIV 2)

Historical Background

The history of HIV/AIDS starts in June 1981 with the identification of an unknown syndrome by epidemiologists of the CDC in Atlanta, Georgia. HIV-1 was identified in 1983 by Luc Montagnier of the Pasteur Institute in Paris from the lymph node of a patient of Willy Rozenbaum in the department of Marc Gentilini at the Pitié-Salpêtrière Hospital. In 1986, HIV-2 was discovered and the first efficient drug, zidovudine (AZT), became available. Worldwide in 2010, there were 34 million people living with HIV, 2.7 million were newly infected, and 1.8 million died from the disease. In 2012, there were more than 3 million children living with HIV. As long as newly infected people outnumber those who have access to a lifelong treatment, the pandemic will grow. Ignorance about the disease remains, particularly in the most endemic countries.

Geographic Distribution

HIV/AIDS is a ubiquitous disease. However, the vast majority of patients and new cases come from low- or middle-income countries. Since the beginning of the epidemic, almost 70 million people have been infected with the HIV virus and about 35 million have died of AIDS. Globally, 34.0 million people

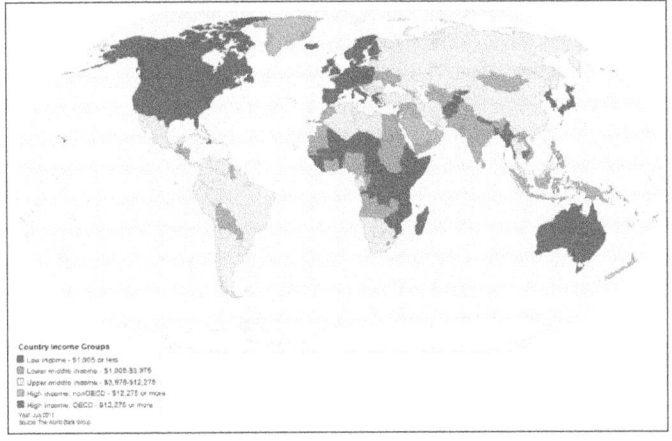

Figure 4.1 Country Income Groups

were living with HIV at the end of 2011. In 2013, an estimated 0.8% of adults aged 15–49 years worldwide are living with HIV, although the burden of the epidemic continues to vary considerably between countries and regions. Sub-Saharan Africa remains most severely affected, with nearly 1 in every 20 adults (4.9%) living with HIV and accounting for 69% of the people living with HIV worldwide.

Main Symptoms

More than 95% of people with HIV infection will develop a fatal illness if left untreated. Descendants of the plague survivors with the delta32 variant of CCR5 (C-C chemokine receptor type 5, which is a protein on the surface of white blood cells) are more resistant to acquiring HIV. The lack of delta32 in the native African population could explain in part, among many other reasons, why that continent has been so hard-hit by the AIDS epidemic. In some patients the progression of the disease is slower than in typical cases. Other very rare patients called "HIV elite high controllers" do not present any symptoms.

The disease evolves in phases.

Initial phase

The virus is transmitted by semen, cervicovaginal secretions, blood, and maternal milk. After infection, about half of adults will have a recognizable acute retroviral syndrome within days to a few weeks. Sometimes they present a mono-like syndrome with or without acute encephalitis, psychiatric symptoms, acute myelitis, lymphocytic meningitis, or polyradiculoneuritis. All symptoms disappear spontaneously. Serology becomes positive 3–6 weeks postinfection and very rarely later (sequentially, radioimmunoprecipitation assay, Western blot, and enzyme-linked immunosorbent assay).

Latency phase

Patients can remain without symptoms or have only chronic lymphadenopathy for years. The latter does not portend a systematically bad prognosis.

AIDS

The CDC and WHO have different classifications to determine the disease. According to the latter, AIDS defining clinical conditions, with a positive HIV serology, are as follows:

- Bacterial infections (multiple or recurrent)
- Candidiasis of bronchi, trachea, or lungs
- Candidiasis of esophagus
- Cervical cancer
- Invasive coccidioidomycosis
- Disseminated or extrapulmonary cryptococcosis
- Extrapulmonary cryptosporidiosis (chronic, duration >1 month, intestinal)
- CMV disease (other than liver, spleen, or lymph nodes; onset at age >1 month)
- CMV retinitis (with vision loss)
- Encephalopathy (HIV-related)
- Herpes simplex chronic (duration >1 month, ulcers or bronchitis; pneumonitis; or esophagitis, onset at age >1 month)
- Histoplasmosis (disseminated or extrapulmonary)
- Isosporiasis (chronic, duration >1 month, intestinal)
- Kaposi sarcoma
- Lymphoid interstitial pneumonia or pulmonary lymphoid hyperplasia complex
- Burkitt lymphoma
- Immunoblastic lymphoma
- Brain primary lymphoma
- *Mycobacterium avium* complex or *Mycobacterium kansasii* (disseminated or extrapulmonary)
- *Mycobacterium tuberculosis* (of any site, pulmonary, disseminated, or extrapulmonary)
- *Mycobacterium* of other species or unidentified species (disseminated or extrapulmonary)
- *Pneumocystis jirovecii* pneumonia
- Recurrent pneumonia
- Recurrent, progressive, multifocal leukoencephalopathy
- *Salmonella* septicemia
- Brain toxoplasmosis (onset at age >1 month)
- Wasting syndrome attributed to HIV

For adults without a CD4 count, the clinical stages are as follows.

One

- Asymptomatic
- Persistent generalized lymphadenopathy

Two

- Moderate unexplained weight loss (under 10% of presumed or measured body weight)

- Recurrent respiratory tract infections (sinusitis, tonsillitis, otitis media, or pharyngitis)
- Herpes zoster
- Angular chelitis
- Recurrent oral ulceration
- Papular pruritic eruptions
- Seborrheic dermatitis
- Fungal nail infections

Three

- Unexplained severe weight loss (over 10% of presumed or measured body weight)
- Unexplained chronic diarrhea for >1 month
- Unexplained persistent fever (intermittent or constant for >1 month)
- Persistent oral candidiasis
- Oral hairy leukoplakia
- Pulmonary tuberculosis
- Severe bacterial infections (e.g., pneumonia, empyema, pyomyositis, bone or joint infection, meningitis, bacteremia)
- Acute necrotizing ulcerative stomatitis, gingivitis, or periodontitis
- Unexplained anemia (<8 g/dl), neutropenia (<0.5 billion/l), and/or chronic thrombocytopenia (<50 billion/l)

Four

- HIV wasting syndrome
- Pneumocystis pneumonia
- Recurrent severe bacterial pneumonia
- Chronic herpes simplex infection (orolabial, genital, or anorectal lasting >1 month or visceral at any site)
- Esophageal candidiasis (or candidiasis of trachea, bronchi, or lungs)
- Extrapulmonary tuberculosis
- Kaposi sarcoma
- CMV infection (retinitis or infection of other organs)
- CNS toxoplasmosis
- HIV encephalopathy
- Extrapulmonary cryptococcosis, including meningitis
- Disseminated nontuberculous mycobacterial infection
- Progressive multifocal leukoencephalopathy
- Chronic cryptosporidiosis
- Chronic isosporiasis
- Disseminated mycosis (extrapulmonary histoplasmosis, coccidiomycosis)
- Recurrent septicemia (including nontyphoidal *Salmonella*)
- Lymphoma (cerebral or B cell non-Hodgkin)
- Invasive cervical carcinoma

- Atypical disseminated leishmaniasis
- Symptomatic HIV-associated nephropathy or HIV-associated cardiomyopathy

For children >4 yr with a positive HIV serology and without a CD4 count, the clinical stages are as follows:

One

- Asymptomatic
- Persistent generalized adenopathy

Two

- Hepatosplenomegaly
- Papular pruritic eruptions
- Seborrheic dermatitis
- Extensive human papillomaviral infection
- Extensive molluscum contagiosum
- Fungal nail infections
- Recurrent oral ulcerations
- Lineal gingival erythema
- Angular cheilitis
- Parotid enlargement
- Herpes zoster
- Recurrent or chronic RTIs (otitis media, otorrhea, or sinusitis)

Three

- Moderate unexplained malnutrition not adequately responding to standard therapy
- Unexplained persistent diarrhea (14 days or more)
- Unexplained persistent fever (intermittent or constant, for >1 month)
- Oral candidiasis (outside neonatal period)
- Oral hairy leukoplakia
- Acute necrotizing ulcerative gingivitis/periodontitis
- Pulmonary TB
- Severe, recurrent presumed bacterial pneumonia

Four

- Unexplained severe wasting or severe malnutrition not adequately responding to standard therapy
- Pneumocystis pneumonia
- Recurrent, severe presumed bacterial infections (e.g., empyema, pyomyositis, bone or joint infection, meningitis, but excluding pneumonia)
- Chronic herpes simplex infection (orolabial or cutaneous lasting >1 month)
- Extrapulmonary TB
- Kaposi sarcoma
- Esophageal candidiasis
- CNS toxoplasmosis (outside the neonatal period)

- HIV encephalopathy

For infants and children <4 yr with a positive HIV serology and without a CD4 count, the following are the clinical conditions:

Presumptive stage 3
- Moderate unexplained malnutrition not adequately responding to standard therapy
- Unexplained persistent diarrhea (14 days or more)
- Unexplained persistent fever (intermittent or constant for >1 month)
- Oral candidiasis (outside neonatal period)
- Oral hairy leukoplakia
- Acute necrotizing ulcerative gingivitis/periodontitis
- Pulmonary TB
- Severe, recurrent presumed bacterial pneumonia

Presumptive stage 4
- Unexplained severe wasting or severe malnutrition not adequately responding to standard therapy
- Pneumocystis pneumonia
- Recurrent, severe presumed bacterial infections (e.g., empyema, pyomyositis, bone or joint infection, meningitis, but excluding pneumonia)
- Chronic herpes simplex infection (orolabial or cutaneous of >1 month duration)
- Extrapulmonary TB
- Kaposi sarcoma
- Esophageal candidiasis
- CNS toxoplasmosis (outside the neonatal period)
- HIV encephalopathy

In African adults, the three most frequent symptoms of AIDS are chronic diarrhea, fever, and weight loss. Others include papular prurigo, alopecia, allergies (in particular to drugs), oral candidiasis, cryptococcal papules, histoplasmic skin eruption, buccal or anal chronic herpes, shingles, hairy leukoplakia, molluscum contagiosum, Kaposi syndrome dysphagia (often due to herpes simplex or CMV), sclerosing pericholangitis (due to *Cryptosporidium* or CMV), cough, pneumonia (due to TB, pneumocystosis, cryptococcosis, coccidioidomycosis, toxoplasmosis, interstitial lymphoid infiltrate, and, late in the disease, CMV and atypical mycobacteria), local or general seizures (due to toxoplasmosis or cryptococcosis), brain function disorders with or without motor or sensory deficit (due to progressive multifocal leukoencephalopathy), myelitis, atypical central neurological picture (due to syphilis), multineuritis, polyradiculoneuritis, polyneuritis (due to CMV), retinitis (due to CMV), retinal nodules, optic vascular lesions, chronic benign lymphadenopathy, other lymphadenopathy (due to cancer, TB, or atypical mycobacteriosis), Kaposi syndrome, systemic mycosis, and kala-azar).

In children, the asymptomatic phase is much shorter, the prognosis worse, and symptoms include stunted growth, thrush, chronic diarrhea, recurring infections with pyogenic germs, lymphadenopathy, hepatomegaly, splenomegaly, parotitis, interstitial lymphoid pneumonia, neurological deficits (loss of acquired knowledge, psychomotor retardation), pyramidal syndrome, ataxia, extrapyramidal rigidity, and seizures.

With the advent of combination therapies, HIV/AIDS has turned into a chronic disease.

Intestinal protozooses

In HIV/AIDS patients and other immunocompromised patients, some intestinal protozooses can cause severe acute or chronic diarrhea often with fever (for 1–4 below), abdominal pain, dehydration, anorexia, asthenia, weight loss, and sometimes malabsorption. The diarrhea can become chronic.

They include (1) cryptosporidiosis (*Cryptosporidium* spp.); (2) cyclosporiasis (*Cyclospora cayetanensis*); (3) isosporiasis or isosporidiosis (*Isospora belli*); (4) sarcosporidiosis, sarcocystosis, or sarcocystitis (*Sarcocystis hominis, Sarcocystis hirsuta, Sarcocystis cruzi*); and (5) microporidiosis (*Encephalitozoon intestinalis, Enterocytozoon bieneusi, Encephalitozoon intestinalis, Encephalitozoon cuniculi, Pleistophora sp., Trachipleistophora hominis, Trachipleistophora anthropophthera, Nosema connori, Nosema ocularum, Brachiola vesicularum, Vittaforma corneae, Microsporidium ceylonensis, Microsporidium africanum, Brachiola algerae*).

Other symptoms include:

Cryptosporidiosis: Biliary involvement with acalculous cholecystitis, sclerosing cholangitis, papillary stenosis, or pancreatitis. All are associated with right upper quadrant pain, nausea, and vomiting. Pulmonary forms have also been described.

Cyclosporiasis: Biliary disease with right upper quadrant pain and thickened gallbladder.

Isosporiasis: Hepatic involvement, acalculous cholecystitis, colitis, reactive arthritis, and tissue invasion and dissemination.

Sarcosporidiosis: Necrotizing enteritis, myalgia, generalized muscle weakness, dysphagia. Cardiac involvement is almost always asymptomatic.

Microsporidiosis: Cholecystitis, renal failure, RTI (with persistent cough, dyspnea, and wheezing), cephalgia, nasal congestion or discharge, sinusitis. Ocular microsporidiosis may occur with foreign body sensation, conjunctivitis, ophthalmalgia, sensitivity to light, hyperlacrimation, blurred vision, or decreased visual acuity. In the musculoskeletal form, the patient may experience myositis with myalgia, generalized muscle weakness, and fever. Microsporidia have been associated with nodular cutaneous lesions. CNS symptoms include seizures and cephalgia. Patients with urinary tract involvement are frequently asymptomatic.

Treatment

- Treatment is for life.
- Monitor allergies and viral resistance. However, with the constant development of new compounds by pharmaceutical companies in new and the same classes of drugs, these events have become less challenging to clinicians.
- Standard antiretroviral therapy consists of a combination of at least three antiretroviral drugs.
- When CD4 cell count is not available, start treatment at clinical stage 3 or 4.

- For adults and adolescents, first-line combinations include zidovudine/lamivudine, tenofovir/lamivudine, tenofovir/emtricitabine, stavudine/lamivudine. All + niverapine, or efavirenz.
- The choice of combination is based on
  - Efficacy
  - Side effects
  - Pregnancy
  - Adherence
  - Cost of drugs
  - Lab monitoring requirements
  - Co-infections (TB, hepatitis, and Kaposi sarcoma)
  - Anemia
  - Continuity of supply
  - Potential future treatment options
- For children or infants, first-line combinations are zidovudine/lamivudine, stavudine/lamivudine + abacavir. All + nevirapine, or efavirenz
- For pregnant women, WHO guidelines recommend an initial regimen of zidovudine + lamivudine + nevirapine.
- Dosing:

In adults

- Zidovudine, 300 mg, po, bid
- Lamivudine, 300 mg, po, once daily, or 150 mg, po, bid
- Stavudine, 30 mg, po, bid
- Efavirenz, 600 mg, po, once daily
- Nevirapine, 200 mg, po, bid, or nevirapine XR, 400 mg, once daily
- Abacavir, 300 mg, po, bid, or 2 tabs, po, once daily
- Embitracine, 200 mg, po, once daily
- Tenofovir, 300 mg, po, once daily

Table 4.2 AIDS treatment regimens for children

Name	Pediatric Use	Precautions
Lamivudine + zidovudine	>12 yr: 1 tab (300 mg zidovudine/150 mg lamivudine), po, bid	Contraindicated in children <12 yr
Emtricitabine	0–3 months: Solution: 3 mg/kg/day 3 months–17 yr: Solution: 6 mg/kg, once daily >33 kg: Cap: 200 mg, po, once daily Solution: 6 mg/kg, po, once daily	Max dosage: Solution: 240 mg/day
Lamivudine	3 months–16 yr: Solution or tab: 4 mg/kg, po, bid >16 yr: refer to adult dosing	Max dosage: 150 mg, bid

(continued)

Table 4.2 (Continued)

Name	Pediatric Use	Precautions
Zidovudine	6 weeks–12 yr: Tab/cap/solution: 160 mg/m^2, q8h For prevention of neonatal transmission <12 h after birth–6 weeks: Solution: 2 mg/kg, q6h, until 6 weeks of age IV: 1.5 mg/kg infused over 30 min, q6h, until 6 weeks of age	Max dosage: 200 mg, q8h
Stavudine	Birth–13 days: Tab/oral solution: 0.5 mg/kg/dose, q12h >14 days and <30kg: Tab/oral solution: 1 mg/kg/dose, q12h >30–< 60kg: 30 mg, q12h >60 kg: 40 mg, q12h	
Abacavir	3 months–16 yr: Tab/oral solution: 8 mg/kg, bid	Max dosage: 300 mg, bid

In children

- Postexposure (HIV/PEP): (1) Treatment should begin as soon as possible, preferably within 1 h of infection, and (2) the antiretroviral regimen is identical to the standard AIDS therapy with two to three antiretroviral medications. To be effective, PEP must begin within 72 h of exposure, before the virus has time to rapidly replicate in the body. PEP should be taken for 28 days.
- Bone marrow transplant can be a last-resort procedure.
- Treat the specific diseases associated with HIV/AIDS, which can be challenging. For example, for intestinal protozooses:
  - *Cryptosporidiosis:* nitazoxanide, 1,000–2,000 mg/day, in divided doses, bid, po, for 14 days. It can only improve symptoms.
  - *Cyclosporiasis:* cotrimoxazole 160 + 800 mg, bid, po, for 7 days, in adults. It reduces diarrhea and eliminates *Cyclospora cayetanansis* from feces.
  - *Isosporiasis:* cotrimoxazole, 160 + 800 mg, bid, po, for 7 days, in adults. Relapses are frequent. Ciprofloxacin is an alternative.
  - *Microsporidiosis:* albendazole, 400 mg/day, once a day, po, for at least 4 weeks
  - *Sarcosporidiosis:* surgical treatment of intestinal complications
- Check for other STDs including syphilis, gonorrhea, chlamydia, HPV, hepatitis B, and hepatitis C.
- Treat sexual partner(s).
- On June 30, 2013, the WHO has issued new guidelines for the early treatment of HIV: http://www.who.int/mediacentre/news/releases/2013/new_hiv_recommendations_20130630/en/index.html

Preventive Measures

- Pre-exposure (PrEP) can reduce transmission of the virus up to 96% when uninfected partners of people infected with HIV take emtricitabine + tenofovir.
- Know the health of your sexual partner(s).
- Use condoms during vaginal or anal intercourse.
- Use only water-based lubricants.

- Screen blood transfusions.
- Treat women predelivery to protect babies.
- Male circumcision reduces a man's risk of becoming infected with HIV during heterosexual intercourse by up to 60%.
- Use clean needles, and do not share needles.
- Consider using tenofovir + emtricitabine while sexually active (1 tab po, 300 mg/200 mg) daily, not more than 3 months.
- No vaccine is available.

Influenza (or Flu)

Influenza A, B, C

Geographic Distribution

Influenza is ubiquitous, but complications are more common in the intertropical zone because of local climatic and socioeconomic conditions. According to the WHO, worldwide, the annual epidemics of the disease result in about 3 to 5 million cases of severe illness, and about 250,000 to 500,000 deaths. In some tropical countries, influenza viruses circulate throughout the year with 1 or 2 peaks during rainy seasons.

Main Symptoms

Interhuman infection occurs (1) directly, by inhaling virus-infected aerosols spread by sneezing or coughing, or (2) indirectly, by touching contaminated objects or surfaces and rubbing the eyes, poking nostrils, or sucking fingers. After an incubation period of 1–5 days, the most frequent symptoms are sudden high fever, pharyngitis, and cough. Chills, myalgia, arthralgia (worse in the back and legs), cephalgia, rhinorrhea, conjunctivitis, fatigue, nausea, emesis, diarrhea, and abdominal pain (in children, more severe with influenza B) can also occur. The data in Table 4.3 are useful for diagnostic purposes.

Table 4.3 Sensitivity and specificity of influenza main symptoms

	Fever	Cough	Nasal Congestion
Sensitivity	68–86%	84–98%	68–91%
Specificity	25–73%	7–29%	19–41%
All findings, especially fever, were less sensitive in patients over 60 yr of age.			

In adults, adolescents, and children ≥2 yr old, serious symptoms include dyspnea, persistent emesis, confusion, and dizziness. In children ≤2 yr old, serious symptoms include high fever, tachypnea, not interacting normally, not eating or drinking as usual, irritability, sleepiness, skin eruption, and bluish color of the lips and/or skin. For all, complications include pneumonia, bronchitis, sinusitis, otitis, Guillain-Barre syndrome, and hemorrhage from mucous membranes.

Groups at risk

Children under 2 yr old, adults over 65 yr old, pregnant women, adults and children with chronic medical conditions, immunodepressed adults and children, residents in senior homes, people in contact with children, health-care workers, people with a body mass index over 40, asthma, diabetes, and heart disease.

Pregnant women

Pregnant women are at increased risk for bacterial pneumonia, dehydration, cardiovascular and neurological complications in their babies. Children born from mothers who contracted influenza during their pregnancy are more likely to develop autism.

Treatment

- Nonspecific:
  - Rest, fluids, paracetamol
  - Avoid taking aspirin, which may cause a potentially fatal Reye's syndrome, particularly with influenza type B.
- Specific:
  - Neuraminidase inhibitors: oseltamivir, zanamivir
  - M2 inhibitors (ineffective against influenza B): amantadine, rimantadine
- Dosing
  * Oseltamivir, 75 mg daily, po, bid, q12h, for adults, for 5 days; for children, see Table 4.4.

Table 4.4 Oseltamivir pediatric regimens for the treatment of influenza

Body Weight	5-Day Regimen
≤15 kg (≤33 lb)	30 mg, po, bid
>15–23 kg (>33–51 lb)	45 mg, po, bid
>23–40 kg (>51–88 lb)	60 mg, po, bid
>40 kg (>88 lb)	75 mg, po, bid

* Treatment should begin within 2 days of symptom onset or exposure.
* Zanamivir, 10 mg, inhaled, bid, for patients 7 yr and older, for 5 days

Preventive Measures

- Oseltamivir (pregnant women in particular), zanamivir
- Dosing:
  * Oseltamivir, 75 mg daily, po, once, for adults, for 10 days; for children, see Table 4.5.

Table 4.5 Oseltamivir pediatric regimens for the prevention of influenza

Body Weight	10-Day Regimen
≤15 kg (≤33 lb)	30mg, po, once daily
>15–23 kg (> 33–51 lb)	45mg, po, once daily
>23–40 kg (> 51–88 lb)	60mg, po, once daily
>40 kg (>88 lb)	75mg, po, once daily

- Zanamivir, 10 mg, inhaled, once a day, for patients 7 yr and older, for 10 days

- Immunization
  - Surface proteins of the virus mutate easily, in particular hemagglutinin and neuraminidase (H1, 2, and 3; N1 and 2); and the H/N combination of the vaccine has to be adjusted iteratively. Therefore, for groups at risk, vaccination should be on a yearly basis.
  - Get immunized to protect yourself, and have your kids immunized to protect others.
  - The vaccine should not be administered within 2 weeks before or 48 h after administration of oseltamivir.
  - The intranasal vaccine should not be administered until 48 h following cessation of zanamivir.
  - Zanamivir should not be taken until 2 weeks following administration of the influenza vaccine.
- Protection

  For self:
  - Wash your hands frequently (for at least 20 sec).
  - Do not shake hands or exchange kisses.
  - Avoid contact with people with flu symptoms (stay >6 ft away).

  For others:

  If you develop sneezing and coughing:
  - Use paper tissues to wipe your nose, and cover your mouth.
  - Throw the used tissues in the trash.
  - Wash your hands again.
  - If no tissues are available, cough or sneeze on the upper part of your sleeve.

  If you are sick:
  - Stay home.
  - When feasible, use a separate bedroom.

Measles

Paramyxovius family, *Morbillivirus* genus

Geographic Distribution

Once a ubiquitous disease, because of immunization campaigns measles is now a serious problem only in developing countries, where it represents one of the top five main causes of mortality for children up to 5 yr old (90% of all cases). According to the WHO, in 2011, there were 158,000 measles deaths globally – about 430 deaths every day or 18 every hour. More than 95% of them occur in low-income countries. If measles morbidity is the same everywhere, its mortality is much higher in challenging environments because of promiscuity (especially in urban areas), poor nutrition (in particular, vitamin A deficiency), comorbidities, and nonaccess or difficult access to health care.

Main Symptoms

Transmission is directly interhuman by Pflügge droplets contaminated by sick persons. The measles virus penetrates the body usually though the URT and rarely via the conjunctivae. In Africa, doctors' waiting rooms are major sources of infection. The incubation period lasts 7–14 days, then the infection develops in sequential stages over a period of 2–3 weeks.

First stage: Nonspecific symptomatology

Measles typically begins with a mild to moderate fever, often accompanied with a persistent cough, coryza, conjunctivitis, and pharyngitis, which may last 2 or 3 days.

Second stage: Acute illness and rash

Enanthema

The sign of Koplik is pathognomonic of measles and consists of white spots on an erythematous base inside the mouth, most often on the cheeks but sometimes on the lips or gingivae.

Exanthema

A skin eruption appears as small red spots, some slightly raised and occurring tightly together, which gives the skin a splotchy appearance. The rash first involves the face, particularly behind the ears and along the hairline, then spreads to the arms and trunk and over the thighs, lower legs, and feet. At the same time, over a few days, fever rises sharply and can reach 104 or 105°F (40 or 40.6°C). The eruption finally fades firstly from the face and lastly from the thighs and feet.

Third stage: Complications

Bronchopulmonary

- Viral superinfections: adenovirus and often herpes virus causing bronchitis, bronchiolitis, and pneumonia
- Bacterial superinfections: *Hemophilus influenzae*, *Staphylococcus aureus*, and *pneumococcus* causing bronchitis, bronchopneumonias, acute respiratory distress, lung or pleura abscesses
- Atelectasias, emphysema (including mediastinal), pneumothorax
- Respiratory complications are the main cause of death related to measles.

Diarrhea and dehydration

They are very common and can lead to vascular collapsus and coma. They contribute to malnutrition.

ENT

They consist of rhinitis, pharyngitis, otitis, mastoiditis, laryngitis, and stomatitis. The latter also contributes to malnutrition.

Neurological

Seizures, alteration of consciousness, motor disturbances, encephalitis.

Ocular

Conjunctivitis, keratitis due to viral or bacterial superinfection, corneal ulcers.

Comorbidities

HIV/AIDS, malaria, malnutrition, TB, salmonellosis, shigellosis, amebiasis worsen the clinical picture.

Pregnancy problems

In pregnant women measles can cause pregnancy loss, preterm labor, or low birth weight.

Thrombocytopenia

Measles may lead to a decrease in platelet number.

The communicable period lasts about 8 days: 4 days before the rash appears and another 4 after it has disappeared.

Treatment

- *Isolation*: Up to 5 days after the rash or during the entire illness in case of malnutrition or immunocompromise.
- *Disinfection*: Particularly the nose, throat, and eyes.
- *Antipyretics*:
  - Acetaminophen, ibuprofen, or naproxen, po, help relieve fever and aches.
  - Avoid aspirin because of the risk of a potentially fatal Reye's syndrome.
- *Antibiotics*: If a bacterial infection develops, choose an antibiotic that covers the bacteria(s) most likely involved.
- *Vitamin A*: Generally, 200,000 IU, po, for 2 days
- *Specific treatment of complications*: Pulmonary, ENT, ocular symptoms, diarrhea, malnutrition, etc.

Preventive Measures

- *Immunization*: Subcutaneous administration of a live attenuated virus (0.5 ml of at least 1,000 viral units) Children and some adults should be vaccinated with the measles, mumps, and rubella (MMR) vaccine. Two doses are needed for complete protection. Children should be given the first dose of MMR vaccine at 12–15 months of age. The second dose can be given 1 month later, but for example in the United States, it is usually given before the start of kindergarten at 4–6 years of age.
- *Postexposure vaccination*: Nonimmunized people, including infants, may be given the measles vaccination within 72 h of exposure to the virus. If measles still develops, the illness usually is milder and shorter.
- *Immune serum globulin*: Pregnant women, infants, and people with weakened immune systems exposed to the virus may receive an injection of immune serum globulin. When given within 6 days of exposure to the virus, it can prevent the disease or make it milder.

Poliomyelitis (or Polio)

Poliovirus 1, 2, and 3

Historical Background

Jakob Heine identified poliomyelitis in 1840. The poliomyelitis virus was isolated in 1908 by Karl Landteiner. For most of human history polio epidemics have crippled and killed scores of people, mostly young children, by causing muscle paralysis. The disease existed as endemic for thousands of years until the 1880s, when major epidemics began to strike Europe, from where it spread to the United States and beyond. By the early 1900s, most of the world saw a dramatic increase in poliomyelitis cases and epidemics occurred on a regular basis, mainly in urban areas and in the summertime. These devastating events triggered the development of a vaccine. Two were developed in the 1950s (parenteral Salk and oral Sabin), and their use reduced the incidence of poliomyelitis dramatically. According to the WHO, polio cases have decreased by over 99% since 1988, from an estimated 350,000 cases to 1,997 cases reported in 2006.

New Problems

Persistent pockets of polio transmission in northern India, in northern Nigeria, and at the border between Afghanistan and Pakistan are the current foci of the polio-eradication initiative.

Nevertheless, three main problems exist.

- As long as a single child remains infected, children in all countries are at risk.
- Between 2003 and 2005, 25 previously polio-free countries were re-infected due to imports of the virus. The possibility of reoccurrence is constant.
- In June 2012, the Taliban prevented the immunization of 161,000 children under 5 yr old in the North Waziristan tribal area of Pakistan. Given the nature of the virus, this poses a threat to other Asian countries.

Geographic Distribution

The poliovirus was ubiquitous but has been eradicated from most of the world. According to the WHO, in 2012, only Afghanistan, Nigeria, and Pakistan remained polio-endemic.

Main Symptoms

The disease is transmitted directly from person to person. It is highly contagious. In a household 90–100% of residents will be infected by a single case. The disease can be caused by any of the serotypes of the poliovirus. Three basic clinical pictures can be seen

Asymptomatic form

This is the form seen in most people with a normal immune system.

Minor illness

It does not involve the CNS. Symptoms include pharyngitis, nausea, emesis, abdominal pain, constipation, diarrhea, and/or a flu-like syndrome.

Major illness

It involves the CNS. It maybe paralytic or nonparalytic and represents about 3% of infections. Overall, approximately 1 in 200 to 1,000 cases progresses to acute flaccid paralysis. However, in most patients it causes nonparalytic aseptic meningitis with cephalgia; neck, back, abdominal, and extremity pain; fever; emesis; lethargy; and irritability. Encephalitis can occur in rare cases, usually in infants. It is characterized by confusion, changes in mental status, headache, fever, and, less commonly, seizures and spastic paralysis.

Depending on the site of paralysis, paralytic poliomyelitis is classified as spinal, bulbar, or bulbospinal.

Spinal

Muscles atrophy and become weak, floppy, poorly controlled, and paralyzed. Progression to maximum paralysis takes 2–4 days and is usually associated with fever and muscle pain. Deep tendon reflexes are absent or diminished. Sensation is not affected.

The extent of paralysis depends on the region of the cord involved (cervical, thoracic, or lumbar). The virus strikes muscles most often unilaterally. Any limb or combination of limbs may be seen: one leg, one arm, both legs, and both arms. Paralysis is often more severe proximally than distally.

Bulbar

It represents 2% of cases of paralytic polio and causes difficulty in breathing, speaking, and swallowing. Secretions of mucus may invade the airway, resulting in suffocation. Other signs and symptoms include facial muscle weakness, diplopia, difficulty in chewing, and irregular respiration, which may lead to respiratory arrest. Pulmonary edema and shock may be fatal.

Bulbospinal

It represents approximately 20% of all paralytic poliomyelitis cases and is also called "respiratory poliomyelitis." The virus affects the upper part of the cervical spinal cord, causing paralysis of the diaphragm. It makes it difficult or impossible for the patient to breathe without artificial ventilation. It may also lead to paralysis of the arms and legs and impact swallowing, and heart function.

Treatment

- There is no cure for poliomyelitis.
- Symptomatic and supportive measures include antibiotics, analgesics, and physical therapy.

Preventive Measures

- Vaccination by
  - Inactivated virus vaccine (Salk), or inactivated polio vaccine (IPV), which is an injected polio vaccine used in most industrialized countries
  - Attenuated virus vaccine (Sabin) or oral polio vaccine (OPV). Three doses of live-attenuated OPV produce protective antibodies against the three poliovirus types in more than 95% of recipients. Four doses are needed (1 dose = 2 drops) and are given at birth, then at 6, 10 and 14 weeks. If the baby has diarrhea at birth, a normal dose is given anyway but an additional dose is included at 18 weeks (1 month after the 4th dose).
  - Because OPV is inexpensive, easy to administer, and produces excellent immunity, it has been the vaccine of choice for controlling poliomyelitis in many developing countries.
  - On very rare occasions (about 1 per 750,000 vaccinations), the attenuated virus reverts into a form that can cause paralysis.

Yellow Fever (or Black Vomit)

Flavivirus

Historical Background

In 1881, Carlos Finlay revealed the role of the *Aedes* mosquito in yellow fever transmission. The Rockefeller and the Pasteur Institutes created the first vaccines for the disease in 1926. In 1932, Fred Soper identified monkeys as the animal reservoirs of the virus. Other names for the disease include "jungle yellow fever," "sylvatic yellow fever," "urban yellow fever," "vomito negro," "bronze John," and "yellow jack."

The best-known epidemic occurred while digging the Panama Canal at the beginning of the 20th century. More recent outbreaks happened in Democratic Republic of Congo (1958); Ethiopia (1960–1962); Senegal (1965); Burkina Faso, Ghana, Mali, Togo, Nigeria, and Angola (1969); and Gambia (1978–1979). Burkina Faso and Ghana were hit again in 1983–1984. In 2010, the number of cases was as shown in Table 4.6.

Table 4.6 Cases of yellow fever in the world in 2010

Global: 737	
Democratic Republic of Congo	289
Ghana	155
Uganda	106
Chad	79
Ivory Coast	49
Peru	18
Cameroon	16
Burkina Faso	7
Central African Republic	6
Bolivia	3
Mali	3
Brazil	2
Guinea	2
Liberia	1
Senegal	1

New Problems

The increase of yellow fever outbreaks in African cities is a serious threat. Recent examples include Ouagadougou (Burkina Faso) in 1983; Jos, Azare, Oju, Ogun, and Ogbormosho (Nigeria) in 1987–1995; Ngaoundere (Cameroon) in 1994; Buchanan (Liberia) in 1995; Luanda (Angola) in 1988 and 1997; Kano (Nigeria) in 2000; Abijan (Ivory Coast) in 2001; Conakry (Guinea) and Dakar and Touba (Senegal) in 2002; and Bobo-Dioulasso (Burkina Faso) in 2004. Moreover, between September 2 and December 3, 2012, yellow fever had killed 164 people in Sudan's Darfur.

Geographic Distribution

Yellow fever is endemic to Africa and Central and South America but is notably absent from Asia. According to the WHO, in 2011, 5,189 suspected cases of yellow fever were reported from 13 countries in Africa.

Main Symptoms

Three to 6 days after being bitten by an infested *Aedes* mosquito, chills, high fever, severe low back pain, myalgia, and intense cephalgia appear suddenly and the patient becomes bedridden. The disease evolves in two phases.

Red

In a few hours the patient becomes agitated and delirious (mainly at night). The face and eyes turn red, and temperature is constantly high but with bradycardia (Faget's sign). The patient's tongue shows a characteristic white, furry coating in the center, surrounded by a swollen, reddened margin. This period can last 2–5 days. Usually, a short remission of 24 h happens on the third day.

Yellow

On the fourth or fifth day, fever reappears and the patient becomes exhausted and mentally confused. Emesis ("black vomit"), excruciating abdominal pain, and moderate to intense icterus are present. Hemorrhage can be seen on the skin and mucous membranes (epistaxis, uterine bleeding) along with hematuria, hematemesis, and hematochezia. Urine output decreases noticeably. This period can last 3–9 days. Death generally occurs from the fourth to the eleventh day from shock, hepatic or renal failure, or coma.

Treatment

- Symptomatic: bed rest, hydration, acetaminophen
- Supportive: IV fluids, emesis, and seizure control
- Hospitalization in severe cases: blood transfusion, ventilator, prevention of secondary pulmonary or urinary tract infection, nursing care

Preventive Measures

- Immunization (a single shot protects for 10 years). It should be given to travelers to endemic areas older than 9 months of age and to people in outbreak areas.
- Stay in air-conditioned rooms.
- Wear long-sleeved clothing and long pants.
- Use insecticide-treated bed netting.
- Use insecticides to kill vectors.
- Use insect repellents containing *N,N*-diethyl-meta-toluamide (DEET) or permethrin on clothes, exposed skin, and bed nets for extra protection. Be aware that they can only provide transitory protection.

Geographic Distribution of the
Animal Reservoir of the Yellow Fever

///// Endemic Areas

Rare Diseases

Arboviral Diseases

Geographic Distribution
Many arboviruses are present in the intertropical area.

Main Symptoms
Arboviruses can be transmitted by mosquitoes, ceratopoganids, ticks, and contact with rodent excrement or urine; but sometimes the mode of transmission is unknown. Interhuman contamination is possible, but it requires contact with blood, secretions, excretions, or cadavers. All arboviruses can initially cause an acute flu-like syndrome including fever, cephalgia, and myalgia (see "Influenza,"). Thereafter, the clinical evolution varies according to the viral species and can be classified into four groups:

1. Dengue-like syndrome with rash and pain (see "Dengue Fever" in Part 3 and Table 4.7)
2. Hemorrhagic syndrome with bleeding (see "Dengue Fever" in Part 3 and Table 4.7)
3. Meningoencephalic syndrome causing various focal neurological symptoms
4. Hepatonephritic syndrome with hepatic and renal disturbances (see above "Yellow Fever" in Part 3 and Table 4.7)

Treatment
- Symptomatic measures for mild cases: analgesics, antipyretics, decongestants, expectorants or antiexpectorants, antiemetics, etc.
- Supportive measures for more severe cases: IV fluids and electrolytes, vasopressors, oxygen, respirator/intubation, etc.

Preventive Measures
- Use repellents containing DEET (15–30%). Be aware that they can only provide transitory protection.
- Treat clothes with insecticides containing permethrin.
- Use insecticides to kill vectors.
- Use insectide-treated mosquito nets.
- Use face shields for patients with cough and/or rhinitis.

Table 4.7 Arboviruses clinical pictures

Dengue-Like Syndrome	Hemorrhagic Syndrome	Meningoencephalic Syndrome	Hepatonephritic Syndrome
• Chikungunya	• Chikungunya	• Eastern equine encephalitis	• Yellow fever
• O'Nyong Nyong	• OHF[a]	• Western equine encephalitis	
• Ross River	• KHF[a]	• Venezuela equine encephalitis	
• Sindbis	• Dengue 1, 2, 3, 4	• Japanese encephalitis	
• Mayaro	• Yellow fever	• Murray Valley encephalitis	
• Dengue 1, 2, 3, 4	• Rift Valley fever	• St. Louis encephalitis	
• West Nile	• CCHF[a]	• West Nile	
• Wesselsbron	• Junin	• Rocio	
• Bunyamwera	• Machupo	• TBE[a]	
• Ilhesha	• Lassa	• Louping Ill[a]	
• Caraparu	• Marburg	• California encephalitis	
• Oriboca	• Ebola	• Tahina	
• Restan		• Lacrosse	
• Marituba			
• Simbu, Bwamba			
• Oropovche			
• Guama, Catu			
• Tahyna			
• Naples			
• Sicily			
• Chagres			
• Candira			
• Rift Valley fever			
• Vesicular stomatitis			
• Tataguine			
• Rocky Mountain spotted fever			
• Zinga			
• Bahanja			
• Bangui			

CCHF = Crimea Congo hemorrhagic fever; KHF = Kyasanur hemorrhagic fever; OHF = Omsk hemorrhagic fever; TBE = tick-borne encephalitis.

[a]Arboviruses mainly transmitted by ticks.

Arenaviral Diseases

Tacaribe Complex

Junin virus, Machupo virus, Guanarito virus

Geographic distribution and historical background

The Junin, Machupo, and Guanarito viruses are responsible for hemorrhagic fevers in Argentina, Bolivia, and Venezuela. The most recent outbreak occurred in Bolivia in July–August 1994. The Sabia virus was identified in São Paulo, Brazil, in 1990.

Main symptoms

A flu-like syndrome (see "Influenza") occurs. Complications include a hemorrhagic syndrome (see "Dengue Fever").

Treatment

- Symptomatic measures for mild cases: analgesics, antipyretics, decongestants, expectorants or antiexpectorants, antiemetics, etc.
- Supportive measures for more severe cases: IV fluids and electrolytes, vasopressors, oxygen, respirator/intubation, etc.

Preventive measures

- Avoid proximity with rodents.

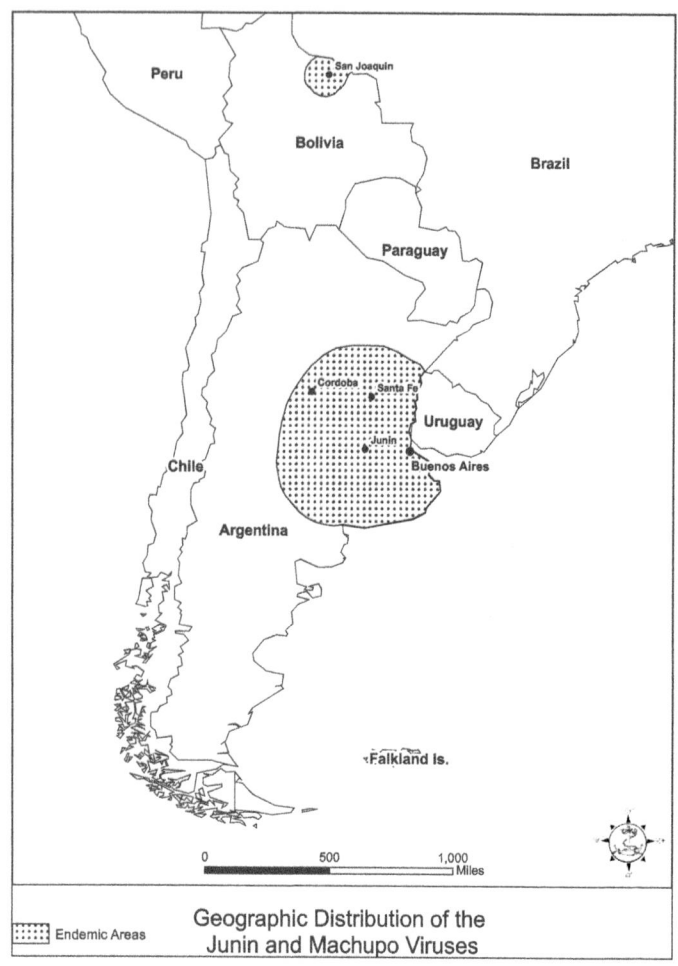

Lassa Fever

Lassa fever virus

Geographic distribution and historical background

First identified in 1969, Lassa fever has been found in Nigeria, Liberia, and Sierra Leone. The disease likely also exists in other West African countries. Rodents are the primary carriers of the virus.

Main symptoms

Transmission rates for Lassa fever are extremely high (50–80%). It is contracted through contact with either an infected person or an infected rodent's urine. Three to 16 days after contamination, the following symptoms appear: fever, myalgia, pharyngitis, chest and/or abdominal pain, emesis, conjunctivitis, and facial edema. Hemorrhage is mild. The association of purulent pharyngitis and proteinuria is highly suggestive of the disease. After 1–3 weeks, in survivors complications include uni- or bilateral deafness, pericarditis, uveitis, and orchitis. In Sierra Leone, the mortality rate was 1–2%, but it can reach 50% in other places.

Treatment

- Complete isolation of the patient is required.
- Ribavirin can limit complications, if taken early.
- Health-care providers must protect themselves (blouse, gloves, mask, and facial screen).
- Precautions must be taken for materials used to take and send biologic samples.
- Symptomatic measures for mild cases: analgesics, antipyretics, decongestants, expectorants or antiexpectorants, antiemetics, etc.
- Supportive measures for more severe cases: IV fluids and electrolytes, blood transfusion, vasopressors, oxygen, respirator/intubation, etc.

Preventive measures

- Complete isolation of the patient
- Avoid all direct contact with Lassa virus–infected patients and infected rodents' urine.
- Wear protective gear in infected areas.

Bunyaviral Diseases

Geographic Distribution

The bunyaviruses and their endemic areas are as follows:

- Bunyamwera, Bwamba, Ilesha, and Germistons: Africa
- Guaroa: South America
- Guama: South and Central America
- Oropouche: South and Central America
- La Crosse: United States
- Phlebovirus: Mediterranean basin, Asia, and Africa
- Nairovirus: Congo, Crimea, and Asia
- Hantaan: Russia, Japan, Korea, China, India, Balkans, Scandinavia, France, Belgium, Africa. See below, page 238.

- Tataguine: central Africa
- Rift Valley fever: Africa, Saudi Arabia, Yemen See below, page 240

Main Symptoms

A flu-like syndrome (see "Influenza").

Treatment

- Symptomatic measures for mild cases: analgesics, antipyretics, decongestants, expectorants or antiexpectorants, antiemetics, etc.
- Supportive measures for more severe cases: IV fluids and electrolytes, vasopressors, oxygen, respirator/intubation, etc.

Preventive Measures

- Use face shields for patients with cough and/or rhinitis.
- Use insecticides to kill vectors.
- Use repellents containing DEET (15–30%). Be aware that they can only provide transitory protection.
- Treat clothes with insecticides containing permethrin.
- Use insectide-treated mosquito nets.
- Wear long sleeves and long pants.

Hantaan Virosis

Hantavirus

Geographic Distribution

Hantavirus is endemic to China, Korea, the Balkans, and North and South America.

Main Symptoms

After 7–30 days of incubation, a flu-like syndrome may occur. Acute myopia is rare but very suggestive of the disease. Complications include a hemorrhagic syndrome. Kidneys, lungs, heart, GI tract, nervous system, and skin may be involved. Death is due to cardiovascular collapse, hemorrhage, hydroelectrolytic imbalance, or encephalitis (in the Balkans). The mortality rate is 5% in Korea and 7–18% in China.

A pulmonary form has been described in the Americas (in particular North America), the "hantavirus pulmonary syndrome," which is caused by the sin nombre virus, or "nameless" virus. Digestive and respiratory symptoms are severe, and their mortality reaches 90%.

Treatment

- Symptomatic measures for mild cases: analgesics, antipyretics, decongestants, expectorants or antiexpectorants, antiemetics, etc.
- Supportive measures for more severe cases: IV fluids and electrolytes, blood transfusion, vasopressors, oxygen, respirator/intubation, etc.

Preventive Measures

- Avoid proximity with rodents.

Geographic Distribution of the Hantaan Virus

////// Endemic Areas

Rift Valley Fever

Phlebovirus genus

Geographic Distribution and Historical Background

Rift Valley fever (RVF) is a zoonosis found occasionally in humans. Many animal species may be affected by the virus (cattle, sheep, camels, goats), with various mosquito species serving as vectors. Humans may become infected by a mosquito bite or contact with body fluids or organs of infected animals through inoculation or inhalation. Since isolation of the virus in 1930, there have been outbreaks in sub-Saharan, North, and East Africa, particularly in Kenya and Somalia. In September 2000, RVF was reported for the first time outside Africa, in Saudi Arabia and Yemen. In 2006, Kenya reported 10 deaths from RVF. From November 30, 2006, to March 3, 2007, a total of 684 cases were reported in Kenya, with 155 deaths (fatality rate 23%), including spread to Tanzania. In 2011, it was reported in South Africa.

Main Symptoms

The incubation period varies from 2–6 days. A flu-like syndrome then appears, with sudden fever, cephalgia, myalgia, and nonspecific back pain. There is occasional neck stiffness and photophobia, nausea, and emesis. Symptoms last 4–7 days. In rare severe cases, retinal lesions (with a 50% rate of permanent loss of vision), meningoencephalitis (with a low death rate), and/or hemorrhage may occur. Deaths are mostly due to the latter, with a 50% mortality rate.

Treatment

- Symptomatic measures for mild cases: analgesics, antipyretics, decongestants, expectorants or antiexpectorants, antiemetics, etc.
- Supportive measures for more severe cases: IV fluids and electrolytes, blood transfusion, vasopressors, oxygen, respirator/intubation, etc.

Preventive Measures

- Vaccination of animals at risk is the most important way of preventing infection in humans.
- Avoid proximity with sick bovines, ovines and caprines.
- Use insecticides to kill vectors.
- Use repellents containing DEET (15–30%). Be aware that they can only provide transitory protection.
- Treat clothes with insecticides containing permethrin.
- Use insectide-treated mosquito nets.

Coronaviral Disease

Severe Acute Respiratory Syndrome (S.A.R.S.)
SARS-CoV

Historical Background and Geographic Distribution

S.A.R.S., a new global threat, first appeared in November 2002 in the Guangdong Province of China. Over the next few months it spread to

32 places in North America, South America, Europe, and Asia, with 8,436 cases and 812 deaths. The areas most affected were mainland China (5,327 cases/348 deaths), Hong Kong (1,755/298), Taiwan (671/84), Singapore (206/32), Vietnam (63/5), and the United States (74/0). The epidemic ended on July 30, 2003, with the last case in Beijing. Masked palm civets were suspected as the origin of the SARS outbreak in 2002/2003 and were confirmed as the direct origin of SARS cases with mild symptoms in 2004 in China. In 2005, horseshoe bats were identified as the natural reservoir of a group of coronaviruses distantly related to SARS-CoV.

Main Symptoms

Two to 10 days after close contact with an infected person (within 3 ft [1 m]) and inhaling Pflügge's droplets, the following symptoms appear: acute pneumonia (sudden onset, high fever, dry cough, chest pain, and dyspnea), myalgia, cephalgia, anorexia, all beginning 24–48 h after the fever. They can progress to respiratory failure and death. The mortality rate is lower for younger patients (6% for those 25–44 yr old vs. >50% for those >65 yr).

Treatment

- The only active drug in vitro is interferon-beta-1b (Betaferon)
- Symptomatic measures for mild cases: analgesics, antipyretics, decongestants, expectorants or antiexpectorants, antiemetics, etc.
- Supportive measures for more severe cases: IV fluids and electrolytes, blood transfusion, vasopressors, oxygen, respirator/intubation, etc.

Preventive Measures

- Wear N95 masks, gloves, and goggles.
- Patient isolation in sterile quarters.
- Quarantine of close contacts.
- Clean and disinfect SARS patient environments.
- Negative pressure in operating rooms.
- Immunization. In China, in 2004, researchers successfully vaccinated people with a SARS vaccine with very few side effects.

Filoviral Diseases

Ebola Virus Disease

Ebola virus

Historical background

The Ebola virus has captured media attention, causing great public concern since reports of the first outbreak. There are five species of the virus, with different host specifications and disease severity. The Zaire, Bundibugyo (western Uganda), and Sudan strains are the most virulent. The mortality rate of Ebola virus averages 83%.

From July to November 1976, Ebola virus epidemics emerged in Africa simultaneously in Sudan and the Democratic Republic of Congo, with another case reported in Kenya in 1980. The virus then spread from western Sudan to the western part of Ivory Coast. In 1995, an outbreak killed 245 people in the Democratic Republic of Congo (Bongo-Yasa, Mosango, Vanga, and Kikwit). Another outbreak struck the northeastern part of Gabon in 1996, claiming at least 10 lives. In November 1996, a nurse contracted Ebola fever in South Africa, after being infected by a doctor coming from Gabon. Further outbreaks occurred in Uganda (2000), the Democratic Republic of Congo (2001–2002, 2003, 2005), Gabon (2002), Sudan (2004), and southern Democratic Republic of Congo (2007). In July 2012, Uganda faced another outbreak. Twenty cases were recorded and at least 14 people died in Kibaale, a district located in the midwest of the country. On August 14, 2012, the WHO reported 31 deaths from an outbreak in the Democratic Republic of Congo.

Geographic distribution

The Ebola virus appears to be endemic to central Africa.

Main symptoms

Two to 21 days after direct contamination from an infected patient's body fluids, the following symptoms often appear: sudden fever, myalgia, cephalgia, pharyngitis, emesis, and diarrhea. Five to 7 days later a maculopapular or a papulovesicular, nonpruritic skin eruption appears. Occasionally, there is a palate enanthema and conjunctival hyperemia. Complications include hepatitis, icterus, hemorrhage, DIC, liver failure, kidney failure, delirium, obnubilation, and coma. Patients usually die from hypovolemic shock on the eighth or ninth day. Recovery is long, occasionally with recurring orchitis, hepatitis, transverse myelitis, uveitis, or parotitis.

Treatment

- Complete isolation of the patient is required.
- Symptomatic measures for mild cases: analgesics, antipyretics, decongestants, expectorants or antiexpectorants, antiemetics, etc.
- Supportive for measures more severe cases: IV fluids and electrolytes, blood transfusion, vasopressors, oxygen, respirator/intubation, etc.

Preventive measures

- Complete isolation of the patient
- Avoid all direct contact with Ebola virus–infected patients.
- Wear protective gear in infected areas (mask, gloves, goggles).

Marburg Virus Disease

Marburg virus

Historical background

The Marburg virus was discovered in 1967, with 32 cases emerging in Germany and the former Yugoslavia (seven deaths). The outbreak was caused by laboratory workers handling green monkeys imported from Uganda. Three cases were reported in 1975 in South Africa with suspected Zimbabwean origins, and in 1980 and 1987, three cases were described in Kenya. From 1998 to 2000, 154 cases were reported in Durba, Democratic Republic of Congo (including 128 deaths). In 2004 and 2005, more than 300 cases were reported in Angola (mainly from the Uige Province) with over 100 deaths. In 2008, Uganda reported one case.

Geographic distribution
In contrast to Ebola, Marburg virus has more geographic and ecologic variations.

Main symptoms
The symptoms and transmission mode are similar to those of Ebola (above). The incubation period is 5–10 days, and the mortality rate approximately 30%.

Treatment
- Complete isolation of the patient is required.
- Symptomatic measures for mild cases: analgesics, antipyretics, decongestants, expectorants or antiexpectorants, antiemetics, etc.
- Supportive measures for more severe cases: IV fluids and electrolytes, blood transfusion, vasopressors, oxygen, respirator/intubation, etc.

Preventive measures
- Complete isolation of the patient
- Avoid all direct contact with Marburg virus–infected patients.
- Wear protective gear in infected areas (mask, gloves, goggles).

Flaviviral Diseases

Flaviviruses are similar to togaviruses.

Geographic Distribution
The flaviviruses and their endemic areas are as follows.

- West: Africa, Mediterranean basin, and India
- Kyasanur Forest: India
- Omsk hemorrhagic fever: Russia
- Spondweni, Wesselsbron, Langat, Zika, Bussuquara, Kunjin, Powassan, Negishi, Ilheus and Bravo: Europe, Africa, South America, and North America, in particular Canada for Powassan
- Yellow fever: Central and South America and Africa. See page 232.
- Dengue fever: intertropical zone. See page 205.

Main Symptoms
A flu-like syndrome (see "Influenza," p. 225). Complications include a hemorrhagic syndrome. The outcome of the diseases they induce is generally favorable; however, the mortality rate of the Omsk hemorrhagic fever virus ranges 1–10%. For dengue fever and yellow fever, please see p. 205 & 232.

Treatment
- Symptomatic measures for mild cases: analgesics, antipyretics, decongestants, expectorants or antiexpectorants, antiemetics, etc.

- Supportive measures for more severe cases: IV fluids and electrolytes, blood transfusion, vasopressors, oxygen, respirator/intubation, etc.
- ICU for hemorrhagic forms
- For dengue fever and yellow fever please see p. 205 & 232.

Preventive Measures

- Use insecticides to kill vectors.
- Use insectide-treated mosquito nets.
- Use repellents containing DEET (15–30%). Be aware that they can only provide transitory protection.
- Treat clothes with insecticides containing permethrin.
- Wear long sleeves and long pants.
- Wear a hat in tick territory.
- Avoid proximity with rodents.
- Immunization (see Yellow Fever, page 232)

Paramyxoviral Diseases

Hendra Virosis

Hendra virus

Geographic distribution

The Hendra virus was first isolated in 1994 from specimens obtained during an outbreak of respiratory and *neurological* disease in 21 horses and three humans in a suburb (Hendra) of Brisbane, Australia. The natural reservoir of the Hendra virus is flying foxes (bats of the *Pteropodidae* family and *Pteropus* genus) found in Australia.

Main symptoms

The virus caused a disease in horses in Australia, and the human infections were due to direct exposure to tissues, secretions, and excretions from animals infected with the virus. No interhuman transmission has been documented. The incubation period ranges 5–14 days. Symptoms vary from mild influenza-like illness to fatal respiratory or neurological disease. Infected people initially develop fever, cephalgia, myalgia, sore throat, and a dry cough. Adenopathy, lethargy, and vertigo can also occur. To date, there have been six confirmed human cases including three deaths. One patient died after developing pneumonitis, respiratory failure, renal failure, arterial thrombosis, and cardiac arrest. Another patient initially had a mild meningoencephalitis with sore throat, cephalgia, drowsiness, emesis, and neck stiffness. After treatment with antibiotics, he fully recovered; but 13 months later the encephalitis recurred and progressed to coma and death. The three infected people who made a full recovery had no residual problems.

Treatment

- No drugs are currently available.

- Symptomatic treatment
- Intensive supportive care, as needed

Preventive measures

- No vaccine is currently available for either people or animals.
- Stay away from sick horses.
- Use appropriate personal protective equipment devices when it is necessary to come into contact with potentially infected animals.

Nipah Virosis

Nipah virus

Geographic distribution

The Nipah virus was first isolated from samples coming from an outbreak of encephalitis and respiratory illness among adult men in Malaysia and Singapore in 1999. Since then, there have been 12 other outbreaks, all in south Asia. Fruit bats of the *Pteropodidae* family and *Pteropus* genus are the natural host of the Nipah virus.

Main symptoms

Humans are infected by close contact with infected pigs. Consumption of fruits or fruit products (e.g., raw date palm juice) contaminated with urine or saliva from infected fruit bats has also been described as a source of infection. In Bangladesh and India, the Nipah virus has spread directly from human to human through close contact with people's secretions and excretions. The incubation period ranges 4–45 days. Symptoms include fever, cephalgia, myalgia, emesis, and sore throat. They can be followed by dizziness, drowsiness, altered consciousness, and neurological signs indicating acute encephalitis. Some patients can also experience severe respiratory problems, including acute respiratory distress and atypical pneumonia. Encephalitis and seizures occur in the most severe cases, progressing to coma within 24–48 h.

Treatment

- No drugs are currently available.
- Symptomatic treatment
- Intensive supportive care, as needed

Preventive measures

- No vaccine is currently available for either people or animals.
- Stay away from sick pigs.
- Use appropriate personal protective equipment devices when it is necessary to come into contact with potentially infected animals.
- Stay away from sick people.

Reoviral Diseases

Geographic Distribution

- Respiratory, enteric, orphan and Kemerovo viruses: Russia and Egypt

- Orungo virus: Africa
- Rotavirus: ubiquitous. See below, page 248.

Main Symptoms

A flu-like syndrome (see "Influenza," p. 225) except for rotavirus (please see below).

Treatment

- Symptomatic measures for mild cases: analgesics, antipyretics, decongestants, expectorants or antiexpectorants, antiemetics, etc.
- Supportive measures for more severe cases: IV fluids and electrolytes, vasopressors, oxygen, respirator/intubation, etc.

Preventive Measures

- Use insectide-treated mosquito nets.
- Use insecticides to kill vectors.
- Use repellents containing DEET (15–30%). Be aware that they can only provide transitory protection.
- Treat clothes with insecticides containing permethrin.
- Wear long sleeves and long pants.
- Wear a hat in tick territory.

Rotavirus Disease

Rotavirus A, B, and C

Geographic Distribution

Rotaviruses are cosmopolitan and are the main cause of diarrhea in infants and very young children. Mortality is significantly higher in children less than 2 yr old. According to the WHO, more than 600,000 children under 5 yr of age die from dehydration due to a rotaviral infection each year in developing countries. By comparison, only 150 die annually in Europe despite the same infection rate. Nonaccess or difficult access to medical care is the main culprit for these dismal statistics.

Main Symptoms

The mode of transmission is via the fecal–oral route. It is a highly contagious disease. The incubation period ranges 1–2 days. Vomiting is often the first symptom. Usually, fever and diarrhea follow. The latter is secretory, lasts 4–8 days, and is more severe than with other viruses. Episodes of diarrhea can continue long after the child starts feeling better, in some cases up to a few weeks, which can lead to malnutrition. Diarrhea along with vomiting can also quickly lead to dehydration in babies and young children. Signs of dehydration include a lack of interest in playing, extreme sleepiness, dry mouth and tongue, sunken and soft fontanel, sunken eyes without tears, tachypnea, tachycardia, and a dry diaper for 12 h or more.

Treatment

- Keep the child comfortable and prevent or treat diaper rash.
- A rehydration drink such as Pedialyte® (manufactured by Abbott Laboratories) is useful in preventing dehydration.
- Plain water does not provide the necessary nutrients, and electrolytes may not be absorbed when a child has diarrhea.
- Rehydration drinks for adults or sports drinks should not be given to children.
- Probiotics may be helpful.
- ICU transfer is needed if dehydration becomes severe.

Preventive Measures

- Keep feeding babies breast milk or formula to prevent dehydration.
- Watch children closely for signs of dehydration.
- Two vaccines against rotavirus A infection are safe and effective in children: Rotarix by GlaxoSmithKline and RotaTeq by Merck. Both are taken orally, made of an attenuated live virus and given after 6 weeks of age. With Rotarix 2 doses are administered, at least 4 weeks apart and the scheme must be completed before 24 weeks of age. With Rotateq, 3 doses are given, at least 4 weeks apart and the scheme must be completed before 26 weeks of age. The protection rates are 90–100% against severe infections and 74–85% against all infections.
- Wash hands thoroughly and often to help prevent the spread of rotaviruses.

Rhabdoviral Diseases

Mossuril Virus Disease

Mossuril virus

Geographic distribution

Central and South Africa

Main symptoms

A flu-like syndrome (see "Influenza").

Treatment

- Symptomatic measures for mild cases: analgesics, antipyretics, decongestants, expectorants or antiexpectorants, antiemetics, etc.
- Supportive measures for more severe cases: IV fluids and electrolytes, vasopressors, oxygen, respirator/intubation, etc.

Preventive measures

- Use insectide-treated mosquito nets.
- Use insecticides to kill vectors.
- Use repellents containing DEET (15–30%). Be aware that they can only provide transitory protection.
- Treat clothes with insecticides containing permethrin.

Lyssavirus Disease

Australian Bat Lyssavirus (ABL)

Historical background

The Australian bat lyssavirus (ABL) emerged in the tropical northern part of Australia in January 1995. It was first isolated from flying foxes in Townsville, Queensland, and has since been isolated from bats in other places in Queensland, New South Wales, Victoria, and the Northern Territory. A woman infected with the virus died in Rockhampton, Queensland, in November 1996. The lyssavirus genus is closely related to the rabies virus.

Main symptoms

Lyssaviruses are usually transmitted to humans via bites or scratches, which provide direct access of the virus in the bat saliva to tissue and nerve endings. Transmission can also occur when the saliva has come in contact with human mucous membranes of the eyes, nose, or mouth. People are not exposed to ABL through tactile contact. Patting bats or exposure to bat urine and feces does not present any risk of infection. Transmission from person to person is theoretically possible, but it has only been documented through corneal transplantation.

The incubation period for lyssavirus is unknown. Symptoms include shoulder pain, emesis, ataxia, difficulty with concentration, palsy (particularly of respiratory muscles), coma, and death.

Treatment

- Full rabies vaccine and hyperimmune rabies globulin regimen (see rabies p. 261).
- Symptomatic measures for mild cases: analgesics, antipyretics, decongestants, expectorants or antiexpectorants, antiemetics, etc.
- Supportive measures for more severe cases: IV fluids and electrolytes, vasopressors, oxygen, respirator/intubation, etc.

Preventive measures

- People in high-risk groups should be fully immunized against rabies.

Togaviral Diseases

Geographic Distribution

- O'Nyong Nyong: Africa
- Marayo: South America
- Sindbis, Pixuna, Mucambo, Ross River, and Chikungunya: Africa, India, and southwest Asia) See below for the latter.

Main symptoms

A flu-like syndrome (see "Influenza, p. 225).

Treatment

- Symptomatic measures for mild cases: analgesics, antipyretics, decongestants, expectorants or antiexpectorants, antiemetics, etc.

- Supportive measures for more severe cases: IV fluids and electrolytes, blood transfusion, vasopressors, oxygen, respirator/intubation, etc.

Preventive measures

- Use insectide-treated mosquito nets.
- Use insecticides to kill vectors.
- Use repellents containing DEET (15–30%). Be aware that they can only provide transitory protection.
- Treat clothes with insecticides containing permethrin.

Chikungunya virus Diseases

Chikungunya virus

Geographic Distribution and Historical Background

The Chikungunya virus is endemic to subequatorial Africa, Madagascar, the Indian subcontinent, Southeast Asia, and the western Pacific islands (including Papua New Guinea and the Solomon Islands). Chikungunya is a word derived from the Makonde language, and it means "which bends up."

In 2005, an epidemic started in the Comoro Islands and spread to all the islands of the south Indian Ocean. From February of that year to November 2006, it struck Reunion Island; 266,000 islanders were infected, and 252 directly or indirectly died from the virus. The unusual large-scale dissemination was made possible by a mutation enabling virus transmission by the mosquito *Aedes albopictus*. In 2011, more than 1,000 cases of Chikungunya virus disease were recorded in the Philippines.

Main Symptoms

Transmission is via the bite of infected *Aedes* mosquitoes, leading to a flu-like syndrome (see "Influenza," p. 225). Evolution of the disease is usually favorable. Complications may occur in infants, the elderly, pregnant women, and sick or immunocompromised patients. Death occurs from hepatitis, myocarditis, or encephalitis.

Treatment

- Symptomatic measures for mild cases: analgesics, antipyretics, decongestants, expectorants or antiexpectorants, antiemetics, etc.
- Supportive measures for more severe cases: IV fluids and electrolytes, blood transfusion, vasopressors, oxygen, respirator/intubation, etc.

Preventive Measures

- Use insectide-treated mosquito nets.
- Use insecticides to kill vectors.
- Use repellents containing DEET (15–30%). Be aware that they can only provide transitory protection.
- Treat clothes with insecticides containing permethrin.
- Wear long sleeves and long pants.

Part 5

Tropical Health Hazards

Animal-Induced Diseases

Bees and Hymenoptera

Geographic Distribution
Bees, wasps, and hornets are found in many parts of the world. They proliferate in some areas of the tropics.

Main Symptoms
Bee, wasp, and hornet stings cause a painful skin reaction. Severity of the symptoms depends on the following factors: (1) extent of allergic reaction—presence or absence of allergic terrain; (2) number of stings—500 or more is lethal; and (3) site of the sting—in the face and mucous areas of the mouth and nose they can trigger Quincke edema and asphyxia.

- *Nonallergic patients* only experience a local reaction: (1) *small*: erythematous skin lesion, painful edema, and/or pruritus—the pain usually disappears over a few hours or (2) *large*: erythema, edema, and pain persist up to 1 week—areas adjacent to the bite site may be involved.
- *Allergic patients* have a systemic reaction including urticaria, nausea, emesis, diarrhea, and dizziness and sometimes anaphylactic, which includes wheezing, dyspnea, suffocation, and hypotension leading to shock.

Treatment
- Mild forms warrant local treatment only (cleaning and dressing of the skin).
- Epinephrine. Allergic patients should always carry EpiPen® (Mylan) with them in infested areas.
- Dosing (see Table 5.1).
- In severe forms, corticosteroids (IV), antihistamines, and calcium may be needed
- Dosing:
  * Prednisone, 20–80 mg, po, daily, for 2–5 days; children, 0.5–1 mg/kg, po, daily for 2–5 days

Table 5.1 Epinephrine doses for severe allergic reactions: 1 mg/ml injection (1:1,000). Use insulin syringes

Newborn	0.1 ml	2 months	0.15 ml	4 months	0.2 ml
1 yr	0.23 ml	3 yr	0.35 ml	5 yr	0.4 ml
7 yr	0.5 ml	12 yr	0.75 ml	Adult	1.0 ml

* Brompheniramine, 4 mg, q4–6h, po, IM, IV or S/C, as many days as needed, or
* Promethazine, 12.5–25 mg, po, IM or IV, as many days as needed
* Prescribe acetaminophen for pain.
- Acetaminophen
- Dosing:
  * See Table 5.2.
- In some cases a tracheotomy may be necessary.
- Advice to telecommunicate to the patient ASAP includes:
  - Remove the stinger.
  - Apply ice or cold packs at 10 minute intervals
  - Clean the bite site area with soap and water.

Preventive Measures

- Avoid areas with hives or nests of bees, wasps, or hornets.

Butterflies

Central and South America *Hylesia* genus, Africa: *Anaphae* genus

Geographic Distribution

Central America: Mexico
South America: Guyana, Venezuela, Brazil, Peru, Argentina
Central Africa: Gabon, Central African Republic

Main Symptoms

Skin eruption, consisting of very itchy papules. It follows penetration of the skin by microscopic "arrows" disseminated in the air by butterflies. It starts in the hour after contact and can last 2–10 days. It is more prominent on uncovered skin areas. Most often there is no contact with the butterfly, and the rash is triggered by manipulation of a contaminated object even days after the butterfly flew in the vicinity.

Treatment

- Avoid scratching.
- Wash the skin with very hot water.
- Topical corticoids and antihistamines po are efficient.

Preventive Measures

- Cover the skin and use a hat in endemic areas.
- Use insecticides to kill vectors

Table 5.2 Acetaminophen doses for infants and children

Weight	Dosage	Infant Drops 80 mg/0.8ml 1 dropper = 0.8 ml	Children Liquid 160 mg/5 ml	Chewable Tabs 80 mg	Junior Strength 160 mg	Adult Tabs 325 mg
5–8 lb	40 mg	0.5 dropper (0.4 ml)	0.25 tsp (1.25 ml)			
9–10 lb	60 mg	0.75 dropper (0.6 ml)	10.33 tsp (1.8 ml)			
11–16 lb	80 mg	1 dropper (0.8 ml)	0.5 tsp (2.5 ml)			
17–21 lb	120 mg	1.5 dropper (1.2 ml)	0.75 tsp (3.75 ml)			
22–26 lb	160 mg	2 droppers (1.6 ml)	1 tsp (5 ml)	2 tabs	1 tab	
27–32 lb	200 mg	2.5 droppers (2 ml)	1.25 tsp (6.25 ml)	2.5 tabs	1 tab	
33–37 lb	240 mg	3 droppers (2.4 ml)	1.5 tsp (7.5 ml)	3 tabs	1.5 tabs	
38–42 lb	280 mg	3.5 droppers (2.8 ml)	1.75 tsp (8.75 ml)	3.5 tabs	1.5 tabs	
43–53 lb	320 mg	4 droppers (3.2 ml)	2 tsp (10 ml)	4 tabs	2 tabs	1 tab
54–64 lb	400 mg	Use liquid or tabs	2.5 tsp (12.5 ml)	5 tabs	2.5 tabs	1 tab
65–75 lb	480 mg		3 tsp (15 ml)	6 tabs	3 tabs	1.5 tabs
76–86 lb	560 mg		3.5 tsp (17.5 ml)	7 tabs	3.5 tabs	1.5 tabs
87–95 lb	640 mg		4 tsp (20 ml)	8 tabs	4 tabs	2 tabs

>96 lb: adult dose = 1,000 mg, q6h, or 650 mg, q4h, with a maximum single dose of 1,000 mg, a minimum dosing interval of 4 h, and a maximum daily dose of 4,000 mg.

Cats

Cats can cause the following diseases by contact, biting, or scratching.

Allergies

Cats can trigger allergic reactions everywhere, with conjunctivitis, lacrimation, rhinitis, cough, urticaria, asthma, etc. Symptoms are the same as in temperate climates, but cats add to the allergen load, which is heavier in hot and humid climates where dust mites and mold thrive.

Cat Bite

Pasteurella multocida

Main symptoms

Between 30% and 50% of cat bites become infected. Bites to the head, face, and neck are less likely to become infected than those to extremities. Puncture wounds are more frequently infected than lacerations. The following symptoms appear rapidly after a bite: fever, chills, cellulitis, and local adenopathy. Any bite history taking should include the following:

- Time and location of event
- Species and breed of the animal and its status (i.e., health, rabies vaccination history, behavior, whereabouts)
- Circumstances of the biting incident (provoked vs. unprovoked)
- Location of bite(s)
- Treatment administered
- Patient's medical history (immunocompromise, peripheral vascular disease, diabetes, tetanus and rabies vaccination)

Treatment

- Local disinfection and wound dressing.
- Avoid suturing.
- Antibiotics are used for infected wounds or to prevent infection, e.g., amoxicillin/clavulanic acid or doxycycline.
- For high-risk wounds start with the IV route.
- Dosing:
  * Amoxicillin/clavulanic acid, adults, po, 875/125 mg, bid, or 500/125 mg, tid, q8h, or IV 1.2 g, q8h; children, po, 90 mg/kg/day divided in two doses, or IV, first week of life 50 mg amoxicillin + 12.5 mg clavulanic acid, q12h; for older children, 50 mg amoxicillin + 12.5 mg clavulanic acid, q6h, all for 10 days.
  * Doxycycline, adults, 100 mg, po, bid, for 10 days; children, 2 mg/kg/day (max 100 mg/day), for 10 days.
  * Doxycycline is contraindicated in children < 8 year old.
- Tetanus immunization must be updated.
- Consider rabies.

Preventive measures

- Stay away from stray cats.

Cat Scratch Disease

Bartonella henselae

Geographic distribution

Cat scratch disease is present everywhere cats can be found. It requires more rapid attention and treatment in the intertropical zone because local conditions are conducive to rapid infection spread and complications.

Main symptoms

A few days after being scratched by an infected cat, about one-third of patients develop an ulcer, nodule, or blister at the scratch site. One to 4 weeks after contamination, the following symptoms often appear: fever, cephalgia, asthenia, and local adenopathy. Lymph nodes may ooze pus. In some cases, the disease is severe and/or can last for weeks. Encephalitis is a possible complication.

Treatment

- Rifampicin is the antibiotic of choice.
- Dosing: 10–20 mg/kg, daily, po or IV (not to exceed 600 mg/day in children), for 10–14 days
- Tetanus immunization must be updated.

Preventive measures

- Stay away from cats, or handle them with great care.

Mycoses

Cats can cause tineas by direct contact (see "Head Ringworm," p. 54).

Rabies

Geographic distribution

Cats are carriers of rabies in parts of northern Europe, Southeast Asia, Africa, and South America.

Main symptoms

See "Rabies" in "Dogs" section, p. 261.

Treatment

See "Rabies" in "Dogs" section, p. 261.

Preventive measures

- Stay away from unknown cats.
- Immunization if risk is high (e.g., travelers who will spend >1 month in highly endemic countries and are likely to come in contact with rabid animals and immediate access to appropriate medical care is limited). See "Rabies" in "Dogs" section, page 261.
- Disinfect wounds adequately.

Scabies

Cats can cause scabies by direct contact (see p. 80).

Taeniasis

Cats can indirectly cause taeniasis (see p. 268).

Tetanus

Cats can cause tetanus (see p. 256) by biting or scratching.

Toxocariasis

Cat can indirectly cause toxocariasis (see p. 103).

Toxoplasmosis

Toxoplasma gondii

Geographic Distribution

In some tropical areas where cats are abundant and the warm and humid climate favors survival of *Toxoplasma gondii* oocysts, the seroprevalence toxoplasmosis is higher than in developed countries. For example, in Panama, it has been reported to be 13% by age 6 years and 90% by age 60 years. It was found to be 78% among pregnant women in Ibadan, Nigeria, and 83% percent in the population of the South Delta in the same country. In a city of south Ivory Coast it was >80%. In Indonesia, and Brazil it ranged from 20.9% to 68.4%. By comparison, in the United States, a National Health and Examination Survey found that from 1999 to 2000, *T. gondii* antibody prevalence was higher among non-Hispanic black persons than among non-Hispanic white persons (age-adjusted prevalence 19.2% vs. 12.1%), and increased with age.

Main Symptoms

Toxoplasmosis is transmitted by the ingestion of mature oocysts of *T. gondii* in water or food contaminated by infected cat feces or by eating live cysts contained in meat that has not been thoroughly cooked. Heart transplant and lab accident transmissions have been described. Diagnosis of toxoplasmosis is only by immunological reaction results from serum, amniotic fluid, or aqueous humor samples.

Various forms have been described:

In immunocompetent patients

Mild
Adenopathy (mostly in the neck), low grade fever, exanthem, myalgia, and asthenia can occur.

Disseminated
High fever lasting more than 10 days, pulmonary involvement with ARDS in 30% of cases, adenopathy, and weight loss >5% can occur.

In immunodeficient patients

Cerebral, with cephalgia, motor or sensitive deficit, fever (only in 50% of cases). Seizures are common.
Ocular. It is associated with the cerebral form in 40% of cases.
Other locations, include the lungs, with symptoms mimicking pneumocystosis. Disseminated forms have been described.

Congenital

It happens when the mother contracts the disease during pregnancy. It can result in miscarriage, or the baby can be born with T. gondii infection in multiple organs, hemorrage, icterus, hepatosplenomegaly, encephalopathy, and rapidly die. If he/she survives, major sequellae can be seen as hydrocephaly, neurological symptoms, intracranial calcifications, and unilateral or peripheral retinochoroiditis. Other sequelae include microphtalmia, strabism, hypotonia, transient somnolence, and icterus. Later, mental retardation, motor deficiencies, seizures and hydrocephaly can be the result of stenosis at the mesencephalic duct level.

Ocular

The retinochoroiditis evolves in an arophic and pigmentary manner. Posterior and pan-uveitis can occur.

Treatment

Immunocompetent patients

- Pyrimethamine (100mg loading dose, po, followed by 25–50 mg/day) plus sulfadiazine (2–4 g/day, divided 4 times daily), po, for 6 weeks, OR
- Pyrimethamine (100-mg loading dose, po, followed by 25–50 mg/day) plus clindamycin, 300 mg, po, qid, for 6 weeks
- Folinic acid, 10–25 mg/day, po, should be given to all patients to prevent hematologic toxicity of pyrimethamine, OR
- Trimethoprim (10 mg/kg/day) sulfamethoxazole (50 mg/kg/day), po, for 4 weeks

Pregnant women

- Spiramycin 1 g, po, q8 h (or 6 MU/day)
- If the amniotic fluid test result for *T gondii* is positive: 3 weeks of pyrimethamine (50 mg/day, po) and sulfadiazine (3 g/day, po, in 2–3 divided doses) alternating with a 3-week course of spiramycin 1 g 3 times daily for maternal treatment OR
- Pyrimethamine (25 mg/day, po) and sulfadiazine (4 g/day, po) divided 2 or 4 times daily until delivery (this agent may be associated with marrow suppression and pancytopenia) AND
- Leucovorin 10–25 mg/day, po, to prevent bone marrow suppression

Immunodeficient patients

- Pyrimethamine 200 mg, po, initially, followed by 50–75 mg/day, po, plus folinic acid 10 mg/day, po, plus sulfadiazine 4–8 g/day, po, for 6 weeks, followed by lifelong suppressive therapy or until immune reconstitution.
- Suppressive therapy for patients with AIDS (CD4 count < 100 cells/µL) is pyrimethamine, 50 mg/day, po, plus sulfadiazine 1–1.5 g/day, po, plus folinic acid 10 mg/day, po, for life or until immune reconstitution.
- Patients with AIDS and CNS toxoplasmosis, and midline shift or increased intracranial pressure may also benefit from steroid therapy.

Preventive Measures

- Cook meat well or freeze it at −18C (= −64.5F) for at least 3 days.
- Avoid contact with cats carrying *Toxoplasma gondii*.
- For immunodeficient patients: Chemoprophylaxis with trimethoprim 160 mg + sulfamethoxazole 800 mg, po, in adults.

Centipedes

Geographic Distribution
Centipedes are common in the intertropical zone.

Main Symptoms
Although their bites are usually harmless and only cause an itching and/or burning skin sensation, some species in the Philippines can be lethal.

Treatment
- Most bites can be treated at home.
- Advice to telecommunicate to the patient ASAP:
  - Wash the bite site with soap and water.
  - Apply a cold compress at 10-min intervals.
  - Monitor allergies; if needed, use antihistamines and corticosteroids.
- Dosing:
  * Prednisone, 20–80 mg, po, daily, for 2–5 days; children, 0.5–1 mg/kg, po, daily for 2–5 days
  * Brompheniramine, 4 mg, q4–6h, po, IM or IV or S/C, as many days as needed, or
  * Promethazine, 12.5–25 mg, po, IM or IV, as many days as needed
  * Contact emergency medical services if severe symptoms appear or pain persists for more than 12 h. Likewise, transfer to ICU, if necessary and feasible.

Dogs

Dog Bite
See "Cat Bite," p. 256.
Pasteurella multocida

- Dog bites become infected only 5% of the time.
- Consider rabies (see below).
- Stay away from stray dogs.

Larva Migrans (Cutaneous)
Dogs can indirectly cause cutaneous larva migrans (see p. 103).

Linguatulosis
Dogs can indirectly cause linguatulosis (see p. 100).

Mycoses
Dogs can cause tineas by direct contact (see "Head Ringworm," p. 54).

Rabies

Rhabdovirus

Geographic distribution

Rabies is a relatively ubiquitous disease, but it occurs more frequently in the intertropical zone because of the higher number of stray dogs and insufficient veterinary surveillance. Dogs are the main source of rabies in South America, Russia, Kazakhstan, Africa, and Southeast Asia.

Some areas are notably exempt of the disease, including Great Britain, Australia, New Zealand, Japan, Singapore, Hong Kong, Tasmania, New Caledonia, Brunei, Greece, Portugal, Sweden, Norway, Finland, Taiwan, Papua New Guinea, Vanuatu, Fiji, Cocos (Keeling) Islands, Norfolk Island, Cyprus, Crete, Hawaii, Malta, Mauritius, Sabah and Sarawak (Malaysia), Seychelles, American Samoa, British Virgin Islands, Christmas Island, Cook Island, French Polynesia, Kimbati, Nauru, Netherlands, West Indies, Niue, Solomon Islands, Tonga, Tuvalu, Wallis and Futuna, and Western Samoa. According to the WHO, rabies occurs in more than 150 countries and territories. More than 55,000 people die of rabies every year mostly in Asia and Africa.

40% of people who are bitten by suspect rabid animals are children under 15 years of age. Dogs are the source of the vast majority of human rabies deaths.

Main symptoms

From 20 to 60 days after being bitten by a rabid dog, the bite site can become itchy or trigger paresthesias. Sometimes, a personality change is the first symptom, followed by one of the two forms of the disease.

Spastic

First, the patient finds it difficult to breathe and experiences spasms immediately after seeing water or after hearing its sound. These spasms reveal an intense repulsion and cause agitation and tremors in the whole body. When rabies progresses, any slight change in surroundings, such as a waft of air, a light being turned on, or a smell, can set off a bout of delusions. Fever and dehydration follow, and death occurs within 3–5 days.

Paralytic

Symptoms begin with excruciating pain along the spine. An upward wave of paralysis follows, which affects the legs, sphincters, torso, arms, and face. If the bite occurs on an arm, it will be the first to become paralyzed. Death occurs within 4–12 days from respiratory failure.

Treatment

- Postexposure immunization (along with specific human immunoglobulins in some cases)
- Dosing
  * A person who is exposed and has never been vaccinated against rabies should get four doses of rabies vaccine: one dose right away and additional doses on the third, seventh, and fourteenth days. Rabies immune globulin should be given at the same time as the first dose.
  * A person who has been previously vaccinated should get two doses of rabies vaccine: one right away and another on the third day.
- Thorough cleaning and flushing of bite wounds with water and soap is necessary.

- No sutures must be made to close up the wound.
- Broad-spectrum antibiotics are needed for associated bacterial infections.
- Tetanus immunization must be updated.
- Hospitalization is indispensable.
- Treatment success rates vary according to the severity of symptoms and which body parts are involved.

Prevention measures
- Avoid stray dogs.
- Preexposure immunization, if the risk level requires it (e.g., travelers who will spend >1 month in highly endemic countries and are likely to come in contact with rabid animals and immediate access to appropriate medical care is limited). Please see below (from the CDC).

Rabies Preexposure Prophylaxis Guide

Risk Category	Nature of Risk	Typical Population	Preexposure Recommendations
Continuous	Virus present continuously, often in high concentrations. Specific exposures likely to go unrecognized. Bite, nonbite, or aerosol exposure.	Rabies research laboratory workers; rabies biologics production workers.	Primary course. Serologic testing every 6 months; booster vaccination if antibody titer is below acceptable level.
Frequent	Exposure usually episodic, with source recognized, but exposure also might be unrecognized. Bite, nonbite, or aerosol exposure.	Rabies diagnostic lab workers, spelunkers, veterinarians and staff, and animal-control and wildlife workers in rabies-enzootic areas. All persons who frequently handle bats.	Primary course. Serologic testing every 2 years; booster vaccination if antibody titer is below acceptable level.
Infrequent	Exposure nearly always episodic with source recognized. Bite or nonbite exposure.	Veterinarians and terrestrial animal-control workers in areas where rabies is uncommon to rare. Veterinary students. Travelers visiting areas where rabies is enzootic and immediate access to appropriate medical care including biologics is limited.	Primary course. No serologic testing or booster vaccination.
Rare (population at large)	Exposure always episodic with source recognized. Bite or nonbite exposure.	U.S. population at large, including persons in rabies-epizootic areas.	No vaccination necessary.

- Primary vaccination: Three 1.0-mL injections of HDCV or PCEC vaccine should be administered intramuscularly (deltoid area)—one injection per day on days 0, 7, and 21 or 28.

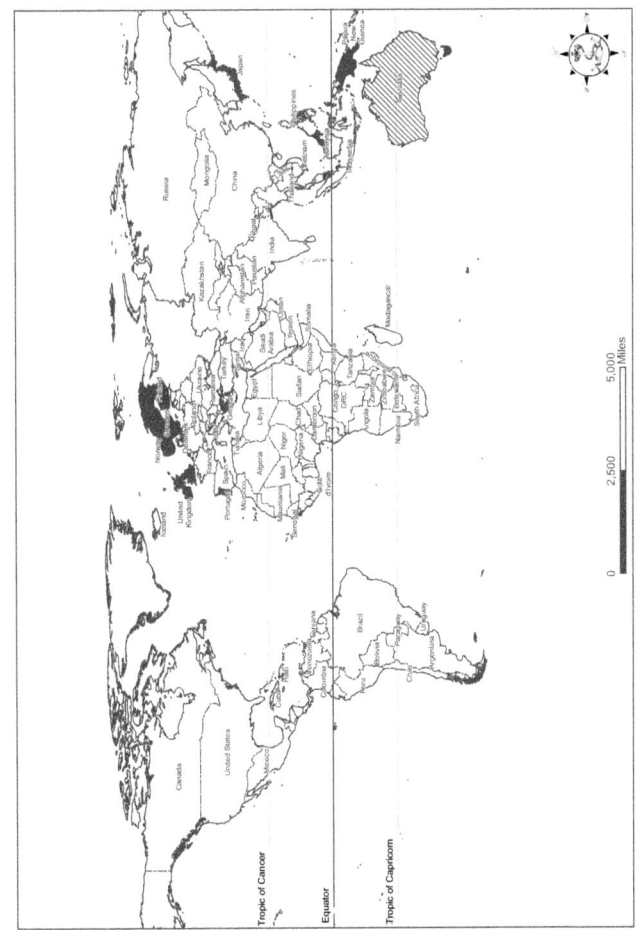

Geographic Distribution of Rabies

Scabies

Dogs can cause scabies by direct contact (see p. 80).

Tetanus (or Lockjaw)

Clostridium tetani

Geographic distribution

Tetanus is found throughout the world, although cases are more common in the intertropical zone, where many people have little or no vaccine coverage. There are also health risks of local practices such as severing the newborn's umbilical cord at birth with unsterilized instruments, women piercing ears for cosmetic purposes without properly disinfecting tools, or male or female circumcision. Tetanus post abortum and post partum when delivery occurs at home are also sources of tetanus infection. Moreover, most people in the intertropical zone are subject to socioeconomic conditions in their daily lives which expose them to tetanus. They often walk barefoot, come into contact with stray animals, use traditional medications (sometimes involving dirty needles and instruments), and may not clean their wounds properly. According to the WHO in 2011, there were 14,132 reported cases of tetanus worldwide.

Main symptoms

Occasionally, on the first days of the disease, tingling at the site of infection and stiffness of the nearby muscles may appear; but usually 5–15 days after contamination, the initial symptoms are stiffness of the jaw and neck with dysphagia and irritability. As tetanus progresses, reflexes are enhanced and the muscles of the face, abdomen, neck, and back start to spasm. The disease ends in death from asphyxiation caused by spasm of the respiratory muscles or cardiac failure.

Treatment

- ICU admission
- Benzodiazepines are the mainstay of symptomatic therapy. To prevent spasms that last longer than 5–10 sec and seizures, administer diazepam, IV, 10–40 mg, q1–8h. Vecuronium (by continuous infusion) and pancuronium (by intermittent injections) are adequate alternatives.
- Supportive therapy includes ventilatory support, and high-calorie nutritional intake.
- Magnesium sulfate at a loading dose of 40 mg/kg, followed by continuous IV infusion of 1.5 g/h if the patient weighs <45 kg or 2g/h if the patient weighs >45 kg, can be used to help control muscle spasms and tetanus-associated autonomic dysfunction.
- Metronidazole, 0.5 g, q6h, po, is used for secondary bacterial infections.
- Sedative hypnotics, narcotics, inhalational anesthetics, neuromuscular blocking agents, and centrally acting muscle relaxants (e.g., intrathecal baclofen) are used as needed.
- Tetanus immune globulin. However, the antitoxin can neutralize only toxin that has not yet bonded to nerve tissue.

Preventive measures

- Immunization by inactivated tetanus anatoxin. In the United States, 5 IM injections are given at 2, 4, 6 and between 15–18 months old with a booster between 4–6 years of age. Thereafter, the Tdap vaccine, which protects adolescents and adults against tetanus as well as pertussis and diphtheria is given only once from 11–64 years of age. In other countries the immunization schedule may differ.
- Disinfect wounds adequately.
- Wear proper shoes.
- Do not use nonsterile materials for traumatic procedures.
- Deliver babies in hospitals
- Stay away from stray animals
- Use disposable syringes

Toxocariasis

Dogs can indirectly cause toxocariasis (see p. 103).

Fish

Geographic Distribution

The intertropical zone.

Main Symptoms

Fish that can cause health problems include the following:

- Zebra fish: The venom in their spines induces pain upon contact.
- Scorpion fish: Their poisonous spines trigger pain upon contact.
- Stonefish (*Pterois voltans*, e.g.): They are difficult to distinguish from their environment because they mimic stones. They have 13 dorsal spines, which can induce excruciating pain upon contact and be lethal. Complications include phlegmon, septicemia, necrosis or gangrene, syncope, convulsions, bradycardia, arrhythmia, hypotension, acute pulmonary edema, and diaphragmatic paralysis.
- Stingrays: The venom in their tails can inflict very painful and serious wounds, occasionally lethal.

Treatment

- Symptomatic
- Specific to fish species. For example, a stonefish serum is available in Australia.
- Surgery is sometimes needed to clean necrotic tissue.

Preventive Measures

- Learn about harmful fish, know the areas where they live, and ask locals.
- Avoid contact with these fish.

Fleas

Fleas can cause the following diseases.

Murine Typhus

Rickettsia typhi

Geographic distribution

Murine typhus is endemic to Texas, Central America, the Mediterranean basin, northern Africa, Madagascar, and Southeast Asia.

Main symptoms

Seven to 14 days after being bitten by an infected flea, high fever may be experienced with cephalgia, intense fatigue, and myalgia. In 6–18 days a whole-body skin eruption appears in 50–79% of cases. GI, respiratory, and neurological involvement may occur. The disease is usually mild and heals spontaneously within a few days. Cerebral and cardiac complications occur in elderly, debilitated patients and Africans (savanna typhus). Without treatment, the mortality rate is 2–3%.

Treatment

- Very high success rates are the norm.
- Cyclines are the drugs of choice.
- Spiramycin is an alternative for young children and pregnant women.
- Dosing:
  * Doxycycline, 200 mg, po, once; in severe cases 200 mg/day, po, children, 2 mg/kg/day (max 100 mg/day) both for up to 7 days or
  * Spiramycin, 2–3 g daily, po, for adults, or 50 mg/kg/day, for children, for 1–7 days

Preventive measures

- Reduce exposure to fleas, mainly through personal hygiene, adequate housing, and by treating pets.
- Use insecticides to kill vectors.
- Use repellent containing DEET (15–30%). Be aware that they can only provide transitory protection.
- Treat clothes with insecticides containing permethrin

Geographic Distribution of Murine Typhus

Endemic Areas

Plague

Fleas can also cause plague (see p. 174).

Taeniasis

Dipylidium caninum

Geographic distribution

This form of taeniasis is found more frequently in the intertropical zone because of insufficient veterinary care of dogs and cats.

Main symptoms

The disease is contracted by unknowingly swallowing an infected flea from a dog or cat. Symptoms are rare and include abdominal pain and BM disturbances.

Treatment

- Unknown

Preventive measures

- Avoid contact with unknown cats and dogs.

Tungiasis

Fleas can also cause tungiasis (see p. 82).

Jellyfish, Sea Anemones, and Physaliae

Geographic Distribution

Jellyfish and sea anemones are abundant in tropical oceans. Men-of-war (physaliae) are very common in Africa and in the West Indies. Some species are very dangerous, especially on the shores of Australia.

Main Symptoms

Coming into contact with jellyfish and sea anemones causes a local allergic reaction with irritation, burning, and/or an itching sensation. Touching a filament of a physalia triggers a whiplash feeling and redness appears where contact was made. Subsequently, in severe cases, fever, asthenia, dyspnea, respiratory arrest, and cardiovascular shock occur. The second contact with a man-of-war always results in worse and more intense symptoms.

Treatment

- Jellyfish and sea anemone lesions can be treated with corticosteroid cream.
- Jellyfish stings can be soothed by any meat tenderizer containing papain.
- Physalia-induced symptoms require calcium gluconate, antihistamines, and corticosteroids (IM or IV).
- Dosing:
  * Prednisone, 20–80 mg, po, daily, for 2–5 days; children, 0.5–1 mg/kg, po, daily for 2–5 days
  * Brompheniramine, 4 mg, q4–6h, po, IM or IV or S/C, as many days as needed, or
  * Promethazine, 12.5–25 mg, po, IM or IV, as many days as needed
- Resuscitation may be necessary in the most severe cases.

Preventive Measures

- Avoid swimming in infested areas.

Leeches

Geographic Distribution

Leeches attach themselves to a person's skin, nose, and/or mouth. They are abundant in aquatic environments of the intertropical zone, particularly in the Mediterranean basin, Asia, South America, and Madagascar. In the Mediterranean basin, certain species like *Limnatis nilotica* fix themselves on URT mucosae.

Main Symptoms

Leeches can cause tetanus (see pp. 264 & 265), skin infection, and anemia when large numbers attach themselves to someone for a long period of time. The main symptoms of anemia include asthenia, dyspnea, tachycardia on exertion, and sometimes a heart murmur. Whitish nails and pale skin are also part of this condition.

Treatment

- Local procaine or lidocaine is used to kill and extract the parasites.
- In case of severe anemia, a blood transfusion is necessary.
- Tetanus immunization must be updated.

Preventive Measures

- Wear boots, long sleeves, and long pants in infested areas.
- Repellants can provide temporary protection (e.g. containing 20% DEET).

Lice

Lice can cause the following diseases.

Epidemic Louse-Borne Typhus

Rickettsia prowazeki

Geographic distribution

Epidemic louse-borne typhus is endemic to the intertropical zone, particularly to Africa (Burundi, Ethiopia, Gambia, Kenya, Mozambique, Nigeria, Rwanda, and Uganda), South America (Bolivia, Columbia, Ecuador, and Peru), and Central America (Costa Rica, Trinidad and Tobago). From 1993 to 2005, the disease killed more than 100,000 people during the civil war in Burundi.

Main symptoms

Ten to 14 days after being bitten by an infected body louse, the following symptoms appear: malaise, sudden fever, chills, myalgia (in 70–100% of cases), arthralgia, spinal pain, cephalgia, congested eyes and face, dehydration, dizziness (from hypotension), dry tongue, nausea, emesis, abdominal pain, mental confusion, stupor, and coma.

Five days after the fever onset, a skin eruption (macular, maculopapular, or petechial exanthem) appears on the trunk and spreads to the limbs but spares the neck, face, palm of the hands, and soles of the feet. Complications include bronchitis, bronchiolitis, interstitial pneumopathy, myocarditis, arteritis, hemiplegia, monoplegia, myelitis, neuritis, encephalitis, hemorrhage, and gangrene of the extremities. Without treatment the mortality rate is 60%. Brill disease is the resurgence of an old typhus infection. It is milder than the initial episode and can occur many years later.

Treatment

- Cyclines are the drugs of choice.
- Spiramycin is an alternative for young children and pregnant women.
- Dosing:
    * Doxycycline, 200 mg, po, once; in severe cases 200 mg, po, children, 2 mg/kg/day (max 100 mg/day) both for up to 7 days or
    * Spiramycin, 2–3 g daily, po, for adults, or 50 mg/kg/day, for children, for 1–7 days

Preventive measures

- Proper personal hygiene
- Use insecticides to kill vectors.
- Use repellents containing DEET (15–30%). Be aware that they can only provide transitory protection.
- Treat clothes with insecticides containing permethrin
- Immunization is no longer used because antibiotics are so efficient

Geographic Distribution of
Epidemic Louse-borne Typhus

Endemic Areas

Pediculosis Capitis, Pediculosis Corporis, Pthiriasis

Lice can also cause pediculosis capitis (see p. 53), pediculosis corporis (see p. 80), and pthiriasis (see p. 54).

Trench Fever (or His-Werner Disease)

Bartonella quintana

Geographic distribution

Trench fever used to be endemic to Europe and Mexico. Fortunately, the disease is slowly disappearing. Other names for trench fever include "5-day fever," "shinbone fever," "Wolhynia fever," and "Quintana fever."

Main symptoms

The disease is transmitted when *Bartonella quintana* found in infected lice feces penetrates the skin, usually through a wound or scratch lesions. Sudden fever appears accompanied with diffuse pain and a morbilliform skin eruption. Fever bouts come back 10–15 times and last 2–3 days, recurring approximately every 5 days. Generally, the disease resolves spontaneously.

Treatment

- Cyclines are the drugs of choice.
- Spiramycin is an alternative for young children and pregnant women.
- Dosing:
  * Doxycycline, 200 mg, po, once; in severe cases 200 mg, po, children 2 mg/kg/day (max 100 mg/day), both for up to 7 days or
  * Spiramycin, 2–3 g daily, po, for adults, or 50 mg/kg/day, for children, for 1–7 days

Preventive measures

- Practice strict personal hygiene.
- Use insecticides to kill vectors.
- Use repellents containing DEET (15–30%). Be aware that they can only provide transitory protection.
- Treat clothes with insecticides containing permethrin.

Ubiquitous Relapsing Fever

Borrelia recurrentis

Geographic distribution

Ubiquitous relapsing fever has been disappearing slowly but can still be found in Ethiopia and Sudan.

Main symptoms

Borrelia recurrentis is found in infected body lice feces. The incubation period ranges 2–14 days after they penetrate through the skin. The disease is divided in 5 phases.

Onset

Symptoms appear very abruptly with chills, constantly high fever, diffuse pain, cephalgia, extreme weakness, and congested eyes and face.

First febrile phase

It lasts 5–7 days, and additional symptoms include anorexia, constipation, abdominal pain, emesis, arthralgia, myalgia, thoracic pain, and splenomegaly. Respiratory symptoms are also often present. Six days after fever onset, body temperature suddenly returns to normal with profuse sweating, urination, and occasionally shock.

Apyretic phase

The patient remains afebrile for the next few days but is very asthenic and sometimes icteric. The spleen size returns to normal ("accordion" spleen).

Second febrile phase

It occurs in 66% of patients, 3–27 days after the apyretic phase. Symptoms are similar but slightly milder than in the first one. They last 3–5 days.

Convalescence

It is usually short.

Benign forms are frequently seen in children. Rare complications include meningitis, hepatitis, nephritis, iritis, optic neuritis, and myocarditis.

Treatment

- Cyclines offer very high success rates and good tolerance. Penicillin is a safe alternative for pregnant women and young children with cerebral symptoms.
- Dosing:
  * Tetracyclines, 2 g, daily, po, in two divided doses, for 5–10 days, or
  * Doxycycline, 200 mg/day, po, for adults, for 5–10 days; for children, 2 mg/kg/day (max 100 mg/day), po, for 5–10 days
  * Penicillin, 1 M IU, daily, IM, for adults, for 8–10 days
  * To avoid serious side effects (Jarisch-Herxheimer reaction), treatment should be started at a low dose to be increased progressively over 3–4 days, until the recommended posology is reached. For children and infants (sodium salt is preferred in children) 100,000–250,000 U/kg/day in divided doses, q4h. Severe infections: up to 400,000 U/kg/day in divided doses, q4h; maximum dose 24 M U/day.

Preventive measures

- Isolation of patients.
- Patients must change clothes.
- Burn or spray patients' old clothes with permethrin powder 1% (spraying to be repeated every 6 weeks).
- Practice strict personal hygiene.
- Use insecticides to kill vectors.
- Use repellents containing DEET (15–30%). Be aware that they can only provide transitory protection.
- Treat clothes with insecticides containing permethrin.
- Doxycycline, 200 mg/day, po, for 4 days, pre-exposure, is efficient.

Mollusks

Geographic Distribution

Gonyaulax-infested mollusks are common on the American Pacific coast. Cones (*Conus textilis*, *Conus aulicus*, and *Conus geographus*) lie on coral reefs or are buried in the sand, mainly in the Indian and Pacific oceans.

Main Symptoms

- After swallowing a mollusk contaminated with *Gonyaulax*, muscle contractions and palsy appear and progress upward. In more severe cases, respiratory arrest and shock may occur.
- After contact with a cone, local or systemic allergic reactions appear. Complications occur in a few hours with muscle paralysis, paresthesia, blurred vision, diplopia, nausea, emesis, diffuse pruritus, respiratory or cardiac arrest, Quincke edema, and asphyxia leading to death.

Treatment

- Symptoms caused by *Gonyaulax* are treated symptomatically and supportively.
- For reactions to cones, corticosteroids and antihistamines can be used.
- Dosing
  * Prednisone, 20–80 mg, po, daily, for 2–5 days; children, 0.5–1 mg/kg, po, daily for 2–5 days
  * Brompheniramine, 4 mg, q4–6h, po, IM or IV or S/C, as many days as needed, or
- Promethazine, 12.5–25 mg, po, IM or IV, as many days as needed
- Advice to telecommunicate to the patient ASAP includes:
  - Immerse the affected area in very hot water.
  - Use the pressure-immobilization technique.
  - Bandage the extremity (sprained ankle type).
  - Bind the limb without blocking the circulation.
  - Avoid movement.
  - CPR by bystander, if necessary.

Preventive Measures

- Avoid eating mollusks.
- Avoid walking and swimming in infested areas.

Muraenae (or Moray Eels)

Geographic Distribution

Moray eels live in the sand and are common in tropical seas and oceans.

Main Symptoms

After a bite on the foot or hand, intense pain spreads throughout the limb. It is so severe that it can cause emesis, tachycardia, sometimes convulsions, and syncope. Toxins exist in the saliva of moray eels, as shown by the persistence of pain after the bite. Secondary bacterial infections are common. Death is extremely rare.

Treatment

- Local wound care (in particular, control hemorrhage and repair tissue, tendon, and nerve damage)
- Symptomatic
- Broad-spectrum antibiotics (ciprofloxacin, cefuroxime, tetracycline, or trimethoprim-sulfamethoxazole) at their usual dosages.
- Update tetanus immunization.
- Monitor lesions until complete healing.

Preventive Measures

- Inquire if moray eels live in the areas where you intend to fish, swim, snorkel, or dive.

Rats

Sodoku (or Rat Bite Fever)

Spirillum minor

Geographic distribution

Rat bite fever is more commonly found in the intertropical zone because of poor housing conditions, particularly in city slums.

Main symptoms

Several weeks after being bitten by a disease-carrying rat, the bite site becomes swollen, hard, painful, and cyanotic; with local adenopathy, fever, chills, emesis, pharyngitis (Haverhill fever), myalgia, arthralgia, asthenia, cephalgia, and a skin eruption consisting of dark red maculae on the torso and limbs. The symptoms subside after a few days but usually return later e.g., normal temperature alternates with fever every 24–48 h, recurring after 4–8 weeks. Without treatment, this cycle may continue for months or years. Other symptoms include regional lymphadenitis and splenomegaly. Complications include myocarditis, endocarditis, hepatitis, and meningitis.

Treatment

- Penicillin is the drug of choice and has very high success rates. In allergic patients, cyclines are a good alternative. Erythromycin can be used in young children.
- Dosing:
  * Mild infection: penicillin V potassium, 500 mg, po, q6h, for 7–10 days
  * Moderate to severe infection: aqueous penicillin G, 3–5 M U, IV, q6h (12–20 M U/day), for 7–10 days
  * Doxycycline, 100 mg, po, bid, q12h, for 7–10 days; children, 2 mg/kg/day (max 100 mg/day)

* Erythromycin, for mild/moderate infections, po, in divided doses, q6h:
  * <10 lb (4.5 kg): 30–50 mg/kg/day
  * 10–15 lb (4.5–6.8 kg): 200 mg/day
  * 16–25 lb (7.3–11.3 kg): 400 mg/day
  * 26–50 lb (11.8–22.7 kg): 800 mg/day
* For more severe infections, the dosage may be doubled.
* All for 7–10 days.
- Cyclines are contraindicated in children < 8 year old.
- Tetanus immunization must be updated.

Preventive measures

- Avoid sleeping in unsanitary environments/conditions.

Tetanus

Rats can cause tetanus (see pp. 264 & 265).

Scorpions

Geographic Distribution

Scorpions are found mainly in hot climates, such as the Mediterranean basin, Africa, Mexico, and in the United States.

Main Symptoms

Most scorpion stings are very painful; however, the symptoms they induce are usually benign. Their severity varies according to the following factors: (1) time of year (worse in the dry season), (2), age of patient (worse in children and elderly people), and (3) species (*Prionurus* in northern Africa and *Centruroides* in the United States and Mexico can both be lethal).

Symptoms include the following:

In children

Pain, hypoesthesia, and paresthesia around the sting site; muscle spasm; abnormal head, neck, and eye motions; diaphoresis; ptyalism; and restlessness.

In adults

Tachypnea, hypertension, tachycardia, fasciculation, and weakness

Treatment

- In mild cases, the patient is comforted. Local anesthetic injections around the sting site may be required.
- In more severe cases, serum (as specific as possible) and corticosteroids (IV) are necessary.
- Dosing:
  * Prednisone, Given as sodium phosphate ester: 5–60 mg prednisolone base, daily, IV infusion. Dose to be individualised based on the severity of the condition and patient's response; for 2–5 days; children. 1–10 yr: 1–2 mg/kg, daily, parenteral for 2–5 days
- Tetanus immunization must be updated.

- Advice to telecommunicate to the patient ASAP includes the following:
  - Wash the sting site with soap and water after cleaning all the skin surface.
  - Apply cool compresses, usually every 10 min alternately.
  - Acetaminophen to relieve pain.
  - Do not cut into the wound or apply suction.

Preventive Measures

- Wear appropriate footwear.
- Become familiar with the scorpion species living in the area where you are traveling or residing.

Snakes

Geographic Distribution

Although snakes live in most areas of the world, the most dangerous species are in the intertropical zone and can be divided into four groups: aglyphous, opisthoglyphous, proteroglyphous, and solenoglyphous. The most notorious venomous snakes are found in the proteroglyphous group and in the Elapidae family:

On land

- United States: mamba, cobra, and coral snakes
- Africa: green mamba and cobra. In the latter, the most famous are *Naja haje* (snake of the pharaohs) and *Naja nigricollis* (spitting snake or ringhal).
- Asia: *Bungarus* sp. and cobras (*Ophiophagus hannah*, *Naja sputatrix*, *Naja kaouthia*)
- Far East: *Naja tripudians*
- Australia: *Pseudonaja* sp., *Notechis* sp., *Acanthophis* sp., *Oxyuranus scutellatus*, and death adders

In the water

- In the Indian and Pacific Oceans: *Enhydrina schitosa*, *Laticauda*, *Maticora*, and *Calliophis*

In the solenoglyphous group, there are two families: vipers and crotalids.

Vipers

- United States: pit viper
- Africa: *Vipera lebetina* (east viper), *Vipera echis carinatus* (viper with scales like a saw), *Bitis gabonica* (Gabon viper), *B. arietans*, and *B. nasicornis*
- Asia: *Daboia russellii* (Russel viper)

Crotalids

- United States: *Crotalus basilicus* (rattlesnake), *Bothrops* (it is also present in the the West Indies where it is known as "Fer de Lance")

Main Symptoms

After a snakebite, the severity of symptoms depends on the following factors: (1) location (the vast majority occur on the arms or legs), (2) quantity of venom injected, and (3) snake species.

Naja

Their venom has toxic effects on the nervous system and possesses curare-like characteristics. Pain at the bite site is minimal, and a feeling of numbness is common in severe cases. Paralysis spreads to the whole body, accompanied with nausea and emesis. In extremely severe cases, death occurs by respiratory arrest.

Crotalids

Their venom causes hemorrhage. There is intense pain at the bite site, with black, hard edema spreading to the entire limb. Surrounding tissues necrotize, while bleeding occurs in various areas including the skin, gums, nose, lungs, and GI tract. Prognosis is reserved and varies on a case-by-case basis.

Vipers

Their venom affects the nervous system and causes profuse bleeding. Pain at the bite site is mild to moderate with purplish edema. General symptoms include dizziness (from hypotension), arrhythmias, nausea, emesis, diarrhea, abdominal pain, anxiety, agitation, and moderate fever. Progression to coma can occur.

Treatment

- Antivenom serum must be given, as specific to the species as possible.
- Tetanus immunization must be updated.
- Advice to telecommunicate to the patient ASAP includes the following:
  - Notice the snake's appearance.
  - Kill the snake or move the person beyond striking distance.
  - Place the wound below heart level.
  - Stay calm.
  - Cover the wound with a loose, sterile bandage.
  - Do not cut the bite wound; attempt to suck out venom; apply tourniquet, ice, or water; or drink alcohol or caffeinated beverages.

Preventive Measures

- Wear adequately protective shoes and hat in endemic areas.

Spiders

Geographic Distribution

Although spiders exist almost everywhere in the world, they are more common and more dangerous in the intertropical zone.

Main Symptoms

The severity of symptoms from a spider bite varies according to the species.

Lactrodectes

They are small (about 2 cm = <1 in) but very venomous, and their bites can cause pain, muscle spasms, profuse sweating, asthma-like symptoms, and extreme fatigue. In this group, the black widow of Amazonia (*Lactrodectus mactans*) can be lethal.

Mygales
Trap door spiders are common in Africa and South America. They are hairy, large (9 cm (= 3 in)), and very aggressive. Their bite can cause a state of excitement, followed by stupor with diaphoresis and overlacrimation. In Australia, *Atrax* and *Hadronyche* are dangerous for humans. The former causes rapidly an erythematous skin reaction, profuse sweating, hypersalivation, colics, nausea, emesis, fasciculation, dyspnea, and occasionally cardiovascular shock leading to death.

Ctenes
These tiny South American spiders live on banana trees and can kill a person in just a few hours.

Lycoses
They have a very deadly bite that causes rapidly progressing gangrene. The brown recluse spider (*Loxosceles reclusa*) belongs to this species.

Treatment

- According to the species:
  - Black widow: muscle relaxants, IV, vasodilators
  - Brown recluse: ICU, if hemolysis or gangrene appears
  - Tarantula: antihistamines and/or glucocorticoids
- In severe cases, hospitalization
- Serum (as specific to the species as possible)
- Broad-spectrum antibiotics
- Antihistamines, corticosteroids, calcium
- Dosing:
  * Prednisone, 20–80 mg, po, daily, for 2–5 days; children, 0.5–1 mg/kg, po, daily for 2–5 days
  * Brompheniramine, 4 mg q4–6h, po or IM or IV or S/C, as many days as needed, or
  * Promethazine, 12.5–25 mg, po or IM or IV, as many days as needed
- Tetanus immunization must be updated.
- Advice to telecommunicate to the patient ASAP includes the following:
  - Clean the bite site with water and soap.
  - Apply ice.
  - Elevate the limb of the bite.

Preventive Measures

- Cover the body and wear appropriate shoes and hat in endemic areas.
- Good housing conditions.

Ticks

Arboviroses
Ticks can cause arboviroses (see p. 235).

Regional Relapsing Fever
Borrelia hispanica, Borrelia persica, Borrelia duttoni, Borrelia venezuelensis

Geographic distribution

Regional relapsing fever occurs sporadically in Spain, Greece, Africa, Iran, Iraq, the Palestinian Territory, Madagascar, the West Indies, the United States, and Central and South America.

Main symptoms

Regional relapsing fever is transmitted by an infected tick bite. The natural reservoirs of the bacteria are wild rodents, pigs, cats, and dogs. The disease has various forms.

Spanish and Moroccan forms

Four to five bouts of an irregular fever generally occur. The meninges are often affected. Complications include hepatitis and nephritis, but the outcome is usually favorable.

Middle Eastern form

The tick bite is always painful, and fever is intermittent rather than relapsing. Convulsions and delirium occur frequently. This form can be fatal despite antibiotic treatment.

Sub-Saharan African form

A local inflammatory reaction at the bite site occurs frequently. Fever onset is gradual with relapsing bouts lasting 3–4 days and recurring up to 10 times. Common complications include hepatitis, nephritis, and eye lesions.

South American form

Almost identical to the sub-Sahara African form, but it has a better prognosis.

North American form

It is always benign.

Treatment

- Cyclines are the drugs of choice.
- For pregnant women and children, penicillin is a safe and effective alternative.
- Dosing:
  * Tetracyclines, 2 g, daily, po, in two divided doses, for 5–10 days or
  * Doxycycline, 200 mg/day, po, for adults, for 5–10 days; for children, 2 mg/kg/day (max 100 mg/day), po, for 5–10 days, or
  * Penicillin, 1 M IU, daily, IM, for adults, for 8–10 days; for children and infants (sodium salt is preferred in children), 100,000–250,000 U/kg/day in divided doses, q4h. Severe infections: up to 400,000 U/kg/day in divided doses, q4h; maximum dose 24 M U/day, for 8–10 days
  * Cyclines are contraindicated in children < 8 year old.

Preventive measures

- Avoid contacts with pigs, rodents and unknown cats and dogs.
- Use insecticides to kill vectors.
- Use repellents containing DEET (15–30%). Be aware that they can only provide transitory protection.
- Treat clothes with insecticides containing permethrin.

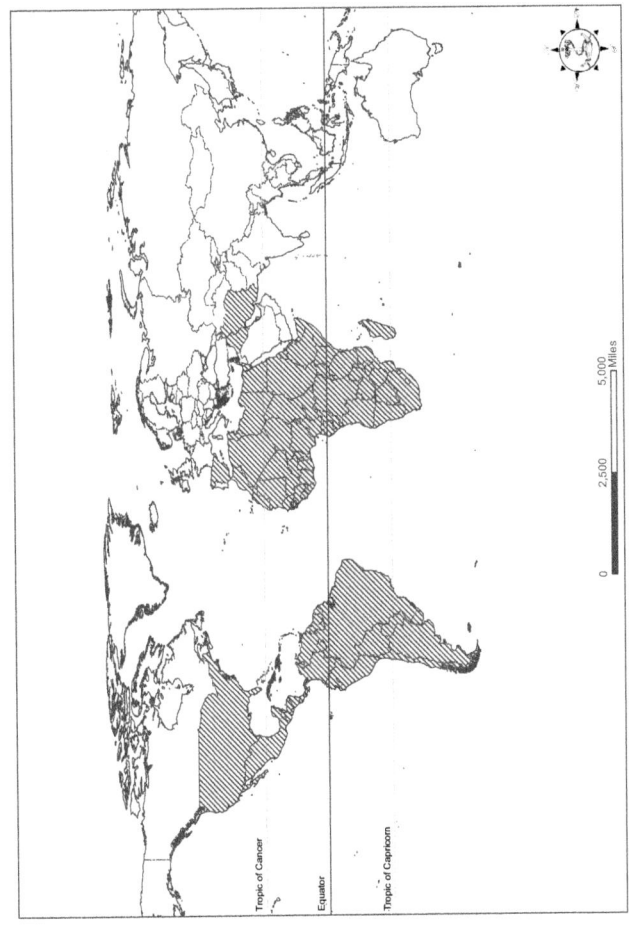

Trombiculidae

Scrub Typhus

Orientia tsutsugamushi

Geographic distribution

Scrub typhus is endemic to the Far East, from India to South Australia. It is transmitted by chiggers (genus *Leptotrombidium*).

Main symptoms

The bacteria causing scrub typhus can be found in wild rodents, rabbits, and dogs. Five to 20 days after contamination by an infected mite bite that leaves an eschar on the skin (in 50% of cases) with local adenopathy, sudden high fever (which will remain in plateau and last for about 10 days), cephalgia, myalgia, polyadenopathy (in 85% of cases), and congested eyes occur. A skin eruption, consisting of macular or maculopapular lesions, slowly appears (in 34% of cases) on various parts of the body but remarkably not on the face, palms of the hands, and soles of the feet. It disappears on the seventh day. Hepatosplenomegaly is found in 30% of cases. Complications include pneumonia, myocarditis, cardiac failure, and rarely encephalitis or DIC. The kidneys and meninges can be involved as well. In mild cases, convalescence takes 2–3 weeks. Without treatment the mortality rates ranges 0–30%.

Treatment

- Cyclines produce high success rates. Chloramphenicol and azithromycin are the recommended drugs for pregnant women and children.
- Dosing:
  * Tetracyclines, 2 g daily, po, in two divided doses, for adults, for 7 days
  * Doxycycline, 100 mg, po, bid, for adults, for 7 days; children 2 mg/kg/day (max 100 mg/day), for 7 days
  * Chloramphenicol, 500 mg, po, qid, for adults, for 7–14 days; for children, 50–100 mg/kg, daily, po, in four divided doses, for 7–14 days. It should not be administered to pregnant women in the last week before parturition.
  * Azythromycin, a single 500-mg dose, po, for pregnant women
- Cyclines are contraindicated in children < 8 year old.
- With chloramphenicol CBC must be monitored.

Preventive Measures

- Avoid contact with wild rodents, rabbits, and dogs.
- Use insecticides to kill vectors.
- Use repellents containing DEET (15–30%). Be aware that they can only provide transitory protection.
- Treat clothes with insecticides containing permethrin.
- Doxycycline, 200 mg, po, once

Geographic Distribution of Scrub Typhus

 Endemic Areas

Exotic Food Poisoning

Ciguatera

Geographic Distribution

Ciguatera is endemic to the West Indies, Polynesia, New Caledonia, and the Indian Ocean region. Many fish can harbor the ciguatera toxin, including barracuda, grouper, loach, parrotfish, and surgeonfish.

Main Symptoms

Minutes to hours after ingesting a contaminated fish, paresthesia in the face, feet, and hands; nausea; cold sweats; and asthenia often appear. One to 2 hours later a skin sensation of burning or electric shock, pain triggered by cold, mydriasis, and hypotonia of the lower limbs occur. Emesis, diarrhea, abdominal cramps, bradycardia, arrhythmias, dizziness (from hypotension), arthralgia, myalgia, cephalgia, asthenia, and chills may also be experienced. On the second day, an itchy skin eruption often appears. All symptoms disappear within days or weeks but sensitivity to cold with burning or electric sensation may continue for months.

Treatment

- Gastric lavage is not recommended.
- Antiemetics to control nausea and vomiting.
- Antihistamines to relieve pruritus.
- Atropine for bradyarrhythmias.
- Dosing:
  * 2–3 mg, IV or S/C or IM, to be repeated no less often than every 20–30 min until signs of poisoning are sufficiently lessened or signs of atropine overdose occur
- In case of hypotension, replace intravascular volume.

Preventive Measures

- Ask about the safety of fish to locals, and if in doubt, do not eat them.
- Cooking does not destroy the ciguatera toxin.

Louis was a 30-year-old French civil servant. He was the only dentist on the island of Lifou, New Caledonia. His passion was snorkeling, diving, and fishing. He came for consultation complaining of "gastrointestinal disturbances." The story of the disease revealed that he had gone fishing in the morning and had eaten the parrotfish he had killed. He was treated symptomatically and successfully. However, the same day he experienced an electric-like discharge in his hand when grabbing an ice cube. A similar sensation appeared on various parts of his body when he took a shower that evening. He was advised to avoid skin contact with cold substances. This nuisance faded slowly, and he recovered completely over several weeks.

DID YOU KNOW THAT:

- Ciguatera prevalence can reach 10% around some tropical islands.
- The toxin probably comes from blue algae, which are ingested by fish.
- It is much more frequent in areas where underwater works have been done (airport, harbor, or pier construction).
- Locals usually give a piece of the fish they caught to cats or ants to eat, and these will show benign, abnormal, and characteristic behavior after a few minutes if the fish is contaminated by the ciguatera toxin.
- The neurological symptoms can last for weeks and be incapacitating.

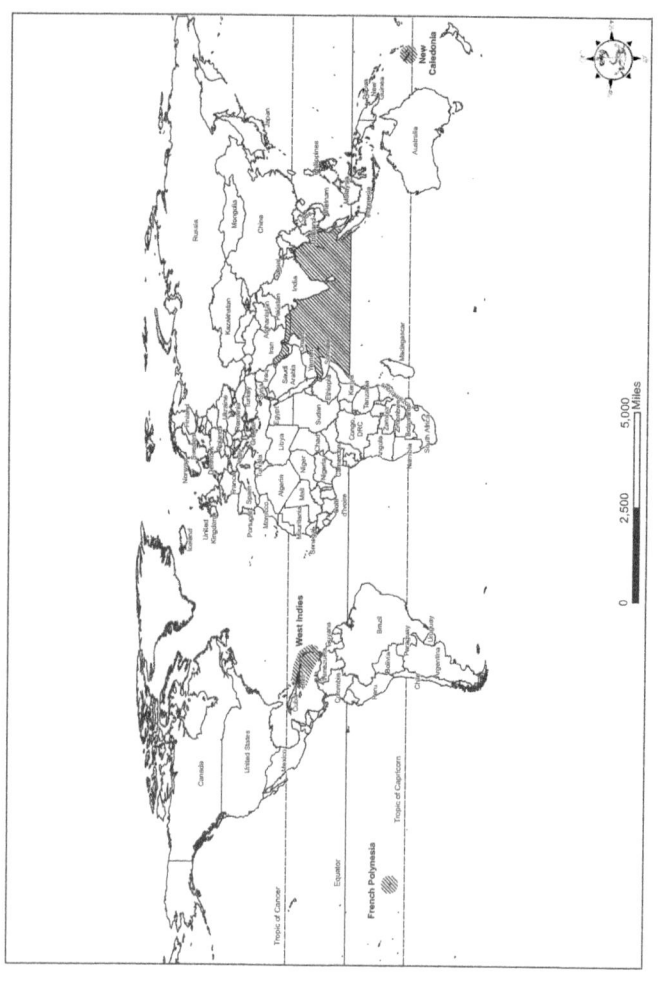

Geographic Distribution of Ciguatera

Ichthyosarcotoxisms (Other)

Geographic Distribution and Symptoms

Ichthyosarcotoxism can be divided into three main categories, according to the toxin location.

Hematotoxism

The blood of eels, conger eels, moray eels, and torpedo fish sometimes contains a toxin that can be lethal to humans.

Ototoxism

The gonads, eggs, and milt (fish sperm) of sturgeon, salmon, pike, carp, and tench sometimes contain a toxin that can cause GI and psychological disturbances.

Sarcotoxism

The skin, flesh, and viscera of some fish can contain a toxin.

Treatment

- Symptomatic and supportive

Preventive Measures

- Avoid eating contaminated fish (ask locals about the risk).

Fish Poisoning

Geographic Distribution

At least 500 species of fish found in tropical oceans and seas can cause food poisoning.

Main Symptoms

- Moonfish can cause paralysis with severe cardiovascular and respiratory disorders, which are often fatal.
- Sharks can induce stomach and bowel disturbances, paresthesia in the hands and feet, and an itchy skin eruption.
- Anchovies, sardines, and herrings can result in acute gastroenteritis, sensory or motor disorders, and sometimes icterus.
- Tuna or mackerel can produce edema of the face, dizziness (from hypotension), and occasionally edema of the larynx.
- Fugu (also know as globefish, blowfish, balloonfish, toadfish, toado, swellfish, botete, fahaka, puffer fish, or tinga) contains a toxin (tetrodotoxin), which can trigger flaccid paralysis, with acute respiratory distress and cardiovascular collapse. Death can occur in a few hours.
- In shellfish, the poisonous ingredients are toxins made by algae-like organisms called *dinoflagellates*. There are different types of shellfish poisoning. The best known are paralytic shellfish poisoning, neurotoxic shellfish poisoning, and amnestic shellfish poisoning. For paralytic shellfish poisoning, about 30 min after eating contaminated seafood, dysesthesia or paresthesia can appear in the mouth. They may spread to the arms and legs. Vertigo, cephalgia, and in some cases temporary paralysis of the arms and legs may be experienced

as well as nausea, emesis, and diarrhea. With neurotoxic shellfish poisoning, symptoms are very similar to those of ciguatera. Amnestic shellfish poisoning begins with nausea, vomiting, and diarrhea, which are followed by short-term memory loss, as well as other, less frequent neurologic symptoms.
- Tuna, mackerel, mahi mahi, and albacore can induce scombroid poisoning. Symptoms include dyspnea (in severe cases), skin erythema, flushing, urticaria, pruritus, nausea, and emesis.

Treatment
- Symptomatic
- Atropine, cholinesterase activators, and high doses of vitamin B_6 are often used.
- For mackerel or tuna ichthyosarcotoxism, antihistamines are useful.
- Dosing:
    * Brompheniramine, 4 mg, q4–6h, po or IM or IV or S/C, as many days as needed, or
    * Promethazine, 12.5–25 mg, po or IM or IV, as many days as needed
- ICU for fugu intoxication
- For scombroid poisoning:
    - Antihistamine, such as diphenhydramine
    - IV fluids (to replace losses from vomiting and diarrhea)
    - Antiemetic
    - Intubation (in rare cases)
- For shellfish poisoning:
    - Antiemetic
    - IV fluids (to replace losses from vomiting and diarrhea)
    - ICU transfer, if paralysis occurs

Mushroom Poisoning

Geographic Distribution
The distribution of poisonous mushrooms in the intertropical zone is patchy. *Amanita*, *Entoloma*, and *Lepiota* have been identified in Africa, Madagascar, Asia, and Central and South America.

Main Symptoms
Symptoms vary according to (1) the quantity ingested and (2) the species.

Amatoxin type: Cyclopetides
Amanita phalloides, *Amanita verna*, *Amanita virosa*, and *Galerina* sp.
After a latent period of 8–12 h, severe abdominal cramps, emesis, diarrhea, hematemesis, hematochezia, renal failure, liver failure (including fulminant hepatitis), and coma may occur.

Gyromitrin type
Gyromitra and *Helvella* sp.
After a latent period of a few hours, vomiting, diarrhea, liver failure (including fulminant hepatitis), convulsions, and coma may occur. Methemoglobinemia and hemolysis are also possible complications.

Muscarinic type
Inocybe and *Clitocybe* sp.
Shortly after eating these mushrooms, emesis, diarrhea, bradycardia, hypotension, diaphoresis, myosis, lacrimation, dyspnea, and, rarely, arrhythmias may occur.

Anticholinergic type
Amanita muscaria and *Amanita pantherina*
One to 2 h after eating these mushrooms, excitement, delirium, mydriasis, flushing, and tremors may occur.

GI irritant type
Boletus and *Cantharellus* sp.
Shortly after ingestion, nausea, emesis, and diarrhea may occur.

Disulfiram type
Coprinus sp.
After ingestion of these mushrooms with alcohol, face flushing, dizziness (from hypotension), and emesis may occur. Sensitivity to alcohol may persist for several days.

Hallucinogenic type
Psilocybe and *Panaeolus* sp.
One to 2 h after ingestion, mydriasis, nausea, emesis, and visual hallucinations may occur.

Treatment
- ICU in severe cases
- Anticholinergic poisoning first aid:
  - Blood pressure support: Dopamine and norepinephrine if crystalloids and colloid infusions fail.
  - Hypoglycemia: Infusions of 10% dextrose with thiamine
  - Cerebral edema: Hyperventilation, fluid restriction, osmotic diuresis, positioning the head of the bed at 30° above horizontal
  - Hemolysis: (1) Large amounts of IV fluids to prevent renal complications and (2) blood transfusions, if needed
  - Agitation: Benzodiazepines. It rarely requires physostigmine.
  - Severe vagal symptoms: Atropine.
- Amatoxin poisoning first aid:
  - Benzyl penicillin, IV, combined with silibinin
  - Cimetidine
- Gyromitrin poisoning first aid:
  - Phenobarbital should be avoided in the treatment of seizures.
  - Hydrazines
- Other symptomatic measures
- Liver transplant in fulminant hepatitis cases

Preventive Measures
- Learn about poisonous mushrooms, and when in doubt, do not eat them.
- Cooking does not prevent symptoms from most poisonous species.

Heat-Related Illnesses

Heat Asthenia (or Tropical Anhidrotic Asthenia)

Geographic Distribution

Very common in hot and humid climates, heat asthenia occurs when people have not yet adjusted to the new climate or when there is a heat wave. It can be aggravated by miliaria.

Main Symptoms

Symptoms are nonspecific and include physical and mental asthenia, cephalgia, nausea, dyspeptic disorders, irritability, anxiety, anorexia, inability to concentrate, drowsiness, vertigo, diaphoresis, polypnea, tachycardia, and insomnia. Heat asthenia can trigger depression and have negative personal and professional consequences.

Treatment

- Rest in a cool (air-conditioned) room.
- Symptomatic (mild analgesics, antiemetic, anxiolytic, if necessary)

Preventive Measures

- Adjust physical exertion progressively and according to local climatic conditions.
- Wear light clothes.
- Use air-conditioning when at work and at night.
- Do not use fans without air conditioning. They would only blow hot air and increase sudation.

Heat Exhaustion

Geographic Distribution

Heat exhaustion occurs when strenuous physical activity is performed in hot environments, particularly when combined with high humidity, which are conditions frequently found in tropical climates.

Main Symptoms

Symptoms can appear suddenly or progressively and include cool, moist skin with goose bumps, paleness, and sometimes cyanosis; cold sweats; diaphoresis; lightheadedness; vertigo; fatigue; tachycardia with a weak pulse; orthostatic hypotension; muscle cramps (by loss of electrolytes); nausea; and cephalgia. Body temperature is normal. Intense vasodilation leads to vascular collapse and loss of consciousness. Dehydration occurs more often in infants and in the elderly. Its signs are as follows:

Mild to Moderate

Slightly sunken eyes, decreased tears, tachypnea, fatigue, restlessness, irritability, coolness of the extremities, dry mouth, thirst (cellular dehydration), and oliguria (extracellular dehydration). In the skinfold test, the skin returns to normal in less than 2 sec after pinching it.

Severe

Parched, dry, or sticky mouth; deeply sunken eyes; no tears when crying; cold or mottled extremities; deep breathing; lethargy; difficultly in waking; difficulty in drinking; and vomiting. In the skinfold test, the skin either remains folded or takes more than 2 sec to return to normal.

Seizures and coma, more common in infants, are rare and appear late in the course of the illness in adults.

Treatment

As soon as the patient is in a supine position with legs elevated in a cool environment he or she will regain consciousness.

- Apply cool water to the skin. If possible, take a cool shower or soak in a cool bath.
- Remove any unnecessary clothing.
- IV fluids, if necessary
- IV electrolytes to replace losses (sodium, bicarbonate)

Preventive Measures

- Wear light clothes.
- Use air-conditioning at work and at night.
- Drink sufficiently (to satisfy thirst).
- If arterial hypertension is not a problem, lightly salt food.
- Sodium chloride supplement for heavy sweaters.
- Do not use fans without air-conditioning. They would only blow hot air and increase sudation.

Heat Stroke

Geographic Distribution

Heat stroke is more frequent in hot and humid climates when ventilation is poor, during a strenuous physical exercise by people who have not adjusted to new climatic conditions. Risk factors include certain medications, drinking alcohol, chronic illnesses, overweight, genetic dispositions, and being a young child or older adult.

Main Symptoms

Heat stroke is the last stage on a continuum of symptoms starting with heat asthenia, followed by heat exhaustion. Heat stroke occurs when the body temperature rises. Its symptoms include temperature of 104°F (40°C) or higher, which is the main sign of heat stroke; dry and flushed skin; nausea and vomiting; tachypnea (Cheyne-Stokes respiration); tachycardia; cephalgia; muscle cramps or weakness; confusion; restlessness; obnubilation; delirium; unconsciousness; and absence of reflexes. Complications range from vascular collapse, asystole, acute respiratory insufficiency, anuria, icterus, tetany, and hemorrhage to coma.

Treatment

- ICU transfer
- Lower body temperature ASAP (ice bath, cool air ventilation, air-conditioning)
- Chlorpromazine
- IV fluids
- Correct acidosis, hypocalcemia, and coagulation disorders.

Preventive Measures

- Wear light clothes.
- Use air-conditioning at work and at night.
- Avoid strenuous exercise when conditions are too hot and humid.
- Get used progressively to a new hot and humid climate.
- Drink sufficiently (to satisfy thirst).
- Do not use fans without air-conditioning. They would only blow hot air and increase sudation.
- Use alcohol with moderation
- Control body weight

Miliaria (or Prickly Heat)

Geographic Distribution

Miliaria is caused by blockage of the sweat gland ducts and can be found in various parts of the world. However, it occurs more frequently in the intertropical zone, where heat and moisture create favorable climatic conditions.

Main Symptoms

Miliaria appears as small blisters on the skin, accompanied with a burning and/or itching sensation, most frequently in the elbow creases, upper chest, neck, and groin. The condition is more common in obese patients. Secondary bacterial infections can result from scratching.

Treatment

- Talcum powder is effective.
- Broad-spectrum antibiotics clear up secondary bacterial infections.

Preventive Measures

- Use air-conditioning at night.
- Wear light garments.
- Dry the skin well after a bath or shower.

Travelers and Tropical Diseases

Overview
Mortality/Morbidity

Mortality

The risk of death linked to travel is estimated at 1 in 100,000/month. The main cause of death directly related to travel is accidents (25% of all cases), primarily due to motor vehicle injury. Cardiovascular diseases are number one on the disease list (50% of cases), but the link to traveling is sometimes indirect or nonexistent. Infectious diseases account for only 1–3% of all deaths. Malaria is the most frequent cause of infectious death among travelers. Between 1989 and 1995, 373 fatalities due to malaria were reported in nine European countries, as well as 25 deaths in the United States. The malaria case fatality rate ranges 0–3.6% in different countries. In 25% of all cases, the cause of death is unknown.

Regarding traveling per se, the CDC's Quarantine Activity Reporting System, which documents morbidity and mortality among travelers, analyzed the epidemiology of deaths during international travel reported from July 1, 2005, to June 30, 2008, in which international travelers died (1) on a United States–bound conveyance, (2) within 72 h after arriving in the United States, or (3) at any time after arriving in the United States from an illness possibly acquired during international travel. Cases were analyzed by age, sex, mode of travel (e.g., by air, sea, land), date, and cause of death; and rates were estimated using generalized linear models. 213 deaths were identified. The median age of deceased travelers was 66 yr (range 1–95); 65% were male. Most deaths (62%) were associated with sea travel; of these, 111 (85%) occurred among cruise ship passengers and 20 (15%) among cargo and cruise ship crew members. Of 81 air travel–associated deaths, 77 occurred among passengers, three among air ambulance patients, and one in a stowaway. One death was associated with land travel. Deaths were categorized as cardiovascular (70%), infectious disease (12%), cancer (6%), unintentional injury (4%), intentional injury (1%), and other (7%). Of 145 cardiovascular deaths with reported ages, 62% were in persons 65 yr of age and older. Nineteen (73%) of 26 persons who died from infectious diseases had chronic medical conditions. There was significant seasonal variation (lowest in July–September) in cardiovascular mortality among cruise ship passengers.

Morbidity

During travel, 15–64% of people become sick. The main symptoms are diarrhea, respiratory disorders, dermatological manifestations, and fever.

Travelers' diarrhea

Turista is still the most frequent illness among travelers who originate from industrialized countries and visit developing countries.

Malaria

Annually, some 20,000 malaria infections are imported by travelers and immigrants to industrialized nations. Travelers to sub-Saharan Africa and Oceania are at highest risk of acquiring malaria. Risk factors include nonimmune travelers, older age, travel to East Africa, and absence of chemoprophylaxis.

Sexually transmitted diseases

In Switzerland, it is estimated that 10% of HIV infections are acquired abroad. In the United Kingdom, the risk of acquiring HIV is considered to be 300 times higher while abroad compared with staying home. Typically, 14–25% of cases of gonorrhea and syphilis diagnosed in Europe are imported from abroad.

Common cold

Common cold is one of the most frequent health problems, with an attack rate of 13%.

Other medical conditions

Senior travelers mostly, may experience a new illness, or complications of a preexisting condition. Of particular concern are cardiovascular diseases. Pulmonary embolism associated with deep vein thrombosis after long-distance air travel may occur in 5 in 1 million travelers. Many of these cases are fatal.

Precautions to Take Before, During, and after Traveling

Before

Immunization

Mandatory

- According to destination: Internationally, only yellow fever and meningitis A, C, Y, W135 may be compulsory.

Recommended

- Everywhere: Booster against diphtheria, tetanus, and polio
- According to destination (many countries) and other factors: Hepatitis B, hepatitis A, typhoid fever, measles, flu, and BCG.
- According to destination (a few countries) and other factors: Rabies, Japanese encephalitis, tick-borne encephalitis

Check with the CDC, for vaccine & immunization information: 1-800-232-4636 (1-800-CDC-INFO) and for information on international travel: 1-877-394-8747.

Malaria

Chemoprophylaxis varies according to the country of destination and other factors. Check with the CDC malaria hotline: 770-488-7788 or 855-856-4713 toll-free.

Mosquito bites

For malaria, avoid mosquito bites between sunset and sunrise by using:

- Insecticide-treated bed mosquito nets (treatment can be predone or self-done)
- Air-conditioning
- Mosquito coils in closed rooms
- Long sleeves and full-length pants
- Insecticide on clothes
- Repellents

These measures are also efficient against fleas, lice, and ticks (for these, wearing a hat is also recommended).

Food and drinks

Food

- Eat only fruits that can be peeled and prepared by oneself or reliable others.
- Avoid ice cubes, ice creams, sherbets, fruits, and fruit juices from street vendors.
- Carefully wash vegetables.

Drinks
- Drink enough water to quench thirst.
- Drink only mineral water from sealed bottles. If this is not possible, boil the drinking/cooking water for 10 min before use; sterilize it at least 1 h before consumption with additives such as iodine tincture (10 drops/l), potassium permanganate, toluene sodium chloramine, or 1,3 dichloro-striazine 2,4,6 trione; or sieve it through resin or microceramic filters.
- Use condensed or powder pasteurized milk.
- Avoid nonpasteurized dairy.
- Cook meat, fish, eggs, shellfish, and crustaceans thoroughly.
- In ciguatera regions ask locals if the origin of the fish you want to eat is safe.

General hygiene
- Keep strict personal hygiene (especially, wash hands before meals).
- Do not bathe in freshwater.
- Do not walk barefoot on wet ground.
- Do not lie directly on sand beaches.
- Avoid contact with unknown animals.
- Dry clothes in places where there are no flies or iron them systematically.

Climate adjustment
- Wear ample and light clothes made out of natural fibers.
- Wear a hat or cap.
- During the hottest hours of the day, rest in the shade.
- If arterial hypertension is not a problem, add a little salt to food the first 10 days of stay, if days are hot.
- Take a shower with soap every day but not more than twice a day.
- At high altitude, rest 48 hours after arrival and start exercising progressively thereafter.

Travel medicine kit
It should include the following (derived from CDC):

Supplies for preexisting medical conditions
Travelers with preexisting medical conditions should carry enough medication for the duration of their trip and an extra supply, in case the trip is extended for any reason. If additional supplies or medications are needed to manage exacerbations of existing medical conditions, these should be carried as well. The clinician managing a traveler's preexisting medical conditions should be consulted for the best plan of action. People with preexisting conditions, such as diabetes or allergies, should consider wearing an alert bracelet (such as those available from www.medicalert.org) and make sure this information is on a card in their wallet and with their other travel documents.

General travel health kit supplies
Medications
- Destination-related, if applicable:
  - Antimalarial medications
  - Medication to prevent or treat high-altitude illness

- Pain or fever (one or more of the following or an alternative):
  - Acetaminophen
  - Aspirin
  - Ibuprofen
- Stomach upset or diarrhea:
  - Over-the-counter antidiarrheal medication (such as loperamide) or bismuth subsalicylate
  - Antibiotics for self-treatment of moderate to severe diarrhea
  - Packets of oral rehydration salts for dehydration
  - Mild laxative
  - Antacid
- Throat and respiratory discomfort:
  - Antihistamine
  - Decongestant, alone or in combination with antihistamine
  - Cough suppressant or expectorant
  - Throat lozenges
- Anti–motion sickness medication
- Epinephrine autoinjector (such as an EpiPen), especially if history of severe allergic reaction; smaller-dose packages are available for children
- Any medications, prescription or over the counter, taken on a regular basis at home

Basic first aid

- Disposable gloves (≥2 pairs)
- Adhesive bandages, multiple sizes
- Gauze
- Adhesive tape
- Elastic bandage wrap for sprains and strains
- Antiseptic
- Cotton swabs
- Tweezers
- Scissors
- Antifungal and antibacterial ointments or creams
- 1% hydrocortisone cream
- Anti-itch gel or cream for insect bites and stings
- Aloe gel for sunburns
- Moleskin or molefoam for blisters
- Digital thermometer
- Saline eye drops
- First aid quick reference card

Other important items

- Sunscreen (≥15 SPF)
- Antibacterial hand wipes or an alcohol-based hand cleaner, containing at least 60% alcohol

Useful items in certain circumstances:

- Extra pair of contact lenses, prescription glasses, or both for people who wear corrective lenses
- Mild sedative (such as zolpidem, other sleep aid, or antianxiety medication)
- Latex condoms
- Water-purification tablets
- Commercial suture or syringe kits to be used by a local clinician. (These items will require a letter from the prescribing physician on letterhead stationery.)
- Insecticide (to kill vectors)
- Repellent containing DEET (15–30%). Be aware that they can only provide transitory protection.

* Note: Air travelers should pack these sharp items in checked baggage since they could be confiscated by airport or airline security if packed in carry-on bags.

Insurance
Make sure that a good insurance will cover all health expenses, in particular very costly medical evacuations in case of emergency.

Contact card
Travelers should carry a contact card with the addresses and phone numbers of the following:

- Family member or close contact remaining in the country of origin
- Place of lodging at the destination
- Health-care provider(s) at home
- Medical insurance information
- Travel insurance and medical evacuation insurance information
- Area hospitals or clinics, including emergency services
- Embassy or consulate in the destination country or countries

During

Long flights
- Drink sufficiently
- Walk and stretch every 2 hours

Long rides
- Beware of dehydration in young children and the elderly when there is no air-conditioning in the vehicle with high temperature outside
- Walk and stretch every 2 hours

After
Upon return, if any symptoms appear (in particular fever) do not procrastinate and consult a specialist in a travel clinic ASAP.

Traveler's Diarrhea (Turista)

Bacteria: *Escherichia coli* (most common), *Salmonella*, *Shigella*, *Yersinia*, *Vibrio*, etc.

Viruses: Rotaviruses, Norwalk-like agents, etc.
Parasites: *Giardia, Entamoeba, Cryptosporidium*

A rapid change in climate and/or food, alcohol consumption, jet lag, fatigue, and different sanitation facilities have all been incriminated as factors causing GI disturbances in travelers. Surprisingly, in 50–70% of cases patients' stool examination does not reveal any virus, bacteria, or parasite that could explain the full clinical picture. Nevertheless, if traveler's diarrhea is suspected, a parasitological stool examination (O and P test) and stool cultures should be performed in order to rule out infectious or parasitic diseases (e.g., typhoid fever, salmonellosis, shigellosis, campylobacteriosis, norovirus, *E. coli*, amebiasis, or giardiasis, or other) because many of them require specific treatment. Furthermore, in 5–15% of cases there are multiple agents involved in the symptoms. Another name for the disease is "Montezuma's revenge."

New Problems

Because of increased travel requirements or options, turista is becoming a growing concern for businesspeople and tourists in many parts of the world.

Geographic Distribution

Traveler's diarrhea is more common in the intertropical zone but can be experienced in any part of the world. Countries can be divided into three groups.

Low-risk

United States, Canada, Australia, New Zealand, Japan, and countries in northern and western Europe

Intermediate-risk

Eastern Europe, South Africa, and some Caribbean islands

High-risk

Asia, the Middle East, Africa, Mexico, Central and South America

Main Symptoms

Two to 10 days after arrival in a new country, diarrhea (up to 10 loose stools per day), abdominal cramps, nausea, emesis, fever, weakness, and occasionally dehydration appear. The illness usually subsides spontaneously within 1–5 days.

Treatment

- Fluids, rest, and a monitored diet (based on rice, banana, chocolate in moderate amounts, and avoiding stomach irritants like alcohol, spices, pepper, citric fruits) are recommended.
- In some cases, loperamide is prescribed for diarrhea. If necessary, metoclopramide can also be dispensed to stop nausea and emesis. Acetaminophen can be prescribed for fever.
- Dosing
  * Loperamide, 4 mg, po, initially, followed by 2 mg after each loose stool (max 16 mg/day), for adults and children 12 yr and older
  * Metoclopramide, 10–15 mg, po or IM, qid, 30 min before each meal, for adults; for children and infants 0.4–0.8 mg/kg/day in four divided doses, po, IM, or IV

* Acetaminophen: (1) immediate-release, 325–650 mg, po, q4h, or 500 mg, po, q8h, or (2), extended-release, 2 caps (1,300 mg), po, q8h, for adults, as long as needed; for children:
  * <12 yr: 10–15 mg/kg, po, divided, q6–8h, not to exceed 2.6 g/day (5 doses/24 h); potential toxic dose <6 yr old = 200 mg/kg
  * >12 yr: 40–60 mg/kg/day, po, divided q6h, not to exceed 3.75 g/day (5 doses/24 h)
  * All as long as needed
* IV fluid replacement is necessary in severe cases.

Preventive Measures

- Intermediate- and high-risk countries
  - Avoid ice cubes and ice cream.
  - Boil or filter tap water or only drink from encapsulated water bottles.
  - Only eat fruits which need to be peeled.
  - Avoid salads and uncooked vegetables, or wash them with water sterilized with potassium permanganate.
- Everywhere
  - Systematically wash hands before meals.

Antibiotic Resistance

Antibiotic resistance presents the following features:

Types
Three types have been described.

Natural
It is the naturally occurring resistance of germs to antibiotics before treatment. It is well known and due to genes called environmental resistomes.

Vertical
It is chromosomal and often involves only one family of antibiotics.

Horizontal
It is extrachromosomal and implies the transfer of resistant genes through plasmids and transposons resulting in spreading of resistance to multiple families of antibiotics. It occurs by conjugation, transduction, or transformation.

New Problems

Aspects of antibiotic resistance in developing tropical countries
Misuse
According to the WHO:

- More than 50% of all medicines are prescribed, dispensed, or sold inappropriately.
- About 50% of all patients fail to take medicines correctly.
- More than 50% of all countries do not implement basic policies to promote rational use of antibiotics.

- Less than 40% of patients in the public sector are treated according to clinical guidelines.

More specifically, this misuse includes the following:

- *Mass use*: The mass use of broad-spectrum antibiotics creates pressure on germs and enables the selection of resistant strains.
- *Insufficient dosage*: As a result, the strongest germs are selected and survive.
- *Inappropriately shortened courses*: It happens for various reasons such as (1) inability of the patient to pay for the full course, (2) rupture of supplier stock, (3) social constraints, and (4) other medical conditions (psychiatric, neurological disorders) and it results in selection of the strongest germs.
- *Self-medication*: The patients' goal is to avoid paying for medical consultation and/or it happens by convenience. Consequently, course length and/or drug dosage are usually inadequate and the strongest germs are selected.
- *Counterfeit or poor-quality drugs*: In Africa, they represent up to 35% of all medications. Lower active ingredient content enables selection of the strongest germs.
- *Erroneous utilization*: For example, using penicillin or cotrimoxazole as cream or ointment, resistance appears more easily, making the subsequent systemic use of these drugs impossible.

Dissemination of resistant strains

Two types have been described:

Community-based: Anarchic urbanization has consequences which facilitate the spread of resistant bacteria, such as:

- Poor or no health-care networks
- Promiscuity
- Poor public hygiene and public health structures

Nosocomial: Nosocomial infections are 2–20 times more frequent in developing countries than in developed countries for various reasons, such as

- Hand carrying of patients
- Lack of asepsis during operations
- Inadequate sterilization of instruments

These shortcomings are due to several factors: (1) insufficient education/training of personnel, (2) budget restrictions, (3) faltering logistics, (4) inadequate or nonexistent isolation of contagious patients, and (5) ineffective or absent protection of health-care providers.

Specific examples

Antibiotic resistance presents serious challenges to medical practitioners in tropical areas, as mentioned in "Buruli's Ulcer" (p. 144), "Chancroid" (p. 146), "Cholera" (p. 147), "Enteric Fever" (pp. 182–184), "Gonorrhea" (p. 154), "Shigellosis" (p. 188), "Syphilis" (p. 190), and "Tuberculosis" (p. 193). Other problems include the following:

- Resistance of *Campylobacter jejuni* to fluoroquinolones in Asia
- Methicillin-resistant *Staphylococcus aureus* (MRSA) in:
  - Sub-Saharan Africa: with high resistance to tetracyclines and cotrimoxazole
- Thailand: >90% additional resistance to fluoroquinolones, aminosides, tetracyclines, and cotrimoxazole

Everywhere, mostl\y quinolones but also glycopeptides and cephalosporins are associated with colonization of infection sites by MRSA.

Moreover, some of these bacteria produce Panton-Valentine leukocidin, a toxin responsible for severe clinical pictures.

Preventive Measures
In order to keep bacteria sensitivity as long as possible, the following measures should be taken:

- *Prevent infections*
  - Immunize patients against infectious diseases.
  - Prevent cross-contamination.
  - Admit patients only for valid medical reasons.
  - Limit invasive procedures in hospitals, as much as possible.
- *Use antibiotics appropriately*
  - Use the correct method of administration.
  - Do not use combined antibiotics when it is not indispensable.
  - Choose the adequate initial antibiotic.
  - Treat infections as early as possible.
  - Prescribe the right regimen (dose and amount of time).
  - Monitor efficacy during treatment, if possible.
  - Replace drugs early in case of inefficiency.
  - Treat only bacterial infections with antibiotics.
- *In the ICU*

In a University of California–Irvine health-care trial conducted in 2010–2011 and involving approximately 75,000 patients, instead of screening ICU patients for the MRSA bacteria and then following protocol with those identified as carriers, all patients were bathed daily using chlorhexidine soap for the duration of their ICU stay and had mupirocin ointment applied inside the nasal passages for 5 days. This strategy resulted in a >33% reduction of patients harboring MRSA and nearly 50% reduction of bloodstream infections caused by MRSA and all other pathogens.

Addendum

Differential Diagnosis

Diarrhea

Acute, with fever

- Anthrax
- Cryptosporidiosis
- Cyclosporiasis
- Hantaan virosis
- Influenza
- Isosporiasis
- Kala-azar
- Malaria
- Pneumococcal pneumonia
- *Salmonella* gastroenteritis
- Shigellosis
- Traveler's diarrhea
- Trichinosis
- Typhoid fever
- Viral hepatitis

Acute, without fever

- Amebiasis
- Balantidiasis
- Cholera
- Cryptosporidiosis
- Cyclosporiasis
- Fish poisoning
- Intestinal amebiasis
- Intestinal distomatosis
- Mushroom poisoning
- Traveler's diarrhea

Chronic, without fever
- Amebiasis
- Ancylostomiasis
- Ascaridiasis
- Balantidiasis
- Giardiasis
- Intestinal distomatosis
- Microsporidiosis
- Murine typhus
- Schistosomiasis
- Strongyloidiasis
- Taeniasis
- Trichuriasis

Fever

Isolated
- Amebic liver abscess
- Malaria

Note: Isolated fever due to malaria and liver amebiasis are parasitic disease emergencies.

With adenopathy
- African trypanosomiasis
- American trypanosomiasis
- Lymphatic filariasis
- Plague
- South American blastomycosis

With diarrhea
- Anthrax
- Cryptosporidiosis
- Cyclosporiasis
- Hantaan viruses
- Influenza
- Isosporiasis
- Kala-azar
- Malaria
- Pneumococcal pneumonia
- *Salmonella* gastroenteritis
- Sarcosporidiosis
- Shigellosis
- Traveler's diarrhea
- Trichinosis
- Typhoid fever
- Viral hepatitis

With icterus
- Leptospirosis
- Viral hepatitis
- Yellow fever

With neurological symptoms
- African trypanosomiasis
- Angiostrongyloidiasis
- Cerebral malaria
- Meningococcal meningitis

With respiratory symptoms
- American histoplasmosis
- Anthrax
- Coccidiodomycosis
- Diphtheria
- Melioidosis
- North American histoplasmosis
- Paragonimiasis
- Pertussis
- Plague
- S.A.R.S.
- South American histoplasmosis
- TB

With skin eruption
- African trypanosomiasis
- American trypanosomiasis
- Dengue
- Leprosy (ENL)
- Rickettsiosis

With splenomegaly
- Bartonellosis
- Borreliosis
- Enteric fever
- Kala-azar
- Leptospirosis
- Malaria
- Septicemia
- Toxocariasis

Pruritus
- Ancylostomiasis

- Candidiasis (vaginal)
- Cutaneous larva migrans
- Dracunculiasis
- Flea bite
- Loiasis
- Myiasis
- Onchocerciasis
- Scabies
- Schistosomiasis
- Strongyloidiasis
- Trichomoniasis (vaginal)

Splenomegaly

Isolated

- Hemoglobinopathy
- Hydatidosis
- Idiopathic collagenosis
- Sarcoidosis

With fever

- African histoplasmosis
- Amebic liver abscess
- American histoplasmosis
- Borreliosis
- Brucellosis
- Enteric fever
- Kala-azar
- Malaria
- Septicemia
- TB
- Toxocariasis

With portal hypertension

- Hepatoma
- Schistosomiasis
- Viral hepatitis

International Generic and Brand Names of Drugs

Abacavir

Abamune, Abavir, Abcavir, Abmune, Virol, Ziagen

Acetaminophen

Actamin, Adprin B, Anacin AF, Apra, Crocin, Doliprane, Efferalgan, Feveral, Mapap, Panadol, Panamax, Panodil, Paracetamol, Paradote, Silapap, Tactinal, Tempra, Triaminic Tycolene, Tylenol, Vitapap

Acyclovir
Accrivir, Aciherpin, Aciv, Acivir, Acivirax, Alovir, Avir, Axovir, Clovirax, Cyclovir, Herpex, Herpovir, Lovir, Rivol, Rovir, Virex, Xovir, Zovir, Zovirax, Zoylex

Adefovir
Hepsera, Preveon

Albendazole
Albazole, Albenza, Alminth, Alworm, Andazol, Anthel, Banthel, Eskazol, Foben, Lupibend, Olban, Tiobend, Vermitel, Vermiz, Wornil, Zencid, Zentel, Zentic

Amikacin
Abiox, Acean, Afcin, Almika, Amcan, Amicin, Amikin, Amizin, Bakacin, Cimikan, Grasil, Ipracin, Kamin, Kindon, Kovex, Lisavin, Mikan, Omobin, Sefkin, Supracal, Zomacin

Amoxicillin
Amoxicot, Amoxil, Amoxin, Biomox, Clamoxyl, Dispermox, Hiconcil, Klavocin, Klavox, Moxatag, Moxilen, Senox, Starmox, Sumox, Trimox, Unimox, Wymox, Zymox

Amoxicillin + Clavulanic Acid
Amok/K Clav, Amoksiklav, Amoxi Clav, AugMaxcil, Augmentin, Augmex, Augpen, Clavamox, Clavulin, Co-amoxiclav, Enhancin, Klamentin, Klavocin, MoxClav, Moxikind, Xiclav

Amphotericin B
Abelcet, AmBisome, Amphocil, Amphotec, Fungilin, Fungisome, Fungizone

Amphotericin B (Liposomal)
AmBisome

Ampicillin
Aldribid, Aletmicina, Alphacin, Amcillin, Amfipen, Amipenix, Ampex, Ampexin, Ampibex, Ampiblan, Ampicher, Ampicin, Ampicyn, Ampidar, Ampifen, Ampiflex, Ampilag, Ampilin, Amsapen, Apo-Ampi

Artemether + Lumefantrine
Arsumet L, Artelum, Artemeter, Coartem, Coartrin, Laristar, Lumefrantrin, Lumether, Lumetrax, Riamet, RTM Forte

Artesunate + Amodiaquine
Artesun-Plus, Coarsucam

Artesunate + Mefloquine
Artequin, Falcigo Plus, Larinate MF, Mefliam Plus

Artesunate + Sulfadoxine-Pyrimethamine
Artesunate, Altinate, Combisunate Forte, Laminate

Atovaquone + Proguanil
Malarone

Atropine
Atreza, Atropen, Atropine Care, Isopto-Atropine, Sal-Tropine

Azithromycin
Abacten, Atromicin, Azadose, Azenil, Azimax, Azomycin, Ribotrex, Ultreon, Zithromax, Z-pak

Aztreonam
Azactam, Azenam, Azom, Azotum, Aztreo, Cayston, Trezam

Benznidazole
Radanil, Rochagan, Ro7-1051

Benzyl Alcohol
Ivy-Dry cream, Ulesfia

Benzyl Benzoate
Ascabiol, Bebesol, Bena, Benzol, Dermin Lotion, Jacutin

Brompheniramine
BPN, Bromfed, Bromfenex, Dimetane, Dimetapp, Lodrane

Cefixime
Arotex, Atocef, Bacitros, Cefi, Cefim, Cefspan, Cemax, Excef, Exime, Nexim, Ocexim, Oxim, Roxim, Saver, Suprax, Topcef, Zotaxime

Cefotaxime
Cefatax, Cefest, Cefotax, Ceftax, Claforan, Obitax, Orgacef, Toxitim

Ceftriaxone
Avrocyn, Cinzy, Corcef, Gentaril, Merigenta, Mogen, Oscagen, Rocephin, Tamiacin, Winceft, Zetox, Zygenta

Chloramphenicol
Alficetyn, Amphicol, Biomicin, Chlornitromycin, Cloranfenicol, Fenicol, Laevomycetin Phenicol, Medicom, Nevimycin, Tifomycine, Vernacetin, Veticol

Chloroquine
Amoquin, Aralen, Avlocor, Cloquin, Emquin, Malaquin, Nivaquine, Reoquin, Resochin,

Chlorpromazine
Chlorecitil Plus, Clozine Plus/Forte, Emetil, Largactil, Megaphen, Megatil, Sun Prazin, Thorazine

Clindamycin
Braclin 300, Braclin 600, Cleocin, Daclin, Dalacin, Lincocin

Clofazimine
Clofaz, Clofozine, Fazim, Feza, Hansepran, Lamprene

Clotrimazole

Candid Vag Tab, Canesten V6 Vag Tab, Clingen Vag Supp, Clocid Vag Tab, Cruex, Decand V3 Vag Tab, Ginal V Vag Tab, Gyne-Lomitrin, Lotril-Lb Vag Tab, Mycelex-G, Myconil-C Vag Tab

2-Dehydroemetine

Dehydroemetine, Tilemetin

Diazepam

Alzepam, Anxol, Calmpose, Campin, Diaclam, Diastat, Diaze, Diazemul-S, Dipax, Dizapam, Dizep, Elpose, Lakpam, Novo-Dipam, Paciquil, Paxum, Ralium, Valium, Val Release, Zeopose, Zycalm

Diethylcarbamazine

Banocide, Carnocide, Filaribits, Filazine, Hetrazan, Notezine, Remazin

Diloxanide Furoate

Amicline, Dilozol, Entamide, Furamide

Dopamine

Cupamin, Domin, Dopacard, Dopacef, Dopamin IV, Dopamin Rotex, Dopan, Dopanis, Dopar, Dopasol, Dopress, Giludop, Intropin, Komidop

Doxycycline

Adoxa, Atridox, Doryx, Doxoral, Doxyhexal, Doxylin, Doxy-1, Microdox, Monodox, Oracea, Periostat, Vibramycin, Vibra-Tabs, Vibrox

Econazole

Ecanol, Ecoderm, Pevaryl, Spectazole

Efavirenz

Sustina

Emtricitabine

Emtriva

Entecavir

Balaclude, Entaliv

Erythromycin

Abboticin, Althrocin, Citamycin, E-Mycin, Erycin, Erymax, Erypar, EryPed, Erythrocot, Erythrocyn, Erythroped, Pediamycin, Propiocyne, Ranbaxy, Robimycin, Stiemycine, Zineryt

Ethambutol

Afimocil, Anvital, Cidanbutol, Dexambutol, EMS-Fasol, Etambin, Etambutyl, Etapiam, Ethambutol, Etibi, Farmabutol, Fimbutol, Inagen, Miambutol, Myambutol, Mycobutol, Mynah, Tibutolo, Tisiobutol

Ethionamide

Ethatyl, Etiocidan, Panathide, Regenicide, Resitran, Theraplix, Thioniden, Trecator, Trecator-SC, Trescatyl, Tubenamide

Famciclovir
Famtrex, Famvir, Microvir, Renvir, Virovir

Flubendazole
Fluvermal

Flucytosin
Acobon

Hydrazines
Hydrazine sulfate, Sehydrin

Ibuprofen
Actron, Adex, Advil, Aktren, Alivium, Brufen, Dolgit, Ibalgin, Ibumetin, Motrin, Nurofen, Spidifen

Imipenem
Primaxin, Tienam

Interferon Beta-1b
Betaferon, Betaseron, Extavia, Ziferon

Iodoquinol
Moebequin, Yodoxin,

Isoniazid
INH, Isonicotinic acid hydrazide, Laniazid,

Itraconazole
Biospore, Candistat, Canditral, Citrol, Fulcover, Fungitrace, Icoz, Itaspor, Itra, Itrole, Sporanox

Ivermectin
Agimect, Biover, Evertin, Hestin, Imec, Imectin, Inover, Ivelop, Iver, Iverkem, Ivermect, Iveron, Kickworm, Mectin, Stromectol, Vermectin, Versil, Zlimetin

Ketoconazole
Can Cream, Derm Keta Cream, Extina, Fungicid Tab, Fungizole Tab, Kenazol Tab, Ketoderm, Ketoz Tab, Kuric, Nizoral, Phytoral Tab, Xolegel

Lamivudine
Epivir, Epivir-HBV, Heptovir, Zeffir, 3TC

Levamisole
Anthelnil, Carisnil, Dewormis, Dicaris, Ergamisol, Levam, Lavasol, Levazole, Solaskil, Vam, Vermisol, Vizole

Levofloxacin
Evo, Glevo, Leon, Levaquin, Levoff, Levoflox, Lotor 500, Quixin

Lidocaine
Duocaine, Xylocaine

Lindane

Aphtiria Poudre, Bexarid Lotion, Elenol Cream, Gab Lotion, Gamaric Lotion, Jacutin, Kwell, Lencide, Scabur Lotion, Swiscab Lotion, Welscab Lotion

Loperamide

Apo-Metoclop, Cerucal, Degan, Maxeran, Maxolon, Nu-Metoclop, Pramin, Primperan, Pylomid, Reglan

Malathion Lotion

Ovide

Mebendazole

Elmin, Helmintol, Idibend, Mabel, Mebex, Mebendex, Mex, Neomex, Vermox, Wormin, Zalzol

Mefloquine

Conflal, Falcigol Plus, Falcital, Lariam, Larinate MF, Mafloma, Mefax, Meflar, Mefloq, Mefly, Meloquine, MQF, Tramef

Meglumine Antimoniate

Glucantim, Glucantime

Melarsoprol

Arsobal, Melarsen Oxide-BAL, Mel B

Metoclopramide

Cerucal, Maxeran, Maxolon, Plasil, Plazilin, Pramin, Primperan, Pulin, Pylomid, Reglan, Tomit

Metronidazole

Aldezole, Aristogyl, Dependal, Dyrade, Filmet, Flagyl, Metro, Metrogyl, Metron, Sprot, Unimezol

Miconazole

Aloe Vesta, Daktarin, Emiconazol, Fungitop, Metazol, Miconit, Mizol, Monistat, Oravig, Sigmazol, Zole, Zole Ovule

Mycostatin

Nystatin

Naproxen

Aleve, Anaprox, Artagen, EC-Naprosyn, Movibon, Naprelan, Naprosyn, Xenal-CR, Xenobid

Nevirapine

Viramune

Nifurtimox

Bayer 2502, Lampit

Nimorazole

Acterol, Esclama, Naxofem, Naxogin, Naxogyn, Nulogyl, Sirled, Vargane Tab

Norepinephrine
Adrenor, Adronis, Epinor, Levophed, Levophed bitartrate, N-Adrin, Noradria, Nor-S, Vescue

Ofloxacin
Alproxen, Aviflox, Bioff, Endif, Floxin, Floxur, Loxin, Odiff, Ofla, Oflox, Tamvid, Verflox, Wisoflox, Zanocin, Zenflox

Ornidazole
Tiberal

Oseltamivir
Antiflu, Fluvir, Tamiflu

Oxamniquine
Mansil, Vansil

Pancuronium
Fancuron, Mioblock, Neocuron, Panconium, Pancuronium Bromide, Pavulon

Paromomycin
Humagel, Humatin

Pegylated Interferon alpha 2A
Pegasys, Reiferon Retard

Pegylated Interferon alpha 2B
PegIntron

Pegylated Interferon alpha 2B + Robavirin
Pegetron

Pentamidine
Lomidin, Pentacarinat, Pentam

Permethrin
Acticin, Alnathrin, Belscab, Elimite, Jolice, Monoscab, Perlice, Permanid, Scabenil, Skabiz, Uniscab

Physostigmine
Anticholium, Eserine, Physostigmine salicylate

Praziquantel
Biltricid, Cest, Cesticid, Helminthex, Prazine

Prednisone
Apo-Prednisolone, Cordrol, Deltasone, Milipred, Orisone, Prednicot, Prednisolone acetate, Predone, Ratio-Prednisolone, Rayos, Sandoz Prednisolone, Sterapred, Winpred

Procaine
Allocaine, Duracaine, Jenacain, Jenacaine, Mericaine Neocane, Novocaine

Promethazine
Atosil, Avomine, Fargan, Farganesse, Lergigan, Phenadol, Phenergan, Promacot, Promethegan, Prothiazine, Receptozine, Romergan, Sominex

Pyrantel
Combantrin, Conbantril

Pyrazinamide
Terazid

Ribavirin
Copegus, Rebetol, Ribavin, Virazide

Rifampicin
Macox, Monocin, Rifacept, Rifacilin, Rifadin, Rimactane, Rimactin, Ripharmed, Taurif, Ticin

Secnidazole
Ambese, Amebin, Amecdal, Bianos, Daksol, Deprozol, Ecuzol, Esnidazol, Flagentyl, Gisistin, Italnidazol, Maxidazol, Pazidol, Sabima, Secdazol, Secnivax, Secnol, Seczol, Strebenzol, Unidazol, Xamex, Yardel

Silibinin
Alepa-Forte, Bilsyl, Carsil, Darsil, Econlin, Eliamine, Enpex, Flavobion, Hepatos, Hepavit, Kenbo, Laragon, Legacel, Legalon SIL, Miltis, Phytohepar, Richem, Silegon, Silimarit, Silybin, Silymarin Dura

Sodium Stibogluconate
Pentostan, Stibanase, Stibanose, Stibatin, Stibinol, Stibotim

Spiramycin
Dicorvin, Osmycin, Rovadin, Rovamycin, Rovamycine, Selectomycin, Spirabiotic, Spiradan, Spiranter, Toxocare, Zyramycin

Stavudine
Zerit, d4T

Sulfadiazine
Adiazine, Lantrisul, Neotrizine, Sulfadiazine, Sulfaloid, Sulfa-Triple #2, Sulfonamides Duplex, Sulfose, Terfonyl, Triple Sulfa, Triple Sulfas, Triple Sulfoid

Sulfadoxine
Fanasil, Fanzil, Solfadossina, Sulfadoxin, Sulfadoxina, Sulfadoxinum, Sulphadoxine

Sulfametoxazole + Trimethoprim
Bactrim, Bactrimel, Bethaprim, Bibactin, Biseptol, Cotrim, Co-trimoxazole, Eusaprim, Graprima Forte Kaplet, Primotren, Septra, Septrin, Sulfatrim, Trisul, Vactrim

Telbivudine
Sebivo, Tyzeka

Tenofovir
Viread

Terbinafine

Anibret, Befine, Conter, Derbina, Exifin, Fungotek, Lamisil, Mycofem, Terbex, Terbinex, Terbo, Terif, Tinafine, Zimig

Terconazole

Gyno-Terazol Vag, Terazol 3, Terazol 7

Tetracyclines

Achromycin, Hostacycline, Idilin, Ingacycline, Lupiterra, Panmycin, Resteclin, Subamycin, Sumycin, Terrapal, Tetracyn

Thalidomide

Asmaval, Distaval, Isomin, Lulanin, Neurodyn, Nevrodyn, Nibrol, Peracon, Softenon, Tensival, Thalidomid, Thalimol, Thalin, Thalinette, Valgis

Thiamine

Betaxin, Thiamilate, Thianomin, Thiason, Thiatab, Thiobion, Thiolex, Thiosinan, Thiovit, Tone, Vita-1, Vitamin B_1

Tiabendazole

Mintezol

Tilliquinol/Tilbroquinol

Intetrix

Tinidazole

Fasigyn

Triclabendazole

Egaten, Fasinex, Tricloben

Valacyclovir

Valcivir, Valtrex, Zelitrex

Vancomycin

Covancin, Forstaph, Lyphocin, Vanacin, Vancocare, Vancocin, Vancogen, Vancoled, Vancomate, Vanking, Vansafe, Vantox, Viovan, Vontox

Vecuronium

Neovec, Norcuron, Ruvec, Survec, Vecuron, Veroni, Verunium, Vibro

Zanamivir

Relenza

Zidovudine

Azydothymidine injection, Compound S, Retrovir, AZT

Contraindications for Drugs

Acetaminophen

- Hypersensitivity to acetaminophen
- Liver failure, liver problems
- Alcoholism

Acyclovir
- Hypersensitivity to acyclovir
- Kidney disease
- Extreme loss of body water

Adefovir
- Hypersensitivity to adenosine analogues
- Drug resistance to antiretroviral therapy
- Enlarged fatty liver
- Kidney damage
- Kidney disease
- Breast-feeding mother
- Hyperlactic acidemia
- Overweight

Albendazole
- Hypersensitivity to benzimidazoles
- Patients should not become pregnant for at least 1 month following cessation of albendazole therapy.
- Use should be discontinued immediately if the patient becomes pregnant during treatment.

Amikacin
- Hypersensitivity to amikacin or other aminoglycoside antibiotics (gentamicin, tobramycin)
- Pregnancy
- Lactation
- Dehydration
- Hearing problems
- Kidney disease
- Myasthenia gravis
- Parkinson's disease
- Cystic fibrosis
- Hypokalemia, hypomagnesemia, hypocalcimeia

Amoxicillin
- Hypersensitivity to amoxicillin or to other β-lactam antibiotics (e.g., penicillins and cephalosporins)

Amoxicillin + Clavulanic Acid
- Hypersensitivity to amoxicillin + clavulanic acid

Amphotericin B
- Hypersensitivity to amphotericin B, liposomal amphotericin B

Ampicillin
- Hypersensitivity to ampicillin

Artemether + Lumefantrine

- Hypersensitivity to artemether
- Hypersensitivity to lumefantrine
- Tachycardia
- Bradycardia
- Torsades de pointes
- Prolonged Q-T
- Congenital Q-T changes
- Hypomagnesemia
- Hypokalemia
- Hypersensitivity to artemisinin analogues

Artesunate + Amodiaquine

- Hypersensitivity to amodiaquine
- Hypersensitivity to artesunate or to other artemisinin derivates
- Liver disease
- Neurological disorders
- Cardiovascular disease
- Glucose-6-phosphate dehydrogenase deficiency

Artesunate + Mefloquine

- Hypersensitivity to artesunate or mefloquine or to their chemically related compounds like other artemisinin derivatives, quinine, quinidine, or chloroquine or to any other ingredient of the stickpack content
- Artequin* pediatric must not be used together with halofantrine

Artesunate + Sulfadoxine-Pyrimethamine

- Hypersensitivity to sulfonamides
- Do not use in combination with cotrimoxazole
- Do not give folic acid on the same day or within 15 days thereafter

Atovaquone + Proguanil

- Hypersensitivity to atovaquone or proguanil hydrochloride or any component of the formulation
- Prophylaxis of *Plasmodium falciparum* malaria in patients with severe renal impairment (creatinine clearance <30 ml/min)

Atropine

- Hypersensitivity to atropine or any component of the formulation
- Narrow-angle glaucoma
- Adhesions between the iris and lens
- Tachycardia
- Obstructive GI disease
- Paralytic ileus
- Intestinal atony of the elderly or debilitated patient
- Severe ulcerative colitis

- Toxic megacolon complicating ulcerative colitis
- Hepatic disease
- Obstructive uropathy
- Renal disease
- Myasthenia gravis (unless used to treat side effects of acetylcholinesterase inhibitor)
- Asthma
- Thyrotoxicosis
- Mobitz type II block
- Pregnancy
- Lactation

Azithromycin

- Hypersensitivity to azithromycin, erythromycin, any macrolide or ketolide antibiotic

Aztreonam

- Hypersensitivity to aztreonam or any other component in the formulation

Benznidazole

- Hypersensitivity to benznidazole
- Early pregnancy

Benzyl Alcohol

- Hypersensitivity to benzyl alcohol
- Pregnancy
- Breast-feeding
- Children younger than 2 yr

Benzyl Benzoate

- Hypersensitivity to benzyl benzoate
- Broken or irritated skin
- Neonates
- Pregnancy

Brompheniramine

- Hypersensitivity to brompheniramine
- Children <6 yr
- Pregnancy
- Lactation
- Narrow-angle glaucoma
- Stenosing peptic ulcer
- Symptomatic prostate hypertrophy
- Lower respiratory tract symptoms (including asthma)
- Monoamine oxidase inhibitor (MAOI) use
- Elderly
- Debilitated patients

Cefixime
- Hypersensitivity to the cephalosporin/penicillin group of antibiotics

Cefotaxime
- Hypersensitivity to the cephalosporin/penicillin group of antibiotics

Ceftirizine
- Hypersensitivity to ceftirizine
- Babies <6 months old
- Lactation
- Kidney disease (severe)
- Liver disease (severe)

Ceftriaxone
- Hypersensitivity to the cephalosporin/penicillin group of antibiotics

Chloramphenicol
- Hypersensitivity to chloramphenicol
- Pregnancy
- Trivial infections
- History of porphyria
- History of bone marrow suppression
- Prevention of systemic bacterial infection
- Inability to monitor complete blood count

Chlorpromazine
- Hypersensitivity to phenothiazines
- Hepatic disease
- Parkinson's disease
- Epilepsy
- Narrow-angle glaucoma
- Myasthenia gravis
- With large amounts of depressants in the CNS (alcohol, barbiturates, narcotics)

Chloroquine
- Hypersensitivity to chloroquine
- Psoriasis
- Epilepsy
- Kidney impairment
- Liver impairment
- G6PD deficiency
- Hearing problems
- Parasitic resistance to chloroquine

Clofazimine
- Hypersensitivity to clofazimine
- Lactation

Clotrimazole

- Hypersensitivity to imidazole
- First trimester of pregnancy

2-Dehydroemetine

- Hypersensitivity to dehydroemetine
- Polyneuritis
- Heart disease
- Renal disease
- Pregnancy

Diazepam

- Hypersensituivity to diazepam or similar drugs
- Myasthenia gravis
- Severe liver disease
- Narrow-angle glaucoma
- Severe breathing problem or sleep apnea
- Children younger than 6 months

Diethylcarbamazine

- Hypersensitivity to diethylcarbamazine
- Pregnancy
- Lactation
- Infants
- Elderly
- Debilitated patients
- Impaired renal function
- Cardiac disease

Diloxanide furoate

- Hypersensitivity to diloxanide furoate
- Pregnancy
- Children <2 yr

Dopamine

- Hypersensitivity to dopamine
- Dopamine must be used with extreme caution in patients who are hypersensitive to sulfites.
- Many, if not all, dopamine preparations are contraindicated in patients with an allergy to corn or corn products due to an ingredient in the product.
- Hypovolemia is a contraindication for dopamine hydrochloride use.
- Dopamine is contraindicated in patients who have cyclopropane or halogenated hydrocarbons in their system. Halogenated hydrocarbons include isoflurane, desflurane, sevoflurane, halothane, methoxyflurane, and enflurane.
- Pheochromocytoma

- Uncorrected tachyarrhythmias or ventricular fibrillation
- Pregnancy
- Lactation
- Safety and effectiveness in children have not been established

Doxycycline

- Hypersensitivity to cyclines
- Women during the last half of pregnancy
- Children <8 yr

Econazole

- Hypersensitivity to econazole

Entecavir

- Hypersensitivity to entecavir
- Children <16 yr
- Lactation

Erythromycin

- Hypersensitivity to erythromycin
- Patients taking terfenadine, astemizole, pimozide, or cisapride

Ethambutol

- Hypersensitivity to ethambutol
- Optic neuritis
- Young children
- Unconscious patients
- Hepatic disease

Ethionamide

- Hypersensitivity to ethionamide

Famciclovir

- Hypersensitivity to famciclovir
- Kidney disease
- Extreme loss of body water

Fenxofenadine

- Hypersensitivity to fenxofenadine
- Children <4 yr
- Kidney disese (severe)
- Liver disease (severe)
- Lactation

Flubendazole

- Hypersensitivity to flubendazole
- Pregnancy

Flucytosin

- Liver problems
- Kidney disease
- Radiation
- Abnormal liver function tests
- Breastfeeding
- Hypokalemia
- Aplastic anemia due to medication
- Thrombocytopenia
- Granulopenia
- Decreased bone marrow function

Hydrazine

- Hypersensitivity to hydrazine
- Pregnancy
- Lactation
- Children

Ibuprofen

- Hypersensitivity to ibuprofen
- Patients who have experienced asthma, urticaria, or allergic-type reactions after taking aspirin or other NSAIDs
- Treatment of perioperative pain in the setting of coronary artery bypass graft surgery
- Active peptic ulcer
- Moderate to severe hepatic disease
- Infants

Imipenem

- Hypersensitivity to imipenem

Iodoquinol

- Hypersensitivity to iodoquinol
- Not for treatment/prophylaxis of traveler's diarrhea or nonspecific diarrhea
- Optic neuropathy
- Renal disease
- Thyroid disease
- Hepatic disease (other than secondary to amebiasis)

Isoniazid

- Hypersensitivity to isoniazid (including drug fever, chills, arthritis)
- Drug-induced hepatitis
- Previous isoniazid-associated hepatic injury
- Acute liver disease of any etiology

Itraconazole

- Hypersensitivity to itraconazole
- Congestive heart failure
- Drug interactions (cisapride, oral midazolam, nisoldipine, felodipine, pimozide, quinidine, dofetilide, triazolam, methadone, levacetylmethadol, lovastatin, simvastatin, dihydroergotamine, ergometrine, ergotamine, and methylergometrine)
- Pregnant patients or women contemplating pregnancy. Adequate contraceptive precautions should be taken by women of childbearing potential during therapy and for one menstrual cycle after stopping therapy
- Lactation
- Not to be used with astemizole, atorvastatin, bepridil, cisapride, eletriptan, ergot alkaloids such as dihydroergotamine, ergometrine, ergotamine, ivabradine, lovastatin, midazolam taken by mouth, mizolastine, nisoldipine, pimozide, quinidine, sertindole, simvastatin, terfenadine, or triazolam
- Not recommended in association with carbamazepine, phenobarbital, phenytoin, rifabutin, rifampicin, the herbal remedy St. John's wort

Ivermectin

- Hypersensitivity to ivermectin
- CNS disorders
- Pregnancy
- Breast-feeding until the infant is at least 3 months old
- Children <5 yr or weighing <15 kg (33 lb)

Ketoconazole

- Hypersensitivity to ketoconazole
- Coadministration of terfenadine, astemizole, cisapride, or triazolam

Lamivudine

- Hypersensitivity to lamivudine

Levamisole

- Hypersensitivity to levamisole
- Hepatic disease
- Severe renal impairment
- Blood disorders
- Rheumatoid arthritis
- Psoriatic arthropathy
- Pregnancy
- Lactation

Levofloxacin

- Hypersensitivity to quinolones
- Children <18 yr

- Pregnancy
- Lactation
- Prolonged Q-T interval
- Hypokalemia
- Myasthenia gravis

Lidocaine

- Hypersensitiviy to lidocaine and class of drugs
- Adams-Stokes syndrome
- WPW syndrome
- Heart block without pacemaker
- Intra-articular continuous infusion

Loperamide

- Hypersensitivity to loperamide
- Conditions when inhibition of peristalsis is undesirable (e.g., ileus or megacolon)
- Antibiotic-induced colitis
- Active inflammatory bowel disease, if abdominal distention develops during use
- Abdominal pain without diarrhea

Loratadine

- Hypersensitivity to loratadine
- Kidney disease (severe)
- Liver disease (severe)
- Children <2 yr
- Lactation

Malathion Lotion

- Hypersensitivity to malathion
- Neonates and infants

Mebendazole

- Hypersensitivity to mebendazole

Mefloquine

- Hypersensitivity to mefloquine
- History of serious psychiatric disorder (e.g., psychosis or severe depression)
- History of seizures

Meglumine Antimoniate

- Hypersensitivity to meglumine antimoniate
- Cardiac disease
- Pregnancy (except risk of maternal death from disease)
- Lactation

Melarsoprol

- Hypersensitivity to melarsoprol
- Pregnancy
- G6PD deficiency

Metoclopramide

- Hypersensitivity to metoclopramide
- GI hemorrhage, obstruction, or perforation
- Pheochromocytoma
- Epilepsy

Metronidazole

- Hypersensitivity to metronidazole
- Pregnancy (first trimester)
- Lactation: Interruption of breast-feeding is recommended during therapy and for 3 days following the last dose.
- Alcohol use during and 72 h after treatment

Miconazole

- Hypersensitivity to miconazole
- Hepatic impairment
- Porphyria
- Pregnancy (first trimester)

Mycostatin

- Hypersensitivity to mycostatin

Naproxen

- People who experience asthma, rhinitis, or nasal polyps after taking aspirin or other NSAIDs
- Aspirin-sensitive patients
- Advanced kidney disease
- Active peptic ulcer
- Severe kidney disease
- Severe liver disease
- Pregnancy (especially the last 3 months)

Nimorazole

- Hypersensitivity to nimorazole
- Liver disease
- Kidney disease
- CNS disease
- Pregnancy
- Lactation
- Children

Nifurtimox

- Hypersensitivity to nifurtimox
- Active or history of peripheral neuropathy
- Active or history of seizures and cerebral impairment, such as behavioral disorders, epilepsy, or psychoses
- Hepatic impairment
- Renal impairment

Norepinephrine

- Hypertension
- Pregnancy
- Patients with peripheral or mesenteric vascular thrombosis unless necessary as a life-saving procedure
- Potentially fatal: increased risk of arrhythmias with cocaine, cyclopropane, or halogenated hydrocarbon anesthetics. Hypertensive crisis may occur with MAOIs.
- Should not be given to patients who are hypotensive from blood volume deficits

Ofloxacin

- Hypersensitivity to quinolones
- Children <18 yr
- Pregnancy
- Lactation
- Prolonged Q-T interval
- Hypokalemia
- Myasthenia gravis

Ornidazole

- Hypersensitivity to ornidazole or to other nitroimidazole derivatives
- Pregnancy (first trimester)
- Lactation: Interruption of breast-feeding is recommended during therapy and for 3 days following the last dose.
- Alcohol use during and 72 h after treatment

Oseltamivir

- Hypersensitivity to oseltamivir
- Patients <1 yr

Oxamniquine

- Hypersensitivity to oxamniquine
- Pregnancy

Pancuronium

- Hypersensitivity to pancuronium
- Renal failure (creatinine clearance <10 ml/min)

- Hepatic failure (>45% hepatic metabolism)
- Unstable cardiovascular status
- Shorter duration of action needed: use another drug
- Neonates
- Infants
- Pregnancy
- Lactation

Paromomycin

- Hypersensitivity to paromycin
- Intestinal obstruction

Pegylated Interferon alpha 2A

- Hypersensitivity to pegylated interferon alpha 2A
- Autoimmune hepatitis
- Decompensated liver disease (Child-Pugh class B, C)
- Neonates, infants (contains benzyl alcohol)
- Pregnancy

Pegylated Interferon alpha 2B

- Hypersensitivity to pegylated interferon alpha 2B
- Autoimmune hepatitis
- Decompensated liver disease (Child-Pugh class B, C)
- Neonates, infants (contains benzyl alcohol)
- Pregnancy

Pegylated Interferon alpha 2B + Robavirin

- Hypersensitivity to pegylated interferon alpha 2B + robavirin
- Autoimmune hepatitis
- Decompensated liver disease (Child-Pugh class B, C)
- Neonates, infants (contains benzyl alcohol)
- Pregnancy

Pentamidine

- Hypersensitivity to pentamidine
- Children weighing <8 kg (17.6 lb)
- Pregnant women (first trimestrer)

Permethrin

- Hypersensitivity to permethrin or to any synthetic pyrethroid or pyrethrin

Physostigmine

- Hypersensitivity to physostigmine
- Hypersensitivity to sulfites
- Asthma
- Gangrene
- Diabetes

- Cardiovascular disease
- Mechanical obstruction of the intestine or urogenital tract or any vagotonic state
- Patients receiving choline esters and depolarizing neuromuscular blocking agents (decamethonium, succinylcholine)
- For postanesthesia, do not use atropine with physostigmine salicylate
- Pregnancy
- Lactation

Prednisone

- Hypersensitivity to prednisone
- Abrupt discontinuation
- Cushing's syndrome
- Fungal infection
- Measles
- Varicella

Procaine hydrochloride

- Hypersensitivity to procaine, drugs of a similar chemical configuration, or para-aminobenzoic acid or its derivatives
- Hypersensitivity to sulfites
- Myasthenia gravis
- Heart and blood vessel disease
- Liver disease
- Kidney disease
- Inadequate amount of cholinesterase enzyme
- Do not take with digoxin.
- Do not take with muscle relaxants including atracurium, pancuronium, and succinylcholine.

Promethazine

- Hypersensitivity to promethazine
- Children <6 yr
- Pregnancy
- Lactation
- Narrow-angle glaucoma
- Stenosing peptic ulcer
- Symptomatic prostate hypertrophy
- Lower respiratory tract symptoms (including asthma)
- MAOI use
- Elderly
- Debilitated patients

Pyrantel

- Hypersensitivity to pyrantel
- Liver disease

Pyrazinamide

- Hypersensitivity to pyrazinamide
- Liver disease
- Kidney disease
- Diabetes mellitus
- Gout
- Hyperuricemia
- Porphyria
- Pregnancy
- Lactation

Praziquantel

- Hypersensitivity to praziquantel
- P450 inducers, such as rifampicin
- Ocular cysticercosis
- Lactation
- Children <4 yr

Ribavirin

- Women who are pregnant or men whose female partners are pregnant
- Hypersensitivity to ribavirin or any component of the product
- Patients with hemoglobinopathies (e.g., thalassemia major or sickle cell anemia); creatinine clearance <50 ml/min (capsules/oral solution)
- Coadministration with didanosine
- Combination therapy with interferon alfa (additional contraindications):
  - Autoimmune hepatitis; in cirrhotic, chronic hepatitis C virus–monoinfected patients with hepatic decompensation (Child-Pugh class B, C) before treatment
  - Cirrhotic, chronic hepatitis C virus–patients coinfected with HIV who have hepatic decompensation (Child-Pugh class B, C) before treatment

Rifampicin

- Hypersensitivity to rifampicin
- Liver disease
- Treatment of meningococcal disease
- Patients who are also receiving ritonavir-boosted saquinavir
- Patients who are also receiving atazanavir, darunavir, fosamprenavir, saquinavir, or tipranavir

Secnidazole

- Hypersensitivity to secnidazole
- Pregnancy (first trimester)
- Lactation: Interruption of breast-feeding is recommended during therapy and for 3 days following the last dose.
- Alcohol use during and 72 h after treatment

Silibinin

- Children <2 yr
- Pregnancy
- Lactation

Sodium Stibogluconate

- Hypersensitivity to sodium stibogluconate
- Cardiac disease
- Pregnancy (except risk of maternal death from disease)
- Lactation

Spiramycin

- Hypersensitivity to spiramycin or another macrolide
- Meningitis
- Disorders of porphyrin metabolism

Sulfadiazine

- Hypersensitivity to sulfadiazine or other sulfas
- Infants <2 months (except as adjunctive therapy with pyrimethamine in the treatment of congenital toxoplasmosis)
- Pregnancy at term
- Lactation
- G6PD deficiency
- Renal disorders
- Liver disorders
- Porphyria
- Anemia from inadequate folic acid

Sulfadoxine

- Hypersensitivity to sulfadoxine or other sulfas
- Infants <2 months
- Pregnancy at term
- Lactation
- G6PD deficiency
- Renal disorders
- Liver disorders
- Porphyria
- Anemia from inadequate folic acid

Sulfametoxazole + Trimethoprime

- Hypersensitivity to sulfas
- Hypersensitivity to pyrimethamine
- Kidney disease
- Liver disease
- Blood dyscrasias

- Documented megaloblastic anemia caused by folate deficiency
- Infants <2 months
- Prophylactic use in pregnancy at term
- Lactation

Telbivudine

- Hypersensitivity to telbivudine
- Combination pegylated interferon alpha 2A is contraindicated because of increased risk of peripheral neuropathy.
- Myopathy

Tenofovir

- Hypersensitivity to tenofovir
- Should not be used in combination with the fixed-dose combination products
- Truvada®, Atripla®, and Complera® since it is a component of these products
- Should not be administered in combination with Hepsera (adefovir dipivoxil)

Terbinafine

- Hypersensitivity to terbinafine
- Terbinafine is an inhibitor of CYP4502D6 isozyme and has an effect on the metabolism of desipramine, cimetidine, fluconazole, cyclosporine, and rifampin.
- Lactation
- Liver disease
- Creatinine clearance <50 ml/min

Terconazole

- Hypersensitivity to terconazole
- Lactation

Tetracyclines

- Hypersensitivity to cyclines
- Pregnancy
- Lactation
- Children <8 yr (except sometimes for inhalational anthrax)

Thalidomide

- Hypersensitivity to thalidomide
- Effective contraception must be used for at least 4 weeks before beginning thalidomide therapy, during thalidomide therapy, and for 4 weeks following discontinuation of thalidomide therapy. Reliable contraception is indicated even where there has been a history of infertility, unless due to hysterectomy or because the patient has been postmenopausal for at least 24 months. Two reliable forms of contraception must be used simultaneously unless continuous abstinence from heterosexual contact is the chosen method. Women of childbearing potential should be referred to a qualified provider of contraceptive methods, if needed. Sexually mature women who have not

undergone a hysterectomy or who have not been postmenopausal for at least 24 consecutive months (i.e., who have had menses at some time in the preceding 24 consecutive months) are considered to be of childbearing potential.
- Before starting treatment, women of childbearing potential should have a pregnancy test (sensitivity of at least 50 mIU/ml). The test should be performed within the 24 h prior to beginning thalidomide therapy. A prescription for thalidomide for a woman of childbearing potential must not be issued by the prescriber until a written report of a negative pregnancy test has been obtained by the prescriber.
- Male patients: Because thalidomide is present in the semen of patients receiving the drug, males receiving thalidomide must always use a latex condom during any sexual contact with women of childbearing potential even if they have undergone a successful vasectomy.
- Once treatment has started, pregnancy testing should occur weekly during the first 4 weeks of use, then repeated at 4 weeks in women with regular menstrual cycles. If menstrual cycles are irregular, pregnancy testing should occur every 2 weeks. Pregnancy testing and counseling should be performed if a patient misses her period or if there is any abnormality in menstrual bleeding.
- If pregnancy does occur during thalidomide treatment, thalidomide must be discontinued immediately.

Thiamine

- Hypersensitivity to thiamine
- Lactation

Tiabendazole

- Hypersensitivity to tiabendazole
- Mixed worm infections involving Ascaris lumbricoides
- Prophylactic treatment for enterobiasis infection

Tilliquinol/Tilbroquinol

- Hypersensitivity to tilliquinol or tilbroquinol
- Pregnancy
- Lactation

Tinidazole

- Hypersensitivity to tinidazole
- Pregnancy (first trimester)
- Nursing mothers: Interruption of breast-feeding is recommended during therapy and for 3 days following the last dose.
- Alcohol use during and 72 h after treatment

Triclabendazole

- Hypersensitivity to triclabendazole
- Pregnancy
- Lactation

Valacyclovir

- Hypersensitivity to valacyclovir
- Kidney disease
- Extreme loss of body water

Vancomycin

- Hypersensitivity to vancomycin
- Hypersensitivity to corn and corn products
- Hearing problem
- Kidney disease
- Severe bloody diarrhea from antibiotics
- Mastocytosis
- Neutropenia

Vecuronium

- Hypersensitivity to vecuronium
- The drug should not be administered unless facilities for intubation, artificial respiration, oxygen therapy, and reversal agents are immediately available. The clinician must be prepared to assist or control respiration. To reduce the possibility of prolonged neuromuscular blockade and other possible complications that might occur following long-term use in the ICU, vecuronium or any other neuromuscular blocking agent should be administered in carefully adjusted doses by or under the supervision of experienced clinicians who are familiar with its actions and with appropriate peripheral nerve stimulator muscle monitoring techniques
- In patients who are known to have myasthenia gravis or the myasthenic (Eaton-Lambert) syndrome, small doses of vecuronium may have profound effects. In such patients, a peripheral nerve stimulator and use of a small test dose may be of value in monitoring the response to administration of muscle relaxants
- Pregnancy
- Lactation

Zanamivir

- Hypersensitivity to zanamivir and milk proteins
- Not recommended in pediatric patients <7 yr
- Lactation

List of FDA-Approved Vaccines

Product Name	Trade Name	Sponsor
Adenovirus type 4 and type 7 vaccine, live, oral	No trade name	Barr Labs
Anthrax vaccine adsorbed	Biothrax	Emergent BioDefense Operations Lansing Inc.
BCG live	BCG vaccine	Organon Teknika
BCG live	TICE BCG	Organon Teknika
Diphtheria and tetanus toxoids adsorbed	No trade name	Sanofi Pasteur
Diphtheria and tetanus toxoids adsorbed	No trade name	Sanofi Pasteur
Diphtheria and tetanus toxoids and acellular pertussis vaccine adsorbed	Tripedia	Sanofi Pasteur
Diphtheria and tetanus toxoids and acellular pertussis vaccine adsorbed	Infanrix	GlaxoSmithKline Biologicals
Diphtheria and tetanus toxoids and acellular pertussis vaccine adsorbed	DAPTACEL	Sanofi Pasteur
Diphtheria and tetanus toxoids and acellular pertussis vaccine adsorbed, hepatitis B (recombinant) and inactivated poliovirus vaccine combined	Pediarix	GlaxoSmithKline Biologicals
Diphtheria and tetanus toxoids and acellular pertussis adsorbed and inactivated poliovirus vaccine	KINRIX	GlaxoSmithKline Biologicals
Diphtheria and tetanus toxoids and acellular pertussis adsorbed, inactivated poliovirus and hemophilus B conjugate (tetanus toxoid conjugate) vaccine	Pentacel	Sanofi Pasteur
Haemophilus B conjugate vaccine (meningococcal protein conjugate)	PedvaxHIB	Merck and
Haemophilus B conjugate vaccine (tetanus toxoid conjugate)	ActHIB	Sanofi Pasteur
Haemophilus B conjugate vaccine (tetanus toxoid conjugate)	Hiberix	GlaxoSmithKline Biologicals
Haemophilus B conjugate vaccine (meningococcal protein conjugate) and hepatitis B vaccine (recombinant)	Comvax	Merck and
Hepatitis A vaccine, inactivated	Havrix	GlaxoSmithKline Biologicals
Hepatitis A vaccine, inactivated	VAQTA	Merck and
Hepatitis A inactivated and hepatitis B (recombinant) vaccine	Twinrix	GlaxoSmithKline Biologicals
Hepatitis B vaccine (recombinant)	Recombivax HB	Merck and
Hepatitis B vaccine (recombinant)	Engerix-B	GlaxoSmithKline Biologicals
Human papillomavirus quadrivalent (types 6, 11, 16, 18) vaccine, recombinant	Gardasil	Merck
Human papillomavirus bivalent (types 16, 18) vaccine, recombinant	Cervarix	GlaxoSmithKline Biologicals

(continued)

List of FDA-Approved Vaccines

Product Name	Trade Name	Sponsor
Influenza A (H1N1) 2009 monovalent vaccine	No trade name	CSL
Influenza A (H1N1) 2009 monovalent vaccine	No trade name	MedImmune
Influenza A (H1N1) 2009 monovalent vaccine	No trade name	ID Biomedical Corporation of Quebec
Influenza A (H1N1) 2009 monovalent vaccine	No trade name	Novartis Vaccines and Diagnostics
Influenza A (H1N1) 2009 monovalent vaccine	No trade name	Sanofi Pasteur
Influenza virus vaccine, H5N1 (for national stockpile)	No trade name	Sanofi Pasteur
Influenza virus vaccine (trivalent, types A and B)	Afluria	CSL
Influenza virus vaccine (trivalent, types A and B)	FluLaval	ID Biomedical Corporation of Quebec
Influenza vaccine, live, intranasal (trivalent, types A and B)	FluMist	MedImmune
Influenza virus vaccine (trivalent, types A and B)	Fluarix	GlaxoSmithKline Biologicals
Influenza virus vaccine (trivalent, types A and B)	Fluvirin	Novartis Vaccines and Diagnostics
Influenza virus vaccine (trivalent, types A and B)	Agriflu	Novartis Vaccines and Diagnostics
Influenza virus vaccine (trivalent, types A and B)	Fluzone, Fluzone High-Dose and Fluzone Intradermal	Sanofi Pasteur
Influenza vaccine, live, intranasal (quadrivalent, types A and B)	FluMist Quadrivalent	MedImmune
Japanese encephalitis virus vaccine, inactivated, adsorbed	Ixiaro	Intercell Biomedical
Japanese encephalitis virus vaccine inactivated	JE-Vax	Research Foundation for Microbial Diseases of Osaka University
Measles virus vaccine, live	Attenuvax	Merck and
Measles and mumps virus vaccine, live	M-M-Vax	Merck and(not available)
Measles, mumps, and rubella virus vaccine, live	M-M-R II	Merck and
Measles, mumps, rubella and varicella virus vaccine live	ProQuad	Merck and
Meningococcal (groups A, C, Y, and W-135) oligosaccharide diphtheria CRM197 conjugate vaccine	Menveo	Novartis Vaccines and Diagnostics

(continued)

List of FDA-Approved Vaccines

Product Name	Trade Name	Sponsor
Meningococcal groups C and Y and hemophilus B tetanus toxoid conjugate vaccine	MenHibrix	GlaxoSmithKline Biologicals
Meningococcal polysaccharide (serogroups A, C, Y, and W-135) diphtheria toxoid conjugate vaccine	Menactra	Sanofi Pasteur
Meningococcal polysaccharide vaccine, groups A, C, Y, and W-135 combined	Menomune-A/ C/Y/W-135	Sanofi Pasteur
Mumps virus vaccine live	Mumpsvax	Merck and
Plague vaccine	No trade name	Greer Laboratories (not available)
Pneumococcal vaccine, polyvalent	Pneumovax 23	Merck and
Pneumococcal 7-valent conjugate vaccine (diphtheria CRM_{197} protein)	Prevnar	Wyeth Pharmaceuticals
Pneumococcal 13-valent conjugate vaccine (diphtheria CRM_{197} protein)	Prevnar 13	Wyeth Pharmaceuticals
Poliovirus vaccine inactivated (human diploid cell)	Poliovax	Sanofi Pasteur (not available)
Poliovirus vaccine inactivated (monkey kidney cell)	IPOL	Sanofi Pasteur
Rabies vaccine	Imovax	Sanofi Pasteur
Rabies vaccine	RabAvert	Novartis Vaccines and Diagnostics
Rabies vaccine adsorbed	No trade name	BioPort (not available)
Rotavirus vaccine, live, oral	ROTARIX	GlaxoSmithKline Biologicals
Rotavirus vaccine, live, oral, pentavalent	RotaTeq	Merck and
Rubella virus vaccine live	Meruvax II	Merck and
Smallpox (vaccinia) vaccine, live	ACAM2000	Sanofi Pasteur Biologics
Tetanus and diphtheria toxoids adsorbed for adult use	No trade name	MassBiologics
Tetanus and diphtheria toxoids adsorbed for adult use	DECAVAC	Sanofi Pasteur
Tetanus and diphtheria toxoids adsorbed for adult use	TENIVAC	Sanofi Pasteur
Tetanus toxoid	No trade name	Sanofi Pasteur
Tetanus toxoid adsorbed	No trade name	Sanofi Pasteur
Tetanus toxoid, reduced diphtheria toxoid and acellular pertussis vaccine, adsorbed	Adacel	Sanofi Pasteur
Tetanus toxoid, reduced diphtheria toxoid and acellular pertussis vaccine, adsorbed	Boostrix	GlaxoSmithKline Biologicals
Typhoid vaccine live oral Ty21a	Vivotif	Berna Biotech
Typhoid VI polysaccharide vaccine	TYPHIM Vi	Sanofi Pasteur
Varicella virus vaccine live	Varivax	Merck and
Yellow fever vaccine	YF-Vax	Sanofi Pasteur
Zoster vaccine, Live (Oka/Merck)	Zostavax	Merck and

List of Vaccines Available in France

Trade Names	Vaccine Type	Sponsors
ACT-HIB	*Haemophilus influenzae* type B (conjugated)	Sanofi Pasteur
Agrippal	Against influenza (inactivated surface antigens)	Novartis Vaccines and Diagnostics
Avaxim 160 U	Against hepatitis A (inactivated, adsorbed)	Sanofi Pasteur
Boostrixtetra	Against diphtheria, tetanus, whooping cough (acellular, conjugate and polio (inactivated, adsorbed))	GlaxoSmithKline
Cervarix	Against type 16, 18 HPV ((recombined, with adjuvant, adsorbed)	GlaxoSmithKline
D.T. Vax	Against diphtheria, and tetanus (adsorbed)	Sanofi Pasteur
Dukoral	Against cholera (recombinant)	Chiron Healthcare
Encepur	Against tick-borne encephalitis	Novartis Vaccines and Diagnostics
Engerix B 10 µg	Against hepatitis B (recombinant adsorbed)	GlaxoSmithKline
Engerix B 20 µg	Against hepatitis B (recombinant adsorbed)	GlaxoSmithKline
Fluarix	Against influenza (inactivated virus fragments)é	GlaxoSmithKline
Gardasil	Against type 6, 11, 16, 18 HPV (recombinant, adsorbed)Vaccin papillomavirus humain [types 6, 11, 16, 18] (recombinant, adsorbé)	Sanofi Pasteur
Genhevac B Pasteur	Against hepatitis B (recombinant).	Sanofi Pasteur
Havrix 1 440 U	Against hepatitis A (inactivated, adsorbed)	GlaxoSmithKline
Havrix 720 U	Against hepatitis A (inactivated, adsorbed)	GlaxoSmithKline
Hbvaxpro 10 µg	Against hepatitis B	Sanofi Pasteur
Hbvaxpro 40 µg	Against hepatitis B	Sanofi Pasteur
Hbvaxpro 5 µg	Against hepatitis B	Sanofi Pasteur
Immugrip	Against influenza (inactivated virus fragments)	Pierre Fabre Medicament
Imovax Polio	Against polio (inactivated)	Sanofi Pasteur
Infanrixhexa	Against diphtheria (D), tetanus (T), whooping cough (acellular multicomposed) (Ca), hepatitis B (DNAr, HepB), polio (inactivated) (P), and type B Hemophylus influenzae (Hib) (combined, adsorbed)	GlaxoSmithKline
Infanrixquinta	Against diphtheria, tetanus, whooping cough (acellular, adsorbed), polio (inactivated) and type B Hemophylus influenzae conjugate	GlaxoSmithKline
Infanrixtetra	Against diphtheria, tetanus, whooping cough, (acellular) polio (inactivated, adsorbed)	GlaxoSmithKline
Influvac	Against influenza (inactivated surface antigens)	Abbott Products
Ixiaro	Against Japanese encephalitis	Novartis Vaccines and Diagnostics

(continued)

List of Vaccines Available in France

Trade Names	Vaccine Type	Sponsors
M-M-Rvaxpro	Against mumps, measles, rubella (live)	Sanofi Pasteur
Menbvac	Against type B: 14 :P1.7, 16 invasive meningococcus infections:	Norwegian Institute of Public Health
Mencevax	Against meningococcus type A, C, W135 (polyosidic) and Y (not conjugate)	GlaxoSmithKline
Meningitec	Against serogroup C meningococcus (oligosidic, conjugate, adsorbed))	Pfizer
Menjugatekit	Against group C meningococcus (oligosidic, conjugate, adsorbed)é).	Novartis Vaccines and Diagnostics
Menveo	Against group A, C. W-135 and Y meningococcus (conjugate)	Novartis Vaccines and Diagnostics
Neisvac	Against group C meningococcus (polyosidic, conjugate, adsorbed))	Baxter Bioscience Division
Nimenrix	Against group A, C, W-135 and Y meningococcus (conjugate)	GlaxoSmithKline
Pentavac	Against diphtheria, tetanus, whooping cough (acellular), polio (inactivated, adsorbed) and type B Hemophylus influenzae (combined).	Sanofi Pasteur
Pneumo 23	Against pneumococcus (polyosidic, 23 valences)	Sanofi Pasteur
Pneumovax 23	Against pneumococcus (polyosidic)	Merck
Prevenar 13	Against pneumococcus (conjugate, polyosidic, 13 valences)	Pfizer
Priorix	Against measles, mumps, rubella (live)	GlaxoSmithKline
Rabipur	Against rabies, for humans (prepared on cell cultures)	Novartis Vaccines and Diagnostics
Repevax	Against diphtheria (reduced antigen content), tetanus, whooping cough (acellular), and polio (inactivated, adsorbed)	Sanofi Pasteur
Revaxis	Against diphtheria, tetanus and polio (inactivated, adsorbed)	Sanofi Pasteur
Rotarix	Against rotaviruses (oral, live)	GlaxoSmithKline
Rotateq	Against rotaviruses (oral, live)	Sanofi Pasteur
Rouvax	Against measles	Sanofi Pasteur
Rudivax	Against rubella (attenuated)	Sanofi Pasteur
Spirolept	Against leptospirosis (inactivated)	IMAXIO
Stamaril	Against yellow fever (live)	Sanofi Pasteur
Tetravac Acellular	Against diphtheria, tetanus, whooping cough (acellular), polio (inactivated, adsorbed)	Sanofi Pasteur
Ticovac Adults	Against tick-borne encephalitis (inactivated)	Baxter Bioscience Division

(continued)

List of Vaccines Available in France

Trade Names	Vaccine Type	Sponsors
Ticovac Children	Against tick-borne encephalitis (inactivated) Vaccin de l'encéphalite à tiques inactivé	Baxter Bioscience Division
Twinrix Adults	Against hepatitis A (inactivated) and hepatitis B (DNAr) HAB (adsorbed)	GlaxoSmithKline
Twinrix Children	Against hepatitis A (inactivated) and hepatitis B (DNAr) HAB (adsorbed) Vaccin de l'hépatite A inactivé et de l'hépatite B (ADNr) HAB, adsorbé	GlaxoSmithKline
Tyavax	Against hepatitis A (inactivared, adsorbed) and typhoid fever (polyosidic)	Sanofi Pasteur
Typherix	Against typhoid fever (Vi polyosidic)	GlaxoSmithKline
Typhim Vi	Against typhoid fever (polyosidic)	Sanofi Pasteur
Vaccin Bcg Ssi	Against tuberculosis	Sanofi Pasteur
Vaccin Encephalite A Tiques	Against tick-borne encephalitis	
Vaccin Encephalite Japonaise	Against Japanese encephalitis	
Vaccin Haemophilus Influenzae B (or Hib)	Against type B Haemophilus influenzae (conjugate)	
Vaccin Hepatite A	Against hepatitis A	
Vaccin Meningococcique A+C	Against A + C meningococcus (polyosidic)	Sanofi Pasteur
Vaccin Rabique Pasteur	Against rabies, for humans (inactivated, prepared on cell cultures)	Sanofi Pasteur
Vaccin Tetanique	Against tetanus	
Vaccin Tetanique Pasteur	Against tetanus (adsorbed)	Sanofi Pasteur MSD
Vaccin Typhoide	Against typhoid fever	
Vaccin Variole	Against smallpox	
Vaccin Zona	Against herpes zoster	
Varilrix	Against chickenpox (live)	GlaxoSmithKline
Varivax	Against chickenpox (live). Chickenpox live vaccine	Sanofi Pasteur
Vaxigrip	Against influenza (inactivated virus fragments)	Sanofi Pasteur
Zostavax	Against herpes zoster	Sanofi Pasteur

Link to Major International Health-Care Organizations

http://www.imva.org/Pages/orgdb/wblstfrm.htm

Map and Table Index

Geographic Distribution Maps

African histoplasmosis, 122
African trypanosomiasis, 18
Amebiasis, 26
American histoplasmosis*, 126
Ancylostomiasis, 29
Angiostrongyliasis, 90
Ascariasis, 31

Bartonellosis, 142
Blastomycoses, 112
Buruli ulcers, 145

Chagas disease, 21
Cholera (1970–1979 epidemic in West Africa), 150
Cholera (1961–1991 pandemic), 151
Cholera, 150, 151
Chromomycosis, 114
Ciguatera, 286
Coccidioidomycosis*, 117
Creutzfeldt-Jakob disease and variant, 204
Cutaneous and mucocutaneous leishmaniases in the Old World, 69
Cutaneous leishmaniasis due to L. tropica and L. aethiopica, 66
Cysticercosis, 93

Dengue fever, 207
Donovan disease, 158
Dracunculiasis, 62

Epidemic louse-borne typhus, 271

Fascioliasis, 36

Gnathostomiasis, 95

Hantaan virus, 241
Hepatitis A, 213
Hepatitis B, 214
Hydatidosis, 98

Intestinal distomatoses, 38

Junin and Machupo viruses, 238

Lobomycosis, 128
Loiasis*, 72
Lymphatic filariasis*, 3

Malaria, 14
Melioidosis, 166
Meningococcal meningitis, 169
Mucocutaneous leishmaniasis in the New World, 68
Murine typhus, 267
Mycetomas*, 131
Myiasis, 75

Nicholas-Favre-Durand disease, 198

Onchocerciasis (in Africa and in the Arabic Peninsula), 78
Opisthorchiases, 34

Paragonimiasis, 51
Pinta, 173
Plague, 176
Pythiosis, 133

Rabies (rabies-free areas in the world), 263
Regional relapsing fever, 281
Rhinosporidiosis, 135

Schistosomiases (in Cameroon)*, 44
Schistosomiases (in Madagascar), 45
Schistosomiases, 43, 44, 45, 87
Scrub typhus, 283
Scytalidiosis, 137
Shigellosis, 189
Sparganosis, 102
Strongyloidiasis, 48

Trichinosis, 106
Tropical mucormycoses, 108, 119
Tungiasis, 84
Typhoid fever, 186

Urinary schistosomiasis (in Northern Africa), 88

Visceral leishmaniasis, 6

Yellow fever (animal reservoir), 234

Tables

1.1 Artesunate suppositories: adult doses, 10
1.2 Artesunate suppositories: children doses, 10
1.3 Malaria presumptive treatment regimens, 10
1.4 Malaria prophylaxis regimens, 12
1.5 Drug regimens for the treatment of Chagas disease in acute phase, 20
1.6 Nitro-imidazole regimens for the treatment of amebiasis, 23
1.7 Itraconazole pulse regimens for the treatment of candidiasis onyxis, 52
1.8 Treatments for scabies and head lice, 81
2.1 Cotrimoxazole adult presentations, 129
2.2 Cotrimoxazole pediatric doses for the treatment of actinomycetomas, 129
3.1 Drug regimens for the treatment of anthrax, 140
3.2 Amoxicillin pediatric doses for the treatment of diphtheria, 153
3.4 Treatment regimens for leprosy, 161
3.5 Treatment regimens for pertussis, 171
3.6 Typhoid fever treatment: antibiotics of choice by disease origin and severity, 184
3.7 TB treatment basic regimens, 194
3.8 Treatment regimens for chlamydial urethritis and cervicitis, 202
4.1 Severity grading for Dengue fever, 207
4.2 AIDS treatment regimens for children, 223–224
4.3 Sensitivity and specificity of influenza main symptoms, 225
4.4 Oseltamivir pediatric regimens for the treatment of influenza, 226
4.5 Oseltamivir pediatric regimens for the preventions of influenza, 226
4.6 Cases of yellow fever in the world in 2010, 232
4.7 Arboviruses clinical pictures, 236
5.1 Epinephrine doses for severe allergic reactions: 1 mg/ml injection (1:1,000)
5.2 Acetaminophen doses for infants and children, 255

* These maps come from the private collection of Prof. Marc Gentilini and were graciously released to Oxford University Press for this book by Lavoisier Publishers, Paris.

Patient Cases Index

African histoplasmosis, 121
African trypanosomiasis, 16
American histoplasmosis, 124
Ancylostomiasis, 27

Ciguatera, 284
Cutaneous larva migrans, 99
Cutaneous leishmaniasis, 64

Dengue fever, 207
Dracunculiasis, 60

Fascioliasis, 32–33–33

Giardiasis, 40

Hepatitis E, 211–212
Hydatidosis, 97

Intestinal amebiasis, 23
Intestinal schistosomiasis, 41

Liver amebiasis, 24
Loiasis, 71

Malaria, 11
Myiasis, 74

Onchocerciasis, 77

Pityriasis versicolor, 73

Scabies, 81
Strongyloidiasis, 47

Trichomoniasis, 57
Tungiasis, 83

Urinary schistosomiasis, 85

Visceral leishmaniasis, 5

Disease Index

African eyeworm, 70–72
Amebiasis (amoeboma), 24–26
Amebiasis (intestinal), 22–24, 26
Amebiasis (liver), 24, 26
Ancylostomiasis, 27–29
Anemone-induced diseases, 269
Angiostrongyliasis, 89–90
Anthrax, 139–141
Antibiotic resistance, 299–301
Arboviral diseases, 235–236, 279
Arenaviral diseases, 237–239
Ascariasis, 30–31

Bacterial diseases, 139–204
Bairnsdale disease, 144–145
Balantidiasis, 35
Bartonellosis, 141–142
Basidiobolomycosis, 107
Beaver fever, 39–40
Bees and hymenoptera-induced diseases, 253–254
Bejel, 143
Biliary fluke diseases, 35–34
Black death, 174–176
Black vomit, 232–234
Blackwater fever, 7–14
Blastomycosis (North American), 109–110, 112
Blastomycosis (South American), 110–112
Body lice, 80
Breakbone fever, 205–207
Bunyaviral diseases, 239–240
Buruli ulcers, 144–145
Butterfly-induced diseases, 254

Candidiasis, 52, 55–56, 58
Carate, 171–173
Carrion disease, 141–142

Cat bite–induced diseases, 256
Cat scratch disease, 257
Centipede-induced diseases, 260
Cenurosis, 91
Chagas disease, 19–21
Chancroid, 146
Chicago disease, 109–110, 112
Chikungunya virus disease, 250–251
Cholera, 146–151
Chromomycosis, 113–114
Ciguatera, 284–286
Clap, 153–155
Coccidioidomycosis, 115–117
Cold sore, 215–216
Conidiobolomycosis, 118–119
Crabs, 54
Creeping eruption, 99
Cryptosporidiosis, 222
Cyclosporiasis, 222
Cysticercosis, 91–93

Daintree disease, 144–145
Darling disease, 123–126
Deep fungal diseases, 107–137
Dengue fever, 205–207
Dermatophytosis, 52–53, 58–59
Differential diagnosis: diarrhea, 303
Differential diagnosis: fever, 303–304
Differential diagnosis: pruritus, 304–306
Differential diagnosis: splenomegaly, 303–305
Diphtheria, 152–153
Distomatosis (intestinal), 37–38
Distomatosis (liver/biliary), 35–34
Dog bite–induced diseases, 260–265
Donovan disease, 155–158
Dracontiasis, 59–62
Dracunculiasis, 59–62
Dum dum disease, 4–6

Ebola virus disease, 243–244
Endemic syphilis, 143
Enteric fever, 182–186
Epidemic louse-borne typhus, 270–271

Fascioliasis, 32–33–36
Fever sore, 215–216
Filariasis (lymphatic), 1–3
Filoviral diseases, 243–245
Fish poisoning, 265, 287–288
Flaviviral diseases, 245–246
Flu, 225–227
Food poisoning by exotic fish, 287–288
Food poisoning by exotic mushrooms, 288–289
Frambesia tropica, 195–196

Giardiasis, 39–40
Gilchrist disease, 109–110, 112
Gonorrhea, 153–155
Gnathostomiasis, 94–95
Granuloma inguinale, 155–158
Guinea worm infection, 59–62
Guinea worm disease, 59–62

Hansen disease, 159–162
Hantaan virosis, 240–241
Hard chancre, 190–192
Head lice, 53
Head ringworm, 54–55
Heat asthenia, 290
Heat exhaustion, 290–291
Heat stroke, 291–292
Heat-related illnesses, 290–292
Hendra virosis, 246–247
Hepatitis, 209–214
Herpes simplex, 215–216
Histoplasmosis (African), 120–122
Histoplasmosis (American), 123–126
HIV/AIDS, 216–225
Hookworm infection, 27–29
Hornet-induced diseases, 253–254
Hydatidosis, 96–98

Ichtyosarcotoxisms, 287
Influenza, 225–227

Jellyfish-induced diseases, 269
Jorge Lobo disease, 127–128

Kala-azar, 4–6

Larva migrans (cutaneous), 99, 260
Lassa fever disease, 239

Leech-induced diseases, 269–270
Leishmaniasis (cutaneous), 63–66, 68, 69
Leishmaniasis (mucocutaneous), 67–69
Leishmaniasis (visceral), 4–6
Leprosy, 159–162
Leptospirosis, 162–163
Linguatulosis, 100, 260
Liver fluke diseases, 35–34
Lobomycosis, 127–128
Loiasis, 70–72
Lung fluke infection, 49–51
Lutz-Splendore-Almeida disease, 110–112
Lymphogranuloma venereum, 196–198
Lyssavirus disease, 250

Madura foot disease, 129–131
Malaria, 7–14
Marburg virus disease, 244–245
Malasseziosis, 73
Measles, 227–229
Melioidosis, 163–166
Meningococcal meningitis, 167–169
Miliaria, 292
Mollusk-induced diseases, 274
Moniliasis, 52, 55–56, 58
Moray eel–induced diseases, 274–275
Mossman disease, 144–145
Mossuril virus disease, 249
Muranae-induced diseases, 274–275
Murine typhus, 266–267
Mushroom poisoning, 288–289
Mycetoma, 129–131
Mycoburuli ulcers, 144–145
Myiasis, 73–75

Nanukayami fever, 162–163
Nicholas-Favre-Durand disease, 196–198
Nipah virosis, 247
Norwegian itch, 80–82

Onchocerciasis, 76–78
Opisthorchiasis, 35–34

Paragonimiasis, 49–51
Paramyxovirus disease, 246–247
Parangi, 195–196
Paru, 195–196
Pediculosis capitis, 53, 272
Pediculosis corporis, 80, 272
Pian, 195–196
Pertussis, 170–171
Physalia-induced diseases, 269
Pinta, 171–173

Pityriasis versicolor, 73
Plague, 174–176, 268
Pneumococcal disease, 177–182
Polio, 229–231
Poliomyelitis, 229–231
Porocephalosis, 100–101
Posadas-Rixford disease, 115–117
Posadas-Wernicke disease, 115–117
Precautions to take before traveling, 294–297
Prickly heat, 292
Pthiriasis, 54, 272
Pythiosis, 132–133

Rabies, 257, 261–263
Rat bite fever, 275–276
Regional relapsing fever, 279–281
Reoviral diseases, 247–248
Rhabdoviral diseases, 249–250
Rhinosporidiosis, 134–135
Rift Valley fever, 242
River blindness, 76–78
Rotavirus disease, 248–249
Roundworm disease, 103–104

Salmonella gastroenteritis, 187
Sarcocystitis, 222
Sarcocystosis, 222
Sarcosporidiasis, 222
SARS, 242–243
Scabies, 80–82, 257, 264
Schistosomiasis (intestinal), 40–45
Schistosomiasis (urinary), 85–88
Scorpion-induced diseases, 276–277
Scrub typhus, 282–283
Scytalidiosis, 136–137
Sea anemone–induced diseases, 269
Searls ulcer, 144–145
Shigellosis, 188–189
Sleeping sickness, 15–18
Snake-induced diseases, 277–278
Sodoku, 275–276
Soft chancre, 146
Sparganosis, 101–102
Spider-induced diseases, 278–279
Strongyloidiasis, 46–48
Syphillis, 190–192

Tacaribe complex diseases, 237–238
Taeniasis, 257, 268
TB, 192–195
Tetanus, 260, 264–265
Tinea capitis, 54–55
Tinea nigra palmis, 82
Tinea nigra plantaris, 82
Tinea versicolor, 73
Togaviral diseases, 250
Toxocariasis, 103–104, 260, 265
Trachoma, 199–200
Travelers and tropical diseases, 292–297
Traveler's diarrhea, 297–299
Trench fever, 272
Trichinosis, 104–106
Trichomoniasis, 56–57
Trichuriasis, 49
Trombiculidae, 282–283
Tropical anhidrotic asthenia, 290
Tumba fly, 73–75
Tungiasis, 82–84, 268
Turista, 297–299
Trypanosomiasis (African), 15–18
Trypanosomiasis (American), 19–21
Typhoid fever, 182–186
Typhus (murine), 266–267
Typhus (scrub), 282–283

Ubiquitous relapsing fever, 272–273
Ulcus molle, 146
Urethritis and cervicitis, 201–202

Variant Creutzfeldt-Jakob disease, 202–204

Wasp-induced diseases, 253–254
Weil disease, 162–163
Whipworm infection, 49
Whitmore disease, 163–166
Whooping cough, 167168

Yaws, 195–196
Yellow fever, 232–234

Symptom Index

abdominal distentions
  Typhoid fever (or Enteric Fever), 183
abdominal mass
  Hydatidosis, 96
abdominal pain/cramps
  Amebiasis, 22, 24
  Ascariasis, 30
  Balantidiasis, 35
  Cholera, 149
  Ciguatera, 284
  Distomatosis, 35, 37
  Epidemic louse-borne typhus, 270
  Giardiasis, 39
  Gonorrhea (or Clap), 154
  Hepatitis, 210
  Histoplasmosis (or Darling Disease), 123
  HIV/AIDS, 222
  Influenza (or Flu), 225
  Lassa fever, 239
  Malaria, 8
  Meningococcal meningitis, 167
  Mushroom poisoning, 288
  Pneumococcal disease, 178
  Poliomyelitis (or Polio), 230
  Salmonella gastroenteritis, 187
  Shigellosis, 188
  Snake-induced diseases, 278
  Sparganosis, 101
  Strongyloidiasis, 46
  Taeniasis, 268
  Toxocasriasis, 103
  Traveler's diarrhea (Turista), 298
  Trichinosis, 104
  Trichomoniasis, 57
  Trichuriasis, 49
  Ubiquitous relapsing fever, 273
  Urethritis and cervicitis, 201
  Yellow fever (or Black vomit), 233

abscesses
  Histoplasmosis (African), 120
  Pneumococcal disease, 177
  Toxocasriasis, 103
adenolymphocele
  Filariasis (lymphatic), 2
adenopathy
  Anthrax, 139
  Bartonellosis (or Carrion disease), 141
  Blastomycosis (or Lutz-Splendore-Almeida disease), 110
  cat bite-induced diseases, 256
  Cat scratch disease, 257
  Dengue fever (or Breakbone fever), 206
  Filariasis (lymphatic), 2
  Hendra virosis, 246
  Leishmaniasis (or Kala-azar, or Dum dum disease), 4
  Plague (or Black death), 174
  Scrub typhus, 282
  Sodoku (or Rat bite fever), 275
  Toxocasriasis, 103
  Trypanosomiasis, 15, 19
adnexal mass/tenderness
  Gonorrhea (or Clap), 154
agitation
  Dengue fever (or Breakbone fever), 206
  Heat asthenia (or Tropical anhidrotic asthenia), 290
  Heat exhaustion, 290
  Influenza (or Flu), 225
  jellyfish-induced diseases, 269
  Pneumococcal disease, 177
  Poliomyelitis (or Polio), 230
  Rabies, 261
  Scabies, 264
  snake-induced diseases, 278
  Yellow fever (or Black vomit), 233

allergic reactions
  bees and hymenoptera-induced
    diseases, 253
  cat bite-induced diseases, 256
  Distomatosis, 35
  Fascioliasis, 32–33
  HIV/AIDS, 221
  jellyfish-induced diseases, 269
  mollusk-induced diseases, 274
  Schistosomiasis, 41
  Trichinosis, 105
alopecia
  Dermatophytosis, 59
  HIV/AIDS, 221
  Leprosy (or Hansen disease), 159
amaurosis
  Cysticercosis, 92
anemia
  Ancylostomiasis, 27
  Bartonellosis (or Carrion disease),
    141
  leech-induced diseases, 269
angina
  Histoplasmosis (or Darling disease),
    123
  Trypanosomiasis, 19–20
angiocholecystitis
  Distomatosis, 35
angiocholitis
  Distomatosis, 35
anhidrosis
  Leprosy (or Hansen disease), 159
anorexia
  Anthrax, 139
  Balantidiasis, 35
  Giardiasis, 39
  Heat asthenia (or Tropical anhidrotic asthenia), 290
  Hepatitis, 210
  HIV/AIDS, 222
  Pneumococcal disease, 177
  S.A.R.S., 243
  Toxocasriasis, 103
  Tuberculosis, 193
  Typhoid fever (or Enteric fever),
    183
  Ubiquitous relapsing fever, 273
anxiety
  Cholera, 149
  Heat asthenia (or Tropical anhidrotic asthenia), 290
  snake-induced diseases, 278
apathy
  Typhoid fever (or Enteric fever), 183
aphonia
  Diphtheria, 152

arrhythmia
  Ciguatera, 284
  fish poisoning, 265
  mushroom poisoning, 289
  snake-induced diseases, 278
  Trypanosomiasis, 19–20
arthralgia
  Bartonellosis (or Carrion disease),
    141
  Ciguatera, 284
  Dengue fever (or Breakbone fever),
    206
  Epidemic louse-borne typhus, 270
  Hepatitis, 210
  Influenza (or Flu), 225
  Leptospirosis (or Weil disease or
    Nanukayami fever), 163
  Malaria, 8
  Schistosomiasis, 41
  Shigellosis, 188
  Sodoku (or Rat bite fever), 275
  Toxocasriasis, 103
  Ubiquitous relapsing fever, 273
arthritis
  Gonorrhea (or Clap), 155
  Pneumococcal disease, 177
ascites
  Anthrax, 139
  Blastomycosis (or Lutz-Splendore-
    Almeida disease), 110
asphyxia
  mollusk-induced diseases, 274
asthenia
  Blastomycosis (or Gilchrist disease
    or Chicago disease), 109
  Blastomycosis (or Lutz-Splendore-
    Almeida disease), 110
  Cat scratch disease, 257
  Ciguatera, 284
  Coccidioidomycosis (or
    Posadas-Wernicke, or Posadas-
    Rixford disease), 115
  Distomatosis, 35, 37
  Heat asthenia (or Tropical anhidrotic asthenia), 290
  Hepatitis, 210
  HIV/AIDS, 222
  jellyfish-induced diseases, 269
  leech-induced diseases, 269
  Pneumococcal disease, 178
  Shigellosis, 188
  Sodoku (or Rat bite fever), 275
  Tuberculosis, 191
  Typhoid fever (or Enteric fever),
    183
  Ubiquitous relapsing fever, 273

asthma-like dyspnea
  Dracunculiasis, 60
  Strongyloidiasis, 46
  Trichinosis, 105
asthma-like symptoms
  spider-induced diseases, 278
ataxia
  HIV/AIDS, 222
  Lyssavirus disease, 250
  Prion disease (Vaiant Creutzfeldt-Jakob disease), 203

back pain
  Coccidioidomycosis (or Posadas-Wernicke, or Posadas-Rixford disease), 115
  Dengue fever (or Breakbone fever), 206
  Meningococcal meningitis, 167
  Poliomyelitis (or Polio), 230
  Rift Valley fever, 242
  Yellow fever (or Black vomit), 233
back rigidity
  Meningococcal meningitis, 167
bacterial infections
  Buruli ulcers (or Bairnsdale, Daintree, Mossman diseases, or Searls ulcers or Mycoburuli ulcers), 144
  Chromomycosis, 113
  Dracunculiasis, 60
  Filariasis (lymphatic), 2
  Larva migrans, 99
  Leishmaniasis, 63
  Miliaria (or Prickly heat), 292
  Muraenae-induced diseases (or Moray eel-induced diseases), 275
  Mycetoma (or Madura foot disease), 129
  Pediculosis capitis, 53
  Pediculosis corporis, 80
balance issues
  Cenurosis, 91
bladder infection
  Trichomoniasis, 57
bleeding. see *also* hemorrhage
  Arboviral diseases, 235
  Gonorrhea (or Clap), 154
blepharitis
  Cysticercosis, 92
blisters
  Cat scratch disease, 257
  Dermatophytosis, 59
  Dracunculiasis, 60

  Herpes simplex (or Cold or Fever sore), 215
  Miliaria (or Prickly heat), 292
bloating
  Amebiasis, 22
bone lesions
  Bejel (or Endemic syphilis), 143
  Blastomycosis (or Gilchrist disease or Chicago disease), 109
  Yaws (Pian, Parangi, Paru, or Frambesia tropica), 196
bowel disturbances
  fish poisoning, 287
  Taeniasis, 268
bradycardia
  Ciguatera, 284
  fish poisoning, 265
  mushroom poisoning, 289
brain abscesses. see abscesses
brain compression
  Linguatulosis, 100
breathing, difficulty with
  Heat exhaustion, 291
  Pneumococcal disease, 178
  Rabies, 261
bronchial compression
  Linguatulosis, 100
Brudzinski's sign
  Meningococcal meningitis, 168
burning sensation
  Candidiasis, 55
  centipede-induced diseases, 260
  Ciguatera, 284
  Dermatophytosis, 59
  Giardiasis, 39
  Herpes simplex (or Cold or Fever sore), 215
  jellyfish-induced diseases, 269
  Miliaria (or Prickly heat), 292
  Trichomoniasis, 56–57

calcification
  Porocephalosis, 101
cardiac arrest
  mollusk-induced diseases, 274
  Paragonimiasis, 50
  Trypanosomiasis, 19–20
cardiac insufficiency
  Histoplasmosis (or Darling disease), 123
  Lymphogranuloma venereum (or Nicholas-Favre-Durand disease), 197
cardiovascular collapse
  fish poisoning, 287

cardiovascular shock
  jellyfish-induced diseases, 269
  spider-induced diseases, 279
cellulitis
  cat bite-induced diseases, 256
  Pneumococcal disease, 177
cephalgia
  Angiostrongyliasis, 89
  Arboviral diseases, 235
  Balantidiasis, 35
  Bartonellosis (or Carrion disease), 141
  Cat scratch disease, 257
  Ciguatera, 284
  Coccidioidomycosis (or Posadas-Wernicke, or Posadas-Rixford disease), 115
  Cysticercosis, 92
  Dengue fever (or Breakbone fever), 206
  Ebola virus disease, 244
  Epidemic louse-borne typhus, 270
  fish poisoning, 287
  Heat asthenia (or Tropical anhidrotic asthenia), 290
  Heat exhaustion, 290
  Heat stroke, 291
  Hendra virosis, 246
  Influenza (or Flu), 225
  Leptospirosis (or Weil disease or Nanukayami fever), 163
  Malaria, 8
  Marburg virus disease, 245
  Meningococcal meningitis, 167
  Murine typhus, 266
  Nipah virosis, 247
  Plague (or Black death), 174
  Poliomyelitis (or Polio), 230
  Rift Valley fever, 242
  S.A.R.S., 243
  Schistosomiasis, 41
  Scrub typhus, 282
  Sodoku (or Rat bite fever), 275
  Toxocasriasis, 103
  Typhoid fever (or Enteric fever), 183
  Ubiquitous relapsing fever, 272
  Yellow fever (or Black vomit), 233
cerebral vasculitis
  Toxocasriasis, 103
cervical lesions
  Chancroid (or Soft chancre or Ulcus molle), 146
  Lymphogranuloma venereum (or Nicholas-Favre-Durand disease), 197

cervical motion tenderness
  Gonorrhea (or Clap), 154
cervicitis
  Herpes simplex (or Cold or Fever sore), 215
chancres
  Pinta (or Carate), 171
  Scabies, 80
  Syphilis (or Hard chancre), 191
  Yaws (Pian, Parangi, Paru, or Frambesia tropica), 196
cheloid nodules
  Lobomycosis (or Jorge Lobo disease), 127
chest pain
  Anthrax, 140
  Filariasis (lymphatic), 2
  Histoplasmosis (or Darling disease), 123
  Lassa fever, 239
  Paragonimiasis, 50
  Plague (or Black death), 174–175
  Pneumococcal disease, 178
  S.A.R.S., 243
chewing, difficulty with
  Poliomyelitis (or Polio), 231
chills
  Blastomycosis (or Gilchrist disease or Chicago disease), 109
  cat bite-induced diseases, 256
  Ciguatera, 284
  Dengue fever (or Breakbone fever), 206
  Epidemic louse-borne typhus, 270
  Gonorrhea (or Clap), 154
  Hepatitis, 210
  Influenza (or Flu), 225
  Lymphogranuloma venereum (or Nicholas-Favre-Durand disease), 197
  Malaria, 8
  Melioidosis (or Whitmore disease), 164
  Meningococcal meningitis, 167
  Plague (or Black death), 174–175
  Pneumococcal disease, 178
  Salmonella gastroenteritis, 187
  Sodoku (or Rat bite fever), 275
  Ubiquitous relapsing fever, 272
  Yellow fever (or Black vomit), 233
chorioretinitis
  Onchocerciasis, 76
chyluria
  Filariasis (lymphatic), 2

cicatricial lesions
  Granuloma inguinale (or Donovan disease), 156
cigarette smoke, distaste for
  Hepatitis, 210
cold
  Buruli ulcers (or Bairnsdale, Daintree, Mossman diseases, or Searls ulcer or Mycoburuli ulcers), 144
cold sweats
  Cholera, 149
  Ciguatera, 284
  Heat exhaustion, 290
colics
  spider-induced diseases, 279
coma
  Dengue fever (or Breakbone fever), 206
  Epidemic louse-borne typhus, 270
  Heat exhaustion, 291
  Lyssavirus disease, 250
  mushroom poisoning, 288
  snake-induced diseases, 278
concentration, difficulty with
  Heat asthenia (or Tropical anhidrotic asthenia), 290
  Lyssavirus disease, 250
confusion
  Heat stroke, 291
  Histoplasmosis (or Darling disease), 123
  Influenza (or Flu), 225
  Poliomyelitis (or Polio), 230
  Typhoid fever (or Enteric fever), 183
congested eyes/face
  Epidemic louse-borne typhus, 270
  Scrub typhus, 282
  Ubiquitous relapsing fever, 272
conjunctival hyperemia
  Ebola virus disease, 244
  Marburg virus disease, 245
  Pertussis (or Whooping cough), 170
conjunctivitis
  Gonorrhea (or Clap), 155
  Influenza (or Flu), 225
  Lassa fever, 239
  Measles, 228
  Pneumococcal disease, 177
  Trachoma (or Granular conjunctivits or Egyptian ophthalmia), 199
  Typhoid fever (or Enteric fever), 183
  Urethritis and cervicitis, 201

consciousness, altered
  Histoplasmosis (or Darling disease), 123
  Nipah virosis, 247
consciousness, loss of
  Heat exhaustion, 290
  Heat stroke, 291
constipation
  Distomatosis, 35
  Hepatitis, 210
  Poliomyelitis (or Polio), 230
  Typhoid fever (or Enteric fever), 183
  Ubiquitous relapsing fever, 273
convulsions
  Dengue fever (or Breakbone fever), 206
  fish poisoning, 265
  Muraenae-induced diseases (or Moray eel-induced diseases), 274–275
  mushroom poisoning, 288
coolness of extremities
  Heat exhaustion, 290, 291
corneal ulcers
  Leprosy (or Hansen disease), 160
  Pythiosis, 132
coryza
  Measles, 228
cough
  Ancylostomiasis, 27
  Anthrax, 140
  Ascariasis, 30
  Blastomycosis (or Gilchrist disease or Chicago disease), 109
  Blastomycosis (or Lutz-Splendore-Almeida disease), 111
  Coccidioidomycosis (or Posadas-Wernicke, or Posadas-Rixford disease), 115
  Hendra virosis, 246
  Histoplasmosis (or Darling disease), 123
  HIV/AIDS, 221
  Influenza (or Flu), 225
  Measles, 228
  Melioidosis (or Whitmore disease), 164
  Paragonimiasis, 50
  Pertussis (or Whooping cough), 170
  Plague (or Black death), 174–175
  Pneumococcal disease, 178
  S.A.R.S., 243
  Schistosomiasis, 41
  Strongyloidiasis, 46

cough (Cont.)
  Toxocasriasis, 103
  Tuberculosis, 191
  Urethritis and cervicitis, 201
cutaneous lesions
  Bejel (or Endemic syphilis), 143
cyanosis
  Anthrax, 140
  Cholera, 149
  Heat exhaustion, 290
  Plague (or Black death), 174–175

death
  Anthrax, 140
  Cholera, 149
  Ichthyosarcotoxisms, 287
  Lyssavirus disease, 250
  Rabies, 261
  snake-induced diseases, 278
  spider-induced diseases, 279
  while traveling, 292–294
  Yellow fever (or Black vomit), 233
dehydration
  Balantidiasis, 35
  Cholera, 149
  Epidemic louse-borne typhus, 270
  Heat exhaustion, 290
  HIV/AIDS, 222
  Plague (or Black death), 174
  Rabies, 261
  Rotavirus disease, 248
  Shigellosis, 188
  Traveler's diarrhea (Turista), 298
delirium
  Filariasis (lymphatic), 1
  Heat stroke, 291
  mushroom poisoning, 289
  Plague (or Black death), 174
  Rabies, 261
  Yellow fever (or Black vomit), 233
dementia
  Prion disease (Variant Creutzfeldt-Jakob disease), 203
  Toxocasriasis, 103
depression
  Heat asthenia (or Tropical anhidrotic asthenia), 290
diaphoresis
  Anthrax, 140
  Heat asthenia (or Tropical anhidrotic asthenia), 290
  Heat exhaustion, 290
  mushroom poisoning, 289
  spider-induced diseases, 278
diarrhea
  Amebiasis, 22
  Ancylostomiasis, 27
  Anthrax, 139
  Ascariasis, 30
  Balantidiasis, 35
  bees and hymenoptera-induced diseases, 253
  Cholera, 149
  Ciguatera, 284
  Distomatosis, 35, 37
  Ebola virus disease, 244
  fish poisoning, 288
  Giardiasis, 39
  Hepatitis, 210
  Histoplasmosis (or Darling disease), 123
  HIV/AIDS, 221, 222
  Influenza (or Flu), 225
  Leishmaniasis (or Kala-azar, or Dum dum disease), 4
  Malaria, 8
  Marburg virus disease, 245
  Melioidosis (or Whitmore disease), 164
  mushroom poisoning, 288, 289
  Plague (or Black death), 174
  Pneumococcal disease, 178
  Poliomyelitis (or Polio), 230
  Rotavirus disease, 248
  Salmonella gastroenteritis, 187
  Schistosomiasis, 41
  Shigellosis, 188
  snake-induced diseases, 278
  Strongyloidiasis, 46
  Toxocasriasis, 103
  Traveler's diarrhea (Turista), 298
  Trichinosis, 104
  Trichuriasis, 49
  Typhoid fever (or Enteric fever), 183
diplopia
  mollusk-induced diseases, 274
  Poliomyelitis (or Polio), 231
dizziness
  bees and hymenoptera-induced diseases, 253
  Ciguatera, 284
  Epidemic louse-borne typhus, 270
  fish poisoning, 287
  Influenza (or Flu), 225
  mushroom poisoning, 289
  Nipah virosis, 247
  snake-induced diseases, 278
  Typhoid fever (or Enteric fever), 183
drinking, difficulty with
  Heat exhaustion, 291

drowsiness
  Heat asthenia (or Tropical anhidrotic asthenia), 290
  Nipah virosis, 247
dysarthria
  Prion disease (Variant Creutzfeldt-Jakob disease), 203
dysesthesia
  fish poisoning, 287
dyskeratosis
  Yaws (Pian, Parangi, Paru, or Frambesia tropica), 196
dyspareunia
  Candidiasis, 55
  Chancroid (or Soft chancre or Ulcus molle), 146
  Trichomoniasis, 57
  Urethritis and cervicitis, 201
dyspeptic disorders
  Heat asthenia (or Tropical anhidrotic asthenia), 290
dysphagia
  Linguatulosis, 100
  Scabies, 264
dysphonia
  Linguatulosis, 100
dyspnea
  Anthrax, 140
  bees and hymenoptera-induced diseases, 253
  Blastomycosis (or Gilchrist disease or Chicago disease), 109
  Dracunculiasis, 60
  fish poisoning, 288
  Histoplasmosis (or Darling disease), 123
  Influenza (or Flu), 225
  jellyfish-induced diseases, 269
  leech-induced diseases, 269
  Linguatulosis, 100
  mushroom poisoning, 289
  Plague (or Black death), 174–175
  S.A.R.S., 243
  Schistosomiasis, 41
  spider-induced diseases, 279
  Strongyloidiasis, 46
  Toxocasriasis, 103
  Trichinosis, 105
dysuria
  Chancroid (or Soft chancre or Ulcus molle), 146
  Gonorrhea (or Clap), 154
  Schistosomiasis, 85
  Urethritis and cervicitis, 201

ear discharge
  Pneumococcal disease, 177
ear lesions
  Leprosy (or Hansen disease), 160
ear pain
  Pneumococcal disease, 177, 178
edema
  Anthrax, 139
  Basidiobolomycosis, 107
  bees and hymenoptera-induced diseases, 253
  Buruli ulcers (or Bairnsdale, Daintree, Mossman diseases, or Searls ulcers or Mycoburuli ulcer), 144
  Diphtheria, 152
  Distomatosis, 37
  Filariasis (lymphatic), 2
  fish poisoning, 287
  Lassa fever, 239
  Loiasis, 70
  mollusk-induced diseases, 274
  Pythiosis, 132
  Schistosomiasis, 41
  snake-induced diseases, 278
  Toxocasriasis, 103
  Trichinosis, 104
  Trypanosomiasis, 15, 19
  Tungiasis, 82
  Yaws (Pian, Parangi, Paru, or Frambesia tropica), 196
elephantiasis
  Chromomycosis, 113
  Filariasis (lymphatic), 2
  Granuloma inguinale (or Donovan disease), 156
embolism
  Trypanosomiasis, 19–20
emesis
  Ancylostomiasis, 27
  Angiostrongyliasis, 89
  Anthrax, 139
  Ascariasis, 30
  Balantidiasis, 35
  bees and hymenoptera-induced diseases, 253
  Cholera, 149
  Ciguatera, 284
  Cysticercosis, 92
  Dracunculiasis, 60
  Ebola virus disease, 244
  Epidemic louse-borne typhus, 270
  fish poisoning, 288
  Gnathostomiasis, 94
  Gonorrhea (or Clap), 154
  Hepatitis, 210

emesis (Cont.)
  Influenza (or Flu), 225
  Lassa fever, 239
  Lyssavirus disease, 250
  Malaria, 8
  Marburg virus disease, 245
  Meningococcal meningitis, 167
  mollusk-induced diseases, 274
  Muraenae-induced diseases (or Moray eel-induced diseases), 274–275
  mushroom poisoning, 288, 289
  Nipah virosis, 247
  Pertussis (or Whooping cough), 170
  Plague (or Black death), 174
  Pneumococcal disease, 178
  Poliomyelitis (or Polio), 230
  Rift Valley fever, 242
  Salmonella gastroenteritis, 187
  Shigellosis, 188
  snake-induced diseases, 278
  Sodoku (or Rat bite fever), 275
  spider-induced diseases, 279
  Traveler's diarrhea (Turista), 298
  Ubiquitous relapsing fever, 273
  Yellow fever (or Black vomit), 233
emotional instability
  Prion disease (Variant Creutzfeldt-Jakob disease), 203
encephalitis
  Cat scratch disease, 257
  Herpes simplex (or Cold or Fever sore), 215
  HIV/AIDS, 217
  Nipah virosis, 247
  Poliomyelitis (or Polio), 230
endocarditis
  Pneumococcal disease, 177
endophthalmitis
  Toxocasriasis, 103
entropion
  Trachoma (or Granular conjunctivits or Egyptian ophthalmia), 199
eosinophilia
  Porocephalosis, 101
epilepsy
  Toxocasriasis, 103
epistaxis
  Conidiobolomycosis, 118
  Linguatulosis, 100
  Typhoid fever (or Enteric fever), 183
  Yellow fever (or Black vomit), 233
eructation
  Giardiasis, 39
erythema
  bees and hymenoptera-induced diseases, 253
  Coccidioidomycosis (or Posadas-Wernicke, or Posadas-Rixford disease), 115
  fish poisoning, 288
  Herpes simplex (or Cold or Fever sore), 215
erythematous lesions
  Diphtheria, 152
  spider-induced diseases, 279
exanthem
  Leptospirosis (or Weil disease or Nanukayami fever), 163
excitement
  mushroom poisoning, 289
  spider-induced diseases, 278
exophtalmia
  Cysticercosis, 92
extrapyramidal rigidity
  HIV/AIDS, 222
eye circles
  Cholera, 149
eye discharge
  Urethritis and cervicitis, 201
eyelids/sockets, swollen
  Sparganosis, 101
eyes, sunken
  Heat exhaustion, 290, 291
  Rotavirus disease, 248

face, flushed
  Dengue fever (or Breakbone fever), 206
  fish poisoning, 288
  mushroom poisoning, 289
face, gaunt
  Cholera, 149
facial muscle weakness
  Poliomyelitis (or Polio), 231
Faget's sign
  Yellow fever (or Black vomit), 233
fasciculation
  scorpion-induced diseases, 276
  spider-induced diseases, 279
fatigue
  Amebiasis, 22
  Filariasis (lymphatic), 1
  Heat exhaustion, 290
  Influenza (or Flu), 225
  Leishmaniasis (or Kala-azar, or Dum dum disease), 4
  Murine typhus, 266
  spider-induced diseases, 278

fever
  Amebiasis, 24
  Angiostrongyliasis, 89
  Anthrax, 139, 140
  Arboviral diseases, 235
  Ascariasis, 30
  Bartonellosis (or Carrion disease), 141
  Blastomycosis (or Gilchrist disease or Chicago disease), 109
  Blastomycosis (or Lutz-Splendore-Almeida disease), 110
  cat bite-induced diseases, 256
  Cat scratch disease, 257
  Coccidioidomycosis (or Posadas-Wernicke, or Posadas-Rixford disease), 115
  Dengue fever (or Breakbone fever), 206
  Distomatosis, 35
  Dracunculiasis, 60
  Ebola virus disease, 244
  Epidemic louse-borne typhus, 270
  Fascioliasis, 32–33
  Filariasis (lymphatic), 1
  Flaviviral diseases, 245
  Gnathostomiasis, 94
  Gonorrhea (or Clap), 154, 155
  Hendra virosis, 246
  Hepatitis, 210
  Herpes simplex (or Cold or Fever sore), 215
  Histoplasmosis (or Darling disease), 123
  HIV/AIDS, 221, 222
  Influenza (or Flu), 225
  jellyfish-induced diseases, 269
  Lassa fever, 239
  Leishmaniasis (or Kala-azar, or Dum dum disease), 4
  Leptospirosis (or Weil disease or Nanukayami fever), 163
  Lymphogranuloma venereum (or Nicholas-Favre-Durand disease), 197
  Malaria, 8–9
  Marburg virus disease, 245
  Measles, 228
  Melioidosis (or Whitmore disease), 164
  Meningococcal meningitis, 167
  Murine typhus, 266
  Nipah virosis, 247
  Paragonimiasis, 50
  Pertussis (or Whooping cough), 170
  Plague (or Black death), 174–175
  Pneumococcal disease, 177, 178
  Poliomyelitis (or Polio), 230, 231
  Rabies, 261
  Regional relapsing fever, 280
  Rift Valley fever, 242
  Rotavirus disease, 248
  Salmonella gastroenteritis, 187
  S.A.R.S., 243
  Schistosomiasis, 41
  Scrub typhus, 282
  Shigellosis, 188
  snake-induced diseases, 278
  Sodoku (or Rat bite fever), 275
  Toxocasriasis, 103
  Traveler's diarrhea (Turista), 298
  Trench fever (or His-Werner disease), 272
  Trichinosis, 104, 105
  Trypanosomiasis, 15, 19
  Tuberculosis, 191
  Typhoid fever (or Enteric fever), 183
  Urethritis and cervicitis, 201
  Yellow fever (or Black vomit), 233
flatulence
  Giardiasis, 39
flu-like syndrome
  Arboviral diseases, 235
  Arenaviral diseases, 237
  Chikungunya virus disease, 251
  Flaviviral diseases, 245
  Hantaan virosis, 240
  Hendra virosis, 246
  Histoplasmosis (or Darling disease), 123
  Meningococcal meningitis, 167
  Mossuril virus disease, 249
  Poliomyelitis (or Polio), 230
  Reoviral diseases, 248
  Rift Valley fever, 242
fontanel, sunken/soft
  Rotavirus disease, 248
foot pain
  Meningococcal meningitis, 167
foot ulcers
  Mycetoma (or Madura foot disease), 129
fourchette lesions
  Lymphogranuloma venereum (or Nicholas-Favre-Durand disease), 197

gait disturbances
  Histoplasmosis (or Darling disease), 123

gangrene
  fish poisoning, 265
  Pythiosis, 132
  spider-induced diseases, 279
gastralgia
  Cholera, 149
  Gnathostomiasis, 94
  Strongyloidiasis, 46
gastroenteritis
  fish poisoning, 287
GI disturbances
  Dengue fever (or Breakbone fever), 206
  Ichthyosarcotoxisms, 287
  Trypanosomiasis, 19
GI tract hemorrhage
  Dengue fever (or Breakbone fever), 206
glaucoma
  Linguatulosis, 100
gonococcal infection
  Gonorrhea (or Clap), 155
goose bumps
  Heat exhaustion, 290
granulomas
  Rhinosporidiosis, 134
growth, stunted
  Giardiasis, 39
  HIV/AIDS, 221
gynecomastia
  Leprosy (or Hansen disease), 160

hairy leukoplakia
  HIV/AIDS, 221
hallucinations
  mushroom poisoning, 289
hand pain
  Meningococcal meningitis, 167
headache
  Histoplasmosis (or Darling disease), 123
  Poliomyelitis (or Polio), 230
hearing problems
  Cenurosis, 91
heart murmur
  leech-induced diseases, 269
heart pumping function, abnormal
  Pneumococcal disease, 178
heart rate, high
  Pneumococcal disease, 178
hematemesis
  Anthrax, 139, 140
  mushroom poisoning, 288
  Yellow fever (or Black vomit), 233
hematochezia
  Anthrax, 139

  mushroom poisoning, 288
  Yellow fever (or Black vomit), 233
hematuria
  Schistosomiasis, 85
  Yellow fever (or Black vomit), 233
hemoptysis
  Blastomycosis (or Gilchrist disease or Chicago disease), 109
  Histoplasmosis (or Darling disease), 123
  Paragonimiasis, 50
hemorrhage. see also bleeding
  Dengue fever (or Breakbone fever), 206
  Lassa fever, 239
  Rift Valley fever, 242
  snake-induced diseases, 278
  Yellow fever (or Black vomit), 233
hemorrhagic mediastinitis
  Anthrax, 140
hepatic colic
  Distomatosis, 35
hepatic disturbances
  Arboviral diseases, 235
hepatitis
  Dengue fever (or Breakbone fever), 207
  Lymphogranuloma venereum (or Nicholas-Favre-Durand disease), 197
hepatomegaly
  Dengue fever (or Breakbone fever), 206
  Distomatosis, 35
  HIV/AIDS, 221
  Hydatidosis, 96
  Leishmaniasis (or Kala-azar, or Dum dum disease), 4
  Toxocasriasis, 103
  Trypanosomiasis, 15
hepatosplenomegaly
  Bartonellosis (or Carrion disease), 141
  Blastomycosis (or Lutz-Splendore-Almeida disease), 110
  Scrub typhus, 282
herpes
  HIV/AIDS, 221
herpetic lesion
  Malaria, 8
hoarseness
  Diphtheria, 152
hydrocele
  Filariasis (lymphatic), 2
hyperemia
  Gonorrhea (or Clap), 155

hyperkeratosis
  Yaws (Pian, Parangi, Paru, or
    Frambesia tropica), 196
hyperkeratotic skin/bone lesions
  Yaws (Pian, Parangi, Paru, or
    Frambesia tropica), 196
hypersalivation
  spider-induced diseases, 279
hypertension
  scorpion-induced diseases, 276
hypertrophic lesions
  Granuloma inguinale (or Donovan
    disease), 156
hypertrophy of nasal bone
  Yaws (Pian, Parangi, Paru, or
    Frambesia tropica), 196
hypoesthesia
  Leprosy (or Hansen disease), 159
  scorpion-induced diseases, 276
hypopigmentation
  Onchocerciasis, 76
hypopyon
  Toxocasriasis, 103
hypotension
  bees and hymenoptera-induced
    diseases, 253
  fish poisoning, 265
  Meningococcal meningitis, 167
  mushroom poisoning, 289
hypotonia
  Ciguatera, 284
hypovolemic shock
  Anthrax, 139
  Cholera, 149

icterus
  Bartonellosis (or Carrion disease), 141
  Distomatosis, 35
  Fascioliasis, 32–33
  fish poisoning, 287
  Hepatitis, 210
  Leptospirosis (or Weil disease or
    Nanukayami fever), 163
  Linguatulosis, 100
  Malaria, 8
  Ubiquitous relapsing fever, 273
  Yellow fever (or Black vomit), 233
inflammation
  Basidiobolomycosis, 107
inflammatory disease
  Lymphogranuloma venereum
    (or Nicholas-Favre-Durand
    disease), 197
insomnia
  Heat asthenia (or Tropical
    anhidrotic asthenia), 290

Pneumococcal disease, 177
interstitial lymphoid pneumonia
  HIV/AIDS, 221
intertrigo
  Scytalidosis, 136
intestinal perforation
  Typhoid fever (or Enteric fever),
    183
iridocyclitis
  Onchocerciasis, 76
iritis
  Cysticercosis, 92
  Toxocasriasis, 103
irritability. see agitation
itching
  butterfly-induced diseases, 254
  centipede-induced diseases, 260
  Ciguatera, 284
  Dermatophytosis, 59
  fish poisoning, 287
  Herpes simplex (or Cold or Fever
    sore), 215
  jellyfish-induced diseases, 269
  Larva migrans, 99
  Miliaria (or Prickly heat), 292
  Pediculosis capitis, 53
  Pediculosis corporis, 80
  Pthiriasis, 54
  Rabies, 261

jaundice
  Hepatitis, 210
jaw stiffness
  Scabies, 264
joint pain
  Histoplasmosis (or Darling disease),
    123

Kala-azar
  HIV/AIDS, 221
Kaposi syndrome
  HIV/AIDS, 221
keratitis
  Leprosy (or Hansen disease), 160
  Onchocerciasis, 76
  Pythiosis, 132
  Toxocasriasis, 103
Kernig's sign
  Meningococcal meningitis, 168

lacrimation
  mushroom poisoning, 289
  Pertussis (or Whooping cough),
    170
  Trachoma (or Granular conjunctivits
    or Egyptian ophthalmia), 199

larva currens
  Strongyloidiasis, 46
lesions. see *specific body parts*
lethargy. see *also* malaise
  Heat exhaustion, 291
  Hendra virosis, 246
  Poliomyelitis (or Polio), 230
leukocoria
  Toxocasriasis, 103
leukomelnoderma
  Pediculosis corporis, 80
lichinification
  Onchocerciasis, 76
lightheadedness
  Heat exhaustion, 290
liver failure
  mushroom poisoning, 288
Loeffler syndrome
  Ascariasis, 30
lung lesions
  Blastomycosis (or Lutz-Splendore-Almeida disease), 110
  Coccidioidomycosis (or Posadas-Wernicke, or Posadas-Rixford disease), 115
lympadenopathy
  HIV/AIDS, 221
lymph nodes, burst
  Plague (or Black death), 174
lymph nodes, oozing
  Cat scratch disease, 257
  Melioidosis (or Whitmore disease), 164
lymph nodes, swollen
  Blastomycosis (or Lutz-Splendore-Almeida disease), 111
  Herpes simplex (or Cold or Fever sore), 215
  Histoplasmosis (African), 120
  Lymphogranuloma venereum (or Nicholas-Favre-Durand disease), 197
lymphadenitis
  Sodoku (or Rat bite fever), 275
lymphadenopathy
  Chancroid (or Soft chancre or Ulcus molle), 146
  Diphtheria, 152
  HIV/AIDS, 221
  Lymphogranuloma venereum (or Nicholas-Favre-Durand disease), 197
  Toxocasriasis, 103
  Yaws (Pian, Parangi, Paru, or Frambesia tropica), 196

lymphangitis
  Anthrax, 139
  Filariasis (lymphatic), 1–2
lymphocytic meningitis
  HIV/AIDS, 217

macular lesions
  Scrub typhus, 282
macular skin eruption
  Toxocasriasis, 103
macules
  Dermatophytosis, 59
  Leprosy (or Hansen disease), 159, 160
  Malasseziosis, 73
  Pediculosis corporis, 80
  Pinta (or Carate), 172
  Tinea nigra palmis, 82
  Yaws (Pian, Parangi, Paru, or Frambesia tropica), 196
maculopapular eruptions
  Ebola virus disease, 244
  Marburg virus disease, 245
  Onchocerciasis, 76
maculopapular lesions
  Scrub typhus, 282
maculopapules
  Yaws (Pian, Parangi, Paru, or Frambesia tropica), 196
malabsorption syndrome
  Giardiasis, 39
  HIV/AIDS, 222
malaise. see *also* lethargy
  Anthrax, 139
  Bartonellosis (or Carrion disease), 141
  Epidemic louse-borne typhus, 270
  Hepatitis, 210
  Herpes simplex (or Cold or Fever sore), 215
  Histoplasmosis (or Darling disease), 123
  Malaria, 8
  Plague (or Black death), 174
  Toxocasriasis, 103
  Trichinosis, 104
membranes
  Diphtheria, 152
memory loss, short-term
  fish poisoning, 288
meningitis
  Cysticercosis, 92
  Dengue fever (or Breakbone fever), 207
  Herpes simplex (or Cold or Fever sore), 215

Lymphogranuloma venereum (or Nicholas-Favre-Durand disease), 197
Pneumococcal disease, 177
Poliomyelitis (or Polio), 230
meningoencephalitis
  Angiostrongyliasis, 89
  Hendra virosis, 246
  Rift Valley fever, 242
  Toxocasriasis, 103
  Trypanosomiasis, 19
mental confusion
  Cysticercosis, 92
  Dengue fever (or Breakbone fever), 206
  Epidemic louse-borne typhus, 270
  Pneumococcal disease, 178
  Poliomyelitis (or Polio), 230
molluscum contagiosum
  HIV/AIDS, 221
mono-like syndrome
  HIV/AIDS, 217
mononeuritis
  Leprosy (or Hansen disease), 160
morbilliform skin eruption
  Trench fever (or His-Werner disease), 272
motor disorders
  fish poisoning, 287
mouth, dry
  Heat exhaustion, 290, 291
  Rotavirus disease, 248
mouth, sticky
  Heat exhaustion, 291
mucous membrane hemorrhage
  Dengue fever (or Breakbone fever), 206
  Yellow fever (or Black vomit), 233
mucous membrane lesions
  Histoplasmosis (or Darling disease), 123
  Syphilis (or Hard chancre), 191
multineuritis
  HIV/AIDS, 221
muscle atrophy
  Poliomyelitis (or Polio), 231
muscle cramps
  Heat exhaustion, 290
  Heat stroke, 291
muscle pain
  Poliomyelitis (or Polio), 231
muscle paralysis
  mollusk-induced diseases, 274
muscle spasms
  mollusk-induced diseases, 274
  spider-induced diseases, 278

muscle stiffness
  Scabies, 264
myalgia
  Arboviral diseases, 235
  Ciguatera, 284
  Dengue fever (or Breakbone fever), 206
  Ebola virus disease, 244
  Epidemic louse-borne typhus, 270
  Hendra virosis, 246
  Hepatitis, 210
  Herpes simplex (or Cold or Fever sore), 215
  Influenza (or Flu), 225
  Lassa fever, 239
  Leptospirosis (or Weil disease or Nanukayami fever), 163
  Malaria, 8
  Marburg virus disease, 245
  Murine typhus, 266
  Nipah virosis, 247
  Rift Valley fever, 242
  S.A.R.S., 243
  Schistosomiasis, 41
  Scrub typhus, 282
  Shigellosis, 188
  Sodoku (or Rat bite fever), 275
  Toxocasriasis, 103
  Trichinosis, 104, 105
  Typhoid fever (or Enteric fever), 183
  Ubiquitous relapsing fever, 273
  Yellow fever (or Black vomit), 233
mycosis
  HIV/AIDS, 221
mydriasis
  Ciguatera, 284
  mushroom poisoning, 289
myelitis
  Herpes simplex (or Cold or Fever sore), 215
  HIV/AIDS, 217, 221
  Toxocasriasis, 103
myocarditis
  Trypanosomiasis, 19
myopia
  Hantaan virosis, 240
myosis
  mushroom poisoning, 289
myositis
  Pneumococcal disease, 177

nail alterations
  Ancylostomiasis, 27
  Candidiasis, 52
  Dermatophytosis, 53
  leech-induced diseases, 269

nasal congestion
  Pertussis (or Whooping cough), 170
nausea
  Ancylostomiasis, 27
  Angiostrongyliasis, 89
  Anthrax, 139
  Ascariasis, 30
  Balantidiasis, 35
  bees and hymenoptera-induced diseases, 253
  Ciguatera, 284
  Cysticercosis, 92
  Dracunculiasis, 60
  Epidemic louse-borne typhus, 270
  fish poisoning, 287–288
  Giardiasis, 39
  Gnathostomiasis, 94
  Gonorrhea (or Clap), 154
  Heat asthenia (or Tropical anhidrotic asthenia), 290
  Heat exhaustion, 290
  Heat stroke, 291
  Hepatitis, 210
  Influenza (or Flu), 225
  Malaria, 8
  Meningococcal meningitis, 167
  mollusk-induced diseases, 274
  mushroom poisoning, 289
  Pneumococcal disease, 177, 178
  Poliomyelitis (or Polio), 230
  Rift Valley fever, 242
  Salmonella gastroenteritis, 187
  snake-induced diseases, 278
  spider-induced diseases, 279
  Toxocasriasis, 103
  Traveler's diarrhea (Turista), 298
neck pain
  Poliomyelitis (or Polio), 230
neck stiffness
  Angiostrongyliasis, 89
  Leptospirosis (or Weil disease or Nanukayami fever), 163
  Meningococcal meningitis, 167
  Rift Valley fever, 242
  Scabies, 264
necrosis
  fish poisoning, 265
  snake-induced diseases, 278
neurological deficits
  Angiostrongyliasis, 89
  Arboviral diseases, 235
  HIV/AIDS, 221–222
neurological lesions
  Leprosy (or Hansen disease), 160, 161

night sweats
  Tuberculosis, 191
nodular lesions
  Granuloma inguinale (or Donovan disease), 156
nodules
  Buruli ulcers (or Bairnsdale, Daintree, Mossman diseases, or Searls ulcer or Mycoburuli ulcers), 144
  Cat scratch disease, 257
  Cysticercosis, 92
  Histoplasmosis (African), 120
  Yaws (Pian, Parangi, Paru, or Frambesia tropica), 196
nose mass
  Conidiobolomycosis, 118
numbness
  snake-induced diseases, 277–278

obnubilation
  Heat stroke, 291
odor, foul
  Diphtheria, 152
odynophagia
  Ancylostomiasis, 27
odynophonia
  Ancylostomiasis, 27
oliguria
  Heat exhaustion, 290–291
  Leptospirosis (or Weil disease or Nanukayami fever), 163
opththalmalgia
  Toxocasriasis, 103
optic neuritis
  Toxocasriasis, 103
optic vascular lesions
  HIV/AIDS, 221
oral candidiasis
  HIV/AIDS, 221
oral lesions
  Candidiasis, 58
orchiepididymitis
  Filariasis (lymphatic), 2
orchitis
  Filariasis (lymphatic), 1
organs, enlargment of
  Trypanosomiasis, 20
orthostatic hypotension
  Heat exhaustion, 290
osteitis
  Yaws (Pian, Parangi, Paru, or Frambesia tropica), 196
osteomyelitis
  Pneumococcal disease, 177

osteoperiostitis
  Yaws (Pian, Parangi, Paru, or Frambesia tropica), 196
otitis media
  Pneumococcal disease, 177
overlacrimation
  spider-induced diseases, 278

pain
  Arboviral diseases, 235
  bees and hymenoptera-induced diseases, 253
  Ciguatera, 284
  Fascioliasis, 32–33
  fish poisoning, 265
  Gnathostomiasis, 94
  Muraenae-induced diseases (or Moray eel-induced diseases), 274–275
  Plague (or Black death), 174
  scorpion-induced diseases, 276
  snake-induced diseases, 277, 278
  spider-induced diseases, 278
  Trench fever (or His-Werner disease), 272
  Tungiasis, 82
  Ubiquitous relapsing fever, 272
palate enanthema
  Ebola virus disease, 244
  Marburg virus disease, 245
palsy
  Lyssavirus disease, 250
  mollusk-induced diseases, 274
pannus
  Trachoma (or Granular conjunctivits or Egyptian ophthalmia), 199
papilledema
  Cysticercosis, 92
papillomas
  Rhinosporidiosis, 134
papular nonpruritic rash
  Coccidioidomycosis (or Posadas-Wernicke, or Posadas-Rixford disease), 115
papular prurigo
  HIV/AIDS, 221
papules
  Blastomycosis (or Gilchrist disease or Chicago disease), 109
  Buruli ulcers (or Bairnsdale, Daintree, Mossman diseases, or Searls ulcer or Mycoburuli ulcers), 144
  butterfly-induced diseases, 254
  Gonorrhea (or Clap), 155
  Histoplasmosis (African), 120
  HIV/AIDS, 221
  Leishmaniasis, 64
  Leprosy (or Hansen disease), 161
  Lymphogranuloma venereum (or Nicholas-Favre-Durand disease), 197
  Pediculosis corporis, 80
  Pinta (or Carate), 171–172
  Pthiriasis, 54
papulonodules
  Leprosy (or Hansen disease), 160
papulovesicular eruption
  Ebola virus disease, 244
  Marburg virus disease, 245
paralysis
  fish poisoning, 265, 287
  Poliomyelitis (or Polio), 231
  Rabies, 261
  snake-induced diseases, 278
parasitic cysts
  Linguatulosis, 100
paresthesia
  Ciguatera, 284
  fish poisoning, 287
  scorpion-induced diseases, 276
parethesia
  fish poisoning, 287
  mollusk-induced diseases, 274
  Rabies, 261
parotitis
  HIV/AIDS, 221
pericarditis
  Pneumococcal disease, 177
pericholangitis
  HIV/AIDS, 221
perihepatitis
  Lymphogranuloma venereum (or Nicholas-Favre-Durand disease), 197
periostitis
  Yaws (Pian, Parangi, Paru, or Frambesia tropica), 196
peripheral hypertrophic neuropathy
  Leprosy (or Hansen disease), 160
peritonitis
  Pneumococcal disease, 177
  Typhoid fever (or Enteric fever), 183
personality changes
  Rabies, 261
petechiae
  Toxocasriasis, 103
pharyngeal infection
  Gonorrhea (or Clap), 155
pharyngitis
  Ebola virus disease, 244
  Gonorrhea (or Clap), 155

pharyngitis (Cont.)
  Hepatitis, 210
  Herpes simplex (or Cold or Fever sore), 215
  Influenza (or Flu), 225
  Lassa fever, 239
  Marburg virus disease, 245
  Measles, 228
  Poliomyelitis (or Polio), 230
  Sodoku (or Rat bite fever), 275
  Typhoid fever (or Enteric fever), 183
phlegmon
  fish poisoning, 265
photophobia
  Dengue fever (or Breakbone fever), 206
  Rift Valley fever, 242
  Trichinosis, 104
photopsia
  Toxocasriasis, 103
plaques
  Bejel (or Endemic syphilis), 143
  Buruli ulcers (or Bairnsdale, Daintree, Mossman diseases, or Searls ulcer or Mycoburuli ulcers), 144
  Lobomycosis (or Jorge Lobo disease), 127
  Pinta (or Carate), 171–172
  Tinea capitis, 54–55
  Yaws (Pian, Parangi, Paru, or Frambesia tropica), 196
pneumonia
  HIV/AIDS, 221
  Pneumococcal disease, 177
  S.A.R.S., 243
polyadenopathy
  Dengue fever (or Breakbone fever), 206
  Leprosy (or Hansen disease), 160
  Scrub typhus, 282
polyneuritis
  HIV/AIDS, 221
  Leprosy (or Hansen disease), 160
polypnea
  Heat asthenia (or Tropical anhidrotic asthenia), 290
polyps
  Rhinosporidiosis, 134
polyradiculoneuritis
  HIV/AIDS, 217, 221
polyuria
  Gonorrhea (or Clap), 154
  Schistosomiasis, 85
post-optic nerve atrophy
  Onchocerciasis, 76

proctitis
  Urethritis and cervicitis, 201
prostration
  Plague (or Black death), 174–175
proteinuria
  Lassa fever, 239
pruritus
  Ancylostomiasis, 27
  bees and hymenoptera-induced diseases, 253
  Candidiasis, 55
  Dracunculiasis, 60
  fish poisoning, 288
  Loiasis, 70
  mollusk-induced diseases, 274
  Onchocerciasis, 76
  Scabies, 80
  Strongyloidiasis, 46
  Toxocasriasis, 103
  Trichomoniasis, 56–57
  Trypanosomiasis, 15
psychiatric disturbances
  HIV/AIDS, 217
psychological disturbances
  Ichthyosarcotoxisms, 287
psychosis
  Typhoid fever (or Enteric fever), 183
pulmonary edema
  fish poisoning, 265
  Poliomyelitis (or Polio), 231
pulmonary involvement
  Lymphogranuloma venereum (or Nicholas-Favre-Durand disease), 197
pulse, weak
  Heat exhaustion, 290
purulent discharge
  Gonorrhea (or Clap), 155
purulent pharyngitis
  Lassa fever, 239
pustules
  Anthrax, 139
  Blastomycosis (or Gilchrist disease or Chicago disease), 109
pyramidal syndrome
  HIV/AIDS, 222
pyrosis
  Giardiasis, 39

rash
  Ancylostomiasis, 27
  Arboviral diseases, 235
  butterfly-induced diseases, 254
  Measles, 228
  Toxocasriasis, 103

rectal discharge
  Urethritis and cervicitis, 201
rectal infection
  Gonorrhea (or Clap), 155
rectal prolapse
  Trichuriasis, 49
rectitis
  Gonorrhea (or Clap), 155
redness, of vulva/vagina/cervix
  Candidiasis, 55
reflexes, absence of
  Heat stroke, 291
renal disturbances
  Arboviral diseases, 235
renal failure
  Anthrax, 139
  mushroom poisoning, 288
respiratory arrest
  jellyfish-induced diseases, 269
  mollusk-induced diseases, 274
  Paragonimiasis, 50
respiratory problems
  Diphtheria, 152
  fish poisoning, 287
  Gonorrhea (or Clap), 155
  Nipah virosis, 247
  Pneumococcal disease, 178
  Poliomyelitis (or Polio), 231
  Toxocasriasis, 103
  Trypanosomiasis, 19
respiratory secretions
  Poliomyelitis (or Polio), 231
restlessness
  Heat exhaustion, 290
  Heat stroke, 291
  Pneumococcal disease, 177
retinal detachment
  Toxocasriasis, 103
retinal granulomas
  Toxocasriasis, 103
retinal lesions
  Rift Valley fever, 242
retinal nodules
  HIV/AIDS, 221
retinitis
  Cysticercosis, 92
  HIV/AIDS, 221
retro-orbital pain
  Dengue fever (or Breakbone fever), 206
  Trichinosis, 104
retroviral syndrome
  HIV/AIDS, 217
rhinitis
  Leprosy (or Hansen disease), 160
rhinorrhea
  Conidiobolomycosis, 118
  Hepatitis, 210
  Influenza (or Flu), 225
  Pertussis (or Whooping cough), 170
  Strongyloidiasis, 46

sacral neuropathy
  Herpes simplex (or Cold or Fever sore), 215
schizotrypanides
  Trypanosomiasis, 19
scrotum lymphangitis and funiculitis
  Filariasis (lymphatic), 1
scrotum pain and swelling
  Urethritis and cervicitis, 201
seizures
  Cysticercosis, 92
  Heat exhaustion, 291
  Histoplasmosis (or Darling disease), 123
  HIV/AIDS, 221, 222
  Meningococcal meningitis, 168
  Nipah virosis, 247
  Poliomyelitis (or Polio), 230
sensitivity to alcohol
  mushroom poisoning, 289
sensory disorders
  fish poisoning, 287
septocemia
  fish poisoning, 265
shingles
  HIV/AIDS, 221
shock
  Anthrax, 140
  bees and hymenoptera-induced diseases, 253
  Dengue fever (or Breakbone fever), 206
  mollusk-induced diseases, 274
  Poliomyelitis (or Polio), 231
  Ubiquitous relapsing fever, 273
shoulder pain
  Lyssavirus disease, 250
Skene's duct infection
  Trichomoniasis, 57
skin, dry and flushed
  Heat stroke, 291
skin, pale
  Heat exhaustion, 290
  leech-induced diseases, 269
  Leishmaniasis (or Kala-azar, or Dum dum disease), 4
skin abscesses. see abscesses
skin blisters
  Scabies, 80

Symptom Index

skin eruptions
- butterfly-induced diseases, 254
- Ciguatera, 284
- Dengue fever (or Breakbone fever), 206
- Ebola virus disease, 244
- Epidemic louse-borne typhus, 270
- fish poisoning, 287
- Gonorrhea (or Clap), 155
- Hepatitis, 210
- HIV/AIDS, 221
- Influenza (or Flu), 225
- Marburg virus disease, 245
- Meningococcal meningitis, 167–168
- Murine typhus, 266
- Schistosomiasis, 40
- Scrub typhus, 282
- Scytalidosis, 136
- Sodoku (or Rat bite fever), 275
- Strongyloidiasis, 46
- Typhoid fever (or Enteric fever), 183

skin infection
- leech-induced diseases, 269

skin lesions
- Bartonellosis (or Carrion disease), 141
- bees and hymenoptera-induced diseases, 253
- Bejel (or Endemic syphilis), 143
- Blastomycosis (or Gilchrist disease or Chicago disease), 109
- Blastomycosis (or Lutz-Splendore-Almeida disease), 110
- Candidiasis, 58
- Chromomycosis, 113
- Coccidioidomycosis (or Posadas-Wernicke, or Posadas-Rixford disease), 115
- Dermatophytosis, 59
- Gonorrhea (or Clap), 155
- Granuloma inguinale (or Donovan disease), 156
- Histoplasmosis (or Darling disease), 123
- Leishmaniasis, 63, 67
- Leprosy (or Hansen disease), 159–160, 161
- Pediculosis capitis, 53
- Pythiosis, 132
- Sparganosis, 101
- Syphilis (or Hard chancre), 191
- Trypanosomiasis, 15
- Tungiasis, 82
- Yaws (Pian, Parangi, Paru, or Frambesia tropica), 196

skin ulcers
- Melioidosis (or Whitmore disease), 164
- Trypanosomiasis, 15, 19

sleepiness
- Influenza (or Flu), 225
- Rotavirus disease, 248

sleeplessness
- Typhoid fever (or Enteric fever), 183

sneezing
- Pertussis (or Whooping cough), 170

somnolence
- Prion disease (Variant Creutzfeldt-Jakob disease), 203

sore throat
- Hendra virosis, 246
- Nipah virosis, 247

spasms
- Rabies, 261

spastic paralysis
- Poliomyelitis (or Polio), 230

spinal pain
- Dengue fever (or Breakbone fever), 206
- Epidemic louse-borne typhus, 270

splenomegaly
- HIV/AIDS, 221
- Leishmaniasis (or Kala-azar, or Dum dum disease), 4
- Sodoku (or Rat bite fever), 275
- Toxocasriasis, 103
- Trypanosomiasis, 15
- Ubiquitous relapsing fever, 273

stomach disturbances
- fish poisoning, 287

stomach pain
- Ancylostomiasis, 27

stools, pale
- Hepatitis, 210

stools, soft
- Giardiasis, 39

stools, watery
- Cholera, 149

strabismus
- Toxocasriasis, 103

stupor
- Epidemic louse-borne typhus, 270
- spider-induced diseases, 278

subconjunctival/subungual hemorrhage
- Trichinosis, 105

suffocation
- bees and hymenoptera-induced diseases, 253

sweating
- Malaria, 8

spider-induced diseases, 278, 279
Ubiquitous relapsing fever, 273
syncope
  fish poisoning, 265
  Muraenae-induced diseases (or Moray eel-induced diseases), 274–275

tachycardia
  Heat asthenia (or Tropical anhidrotic asthenia), 290
  Heat exhaustion, 290
  Heat stroke, 291
  leech-induced diseases, 269
  Meningococcal meningitis, 167
  Muraenae-induced diseases (or Moray eel-induced diseases), 274–275
  Pneumococcal disease, 178
  Rotavirus disease, 248
  scorpion-induced diseases, 276
  Shigellosis, 188
  Trichinosis, 105
  Trypanosomiasis, 19
tachypnea
  Anthrax, 140
  Heat exhaustion, 290
  Heat stroke, 291
  Influenza (or Flu), 225
  Meningococcal meningitis, 167
  Plague (or Black death), 174–175
  Pneumococcal disease, 178
  Rotavirus disease, 248
  scorpion-induced diseases, 276
  Typhoid fever (or Enteric fever), 183
tears, lack of
  Heat exhaustion, 290, 291
tenesmus
  Amebiasis, 22
  Shigellosis, 188
  Trichuriasis, 49
tenosynovitis
  Gonorrhea (or Clap), 155
tetanus
  leech-induced diseases, 269
thirst
  Heat exhaustion, 290
thoracic pain
  Ubiquitous relapsing fever, 273
thrombocytopenia
  Pneumococcal disease, 178
thrombosis
  Trypanosomiasis, 19–20
thrush
  HIV/AIDS, 221

tingling
  Herpes simplex (or Cold or Fever sore), 215
  Linguatulosis, 100
  Scabies, 264
tongue, dry
  Epidemic louse-borne typhus, 270
  Rotavirus disease, 248
tongue changes
  Yellow fever (or Black vomit), 233
tremors
  mushroom poisoning, 289
  Prion disease (or Creutzfeldt-Jakob disease), 203
  Rabies, 261
trichiasis
  Trachoma (or Granular conjunctivits or Egyptian ophthalmia), 199
tumor-like masses
  Rhinosporidiosis, 134

ulcerated papule
  Blastomycosis (or Lutz-Splendore-Almeida disease), 111
  Cat scratch disease, 257
ulcerating rhinophryngitis
  Yaws (Pian, Parangi, Paru, or Frambesia tropica), 196
ulcerovegetative lesions
  Granuloma inguinale (or Donovan disease), 156
ulcers
  Chancroid (or Soft chancre or Ulcus molle), 146
  Mycetoma (or Madura foot disease), 129
  Yaws (Pian, Parangi, Paru, or Frambesia tropica), 196
upper respiratory tract infection
  Pertussis (or Whooping cough), 170
urethra infection
  Trichomoniasis, 57
urethral discharge
  Gonorrhea (or Clap), 154
  Herpes simplex (or Cold or Fever sore), 215
  Urethritis and cervicitis, 201
urination, dark
  Hepatitis, 210
urination, decreased
  Pneumococcal disease, 178
  Yellow fever (or Black vomit), 233
urination, frequent
  Ubiquitous relapsing fever, 273

urticaria
  bees and hymenoptera-induced diseases, 253
  fish poisoning, 288
  Gnathostomiasis, 94
  Toxocasriasis, 103
  Trichinosis, 105
uterine bleeding
  Yellow fever (or Black vomit), 233
uveitis
  Toxocasriasis, 103

vaginal bleeding, abnormal
  Urethritis and cervicitis, 201
vaginal discharge
  Candidiasis, 55
  Gonorrhea (or Clap), 154
  Herpes simplex (or Cold or Fever sore), 215
  Trichomoniasis, 56
  Urethritis and cervicitis, 201
vaginal lesions
  Chancroid (or Soft chancre or Ulcus molle), 146
  Lymphogranuloma venereum (or Nicholas-Favre-Durand disease), 197
  Sparganosis, 101
vaginal pruritus
  Trichomoniasis, 56–57
valvular disease
  Histoplasmosis (or Darling disease), 123
varicose lymphatic vessels
  Filariasis (lymphatic), 2
vascular lesions
  Pythiosis, 132
vasodilation
  Heat exhaustion, 290
verrucous lesions
  Granuloma inguinale (or Donovan disease), 156
vertebral lesions
  Histoplasmosis (African), 120
vertigo
  fish poisoning, 287
  Heat asthenia (or Tropical anhidrotic asthenia), 290
  Heat exhaustion, 290
  Hendra virosis, 246
vision problems
  Cenurosis, 91
  Histoplasmosis (or Darling disease), 123
  mollusk-induced diseases, 274
  Toxocasriasis, 103
vitreous abscesses. see abscesses
vomiting
  fish poisoning, 288
  Heat exhaustion, 291
  Heat stroke, 291
  mushroom poisoning, 288
  Rotavirus disease, 248
  Toxocasriasis, 103
vulva lesions
  Chancroid (or Soft chancre or Ulcus molle), 146
  Lymphogranuloma venereum (or Nicholas-Favre-Durand disease), 197

waking, difficulty with
  Heat exhaustion, 291
weakness
  Cholera, 149
  Heat stroke, 291
  scorpion-induced diseases, 276
  Traveler's diarrhea (Turista), 298
  Ubiquitous relapsing fever, 272
weight loss
  Amebiasis, 22
  Ancylostomiasis, 27
  Balantidiasis, 35
  Blastomycosis (or Gilchrist disease or Chicago disease), 109
  Blastomycosis (or Lutz-Splendore-Almeida disease), 110
  Distomatosis, 37
  Histoplasmosis (or Darling disease), 123
  HIV/AIDS, 221, 222
  Leishmaniasis (or Kala-azar, or Dum dum disease), 4
  Melioidosis (or Whitmore disease), 164
  Tuberculosis, 191
  Typhoid fever (or Enteric fever), 183
wheezing
  bees and hymenoptera-induced diseases, 253
  Toxocasriasis, 103

Meaning of Abbreviations

ABL	Australian bat lyssavirus
AIDS	acquired immunodeficiency syndrome
ARDS	acute respiratory distress syndrome
ASA	acetylsalicylic acid
ASAP	as soon as possible
BCG	bacillus Calmette-Guérin
bid	twice a day
BM	bowel movement
BP	blood pressure
BSE	bovine spongiform encephalopathy
cap	capsule
CBC	complete blood count
CD4	cluster of differentiation 4
CDC	centers for disease control and prevention
CMV	cytomegalovirus
CNS	central nervous system
CPR	cardiopulmonary resuscitation
CSF	cerebrospinal fluid
CV	cardiovascular
DEC	diethylcarbamazine
DEET	N,N-diethyl-m-toluamide
DHE	dehydroemetine
DIC	disseminated intravascular coagulation
e.g.	for example
EEG	electroencephalogram
EKG	electrocardiogram
ELISA	enzyme-linked immunosorbent assay
ENL	erythema nodosum leprosum
ENT	ears, nose, and throat
FDA	food and drug administration
GI	gastrointestinal
h	hours
HDCV	human diploid cell vaccine
HIV	human immunodeficiency virus
HPV	human papillomavirus
HSV	herpes simplex virus
ICU	intensive care unit

i.e.	that is
IM	intramuscularly
IU	international unit
IV	intravenously
M	million
min	minutes
mo	month
MRSA	methicillin-resistant *Staphylococcus aureus*
NSAID	nonsteroidal anti-inflammatory drug
PCEC	purified chick embryo cell
PEP	postexposure prophylaxis
PID	pelvic inflammatory disease
po	orally
PCV13	pneumococcal conjugate vaccine
PPSV23	pneumococcal polysaccharide vaccine
PrEP	pre-exposure prophylaxis
prn	as needed
q	every
qid	four times a day
RIPA	radioimmunoprecipitation assay
RTI	respiratory tract infection
RVF	Rift Valley fever
SARS	severe acute respiratory syndrome
S/C	subcutaneously
sec	seconds
sp.	species
STD	sexually transmitted disease
subsp.	subspecies
suppo	suppository
tab	tablet
TB	tuberculosis
tid	three times a day

TORCH complex =

T – toxoplasmosis
O – other infections*
R – rubella
C – cytomegalovirus
H – herpes simplex virus-2

UN	united nations
URT	upper respiratory tract
URTI	upper respiratory tract infection
vag	vaginal
var	variety
vs.	versus
WBC	white blood cells
WHO	world health organization
WPW	Wolff-Parkinson-White syndrome
yr	year

* coxsackievirus, syphilis, varicella-zoster virus, HIV, and parvovirus B19

References

General References

Agreges du Pharo. Therapeutique en medecine tropicale. Marseille, France: Maloine; 1980.

American Public Health Association. Control of Communicable Diseases in Man. 15th ed. Washington, DC: American Public Health Association; 1990.

Aryand OP, Hart CA, eds. Sexually Transmitted Infections and AIDS in the Tropics. New York, NY: Oxford University Press; 1998.

Association des Professeurs de Pathologie Infectieuse. Le POPI, Guide de poche deconduit therapeutique en pathologie infectieuse. Paris, France: Editions Janvier; 1990.

Auerbach PS, Donner HJ, Weiss EA. Field Guide to Wilderness Medicine. 3rd ed. Philadelphia, PA: Mosby Elsevier; 2008.

Bethony J, Brooker S, Albonico M, et al. Soil-transmitted helminth infections: ascariasis, trichuriasis, and hookworm. Lancet. 2006;367(9521):1521–1532.

Boyer J. Precis de medicine preventive et d'hygiene. 5th ed. Paris, France: J.B. Bailliere, 1973.

Cahill KM. Tropical Medicine: A Clinical Text. 8th ed. New York, NY: Center for International Humanitarian Cooperation; 2005.

Cecil L. Textbook of Medicine. 13th ed. Philadelphia, PA: W.B. Saunders, 1971.

Centers for Disease Control and Prevention. CDC Health Information for International Travel 2012: The Yellow Book. New York NY: Oxford University Press; 2012.

Cheesbrough M. District Laboratory Practice in Tropical Countries. Part 1. Norfolk, UK: Tropical Health Technology; 1998.

Clinical Tropical Medicine, Infectious Diseases Training and Research Center (IDTRC), Christian Medical College, Vellore, India. Clinical cases. Accessed on 5/29/13 http://www.cmctropmed.com/clinicalcasecontinue.

Cook G, Zumla A. Manson's Tropical Diseases. 22nd ed. Philadelphia, PA: Saunders Elsevier; 2008.

Dictionnaire Vidal. Paris, France: Editions du Vidal: 2001.

Eddleston M, Davidson R, Wilkinson R, Pierini S. Oxford Handbook of Tropical Medicine. 2nd ed. Oxford, UK: Oxford University Press; 2004.

Fitzpatrick TB, Johnson RA, Polano MK, Suurmoud D, Wolff K. Color Atlas and Synopsis of Clinical Dermatology. 2nd ed. New York, NY: McGraw-Hill; 1992.

Garnier M, Delamare V, Delamare J, Delamare T. Dictionnaire des termes de medecine. 26th ed. Paris, France: Maloine; 2001.

Gentilini M. Medicine tropicale. 5th ed. Paris, France: Flammarion Medecine-Sciences; 1995.

Gill GV, Beeching N, eds. Lectures Notes: Tropical Medicine. 6th ed. Hoboken, NJ: John Wiley & Sons; 2009.

Gorgas Courses in Clinical Tropical Medicine. Selected Cases Seen by 2012 Course Participants. http://gorgas.dom.uab.edu/2012cases/120305.html.

Guerrant RL, Walker DH, Weller PF, eds. Essentials of Tropical Infectious Diseases. Philadelphia, PA: Churchill Livingstone; 2001.

Haider BA, Humayun Q, Bhutta ZA. Effect of administration of antihelminthics for soil transmitted helminths during pregnancy. Cochrane Database Syst Rev. 2009;2:CD005547.

Hamburger J. Petite encyclopedie medicale. 4th ed. Paris, France: Flammarion; 1972.

Harries JRR, Harries AD, Cook GC. Clinical Problems in Tropical Medicine. 2nd ed. London, UK: W.B. Saunders; 1999.

Heymann DL, ed. Control of Communicable Diseases Manual. 19th ed. Washington, DC: American Public Heath Association, 2008.

Institut de Veille Sanitaire. Accessed on 5/29/13 http://www.invs.sante.fr/

Jeffs B. A clinical guide to viral haemorrhagic fevers: Ebola, Marburg and Lassa. Trop Doct. 2006;36(1):1–4.

Jong EC, Stevens DL. Netter's Infectious Diseases. Philadelphia, PA: Saunders; 2011.

Keiser J, Utzinger J. Efficacy of current drugs against soil-transmitted helminth infections: systematic review and meta-analysis. JAMA. 2008;299(16):1937–1948.

Kernbaum S. Elements de pathologie infectieuse. Paris, France: SIMEP/SPECIA; 1985.

Keystone JS, Freedman DO, Kozarsky P, Nothdurft HD, Connor BA. Travel Medicine. 3rd ed. Philadelphia, PA: Elsevier Saunders; 2013.

Kwan-Gett TS, Kemp C, Kovarik C. Infectious and Tropical Diseases: A Handbook for Primary Care. Philadelphia, PA: Mosby Elsevier; 2005.

Lapeyssonle L. Des epidemics. Lyon, France: Fondation Marcel Merieux, 1979.

Lawson CJ, Dykewicz CA, Molinari NA, Lipman H, Alvarado-Ramy F. Deaths in international travelers arriving in the United States, July 1, 2005 to June 30, 2008. J Travel Med. Mar–Apr;19(2):96–103.

Leach M, Scoones I, Stirling A. Governing epidemics in an age of complexity: narratives, politics and pathways to sustainability. Glob Environ Change. 2010;20(3)(special issue):369–377.

Longo D, Fauci A, Kasper D, Hauser S, Jameson J, Loscalzo J. Harrison's Principles of Internal Medicine. Vols. 1 and 2, 18th ed. New York, NY: McGraw Hill Medical; 2013.

Magill AJ, Ryan ET, Solomon T, Hill DR. Hunter's Tropical Medicine and Emerging Infectious Diseases. 9th ed. New York, NY: Elsevier Saunders; 2013.

Main common and tropical diseases. In Encyclopedie Jeune Afrique. Vol. 4. Paris, France: Editions Jeune Afrique publisher, 1980; 217–261.

Mandell GL, Douglas RG, Bennett JE, eds. Principles and Practice of Infectious Diseases. 7th ed. Philadelphia, PA: Churchill Livingstone-Elsevier; 2010.

McMullen WR, Thomson M. The Travel and Tropical Medicine Manual. 4th ed. Philadelphia, PA: Saunders; 2008.

Meunier YA. Cancer and tropical disease therapeutic research: a call for deeper and wider ties. Internet Journal of Tropical Diseases. 2007;4(1). DOI: 10.5580/392.

Meunier YA. Essential drugs and compliance: the example of anti-parasitic drugs. Med Chir Dig. 1987;16:329–330.

Meunier YA. Global Health: Welcome to the Unexpected. Los Gatos, CA: Robertson; 2011.

Meunier YA. Globalization: health challenges for multinational corporations. Journal of International Business and Law. 2007;6(1):1–16.

Meunier YA. Review of Medical Aspects of Homosexuality [dissertation]. Paris, France: Pitie-Salpetriere Faculty of Medicine; 1982.

Meunier YA. Tropical Diseases: 20 Case Studies. Los Gatos, CA: Robertson; 2012.

Meunier YA, Gentilini M, Brucker G. Urbanization and public health. Bull Soc Path Exot. 1983;76:276–284.

Compendium of full prescribing information: MIMS Annual Singapore DIMS. 15th ed. 2003, 2004.

Ministerio da Saude do Brasil. Protocolos clinicos e diretrizes terapeuticas. Vol. 1. São Leopoldo, Brazil: Grafica Editora Palotti; 2010.

Nelson AL, Woodward JA, eds. Sexually Transmitted Diseases: A Practical Guide for Primary Care. Totowa, NJ: Humana Press; 2006.

Organizacao Pan Americana de Saude (Pan American Health Organization) Profilaxia das doencas transmissiveis Dr. Abram S. Benenson, editor, 1973.

Pande JN, ed. Respiratory Medicine in the Tropics. Delhi, India: Oxford University Press; 1998.

Peard JG. Race, Place, and Medicine: The Idea of the Tropics in Nineteenth Century Brazilian Medicine. Durham, NC: Duke University Press; 2000.

Peters W, Pasvol G. Atlas of Tropical Medicine and Parasitology. 6th ed. New York, NY: Mosby Elsevier; 2011.

Physician's Desk Reference. Montvale, NJ: Thomson Healthcare; 2001.

Power HJ. Tropical Medicine in the Twentieth Century: A History of the Liverpool School of Tropical Medicine 1898–1990. London, UK: Keegan Paul International; 1999.

Ranjan FL, Sujathat FSE, Leong ASY. Tropical Infectious Diseases: Epidemiology, Investigation, Diagnosis, and Management. San Francisco, CA: Greenwich Medical Media; 2001.

Reddy M, Gill SS, Kalkar SR, Wu W, Anderson PJ, Rochon PA. Oral drug therapy for multiple neglected tropical diseases: a systematic review. JAMA. 2007;298(16):1911–1924.

Rodriguez-Morales AJ, ed. Current Topics in Tropical Medicine. New York, NY: InTech; 2012.

Snowden FM. Emerging and reemerging diseases: a historical perspective. Immunol Rev. 2008;225:9–26.

Steffen R, Dupont HL, Wilder-Smith A. Manual of Travel Medicine and Health. 2nd ed. Hamilton, Canada: BC Decker; 2003.

Taylor-Robinson DC, Maayan N, Soares-Weiser K, Donegan S, Garner P. Deworming drugs for soil-transmitted intestinal worms in children: effects on nutritional indicators, haemoglobin and school performance. Cochrane Database Syst Rev. 2012;11:CD000371.

Tierney LM Jr, McPhee SJ, Papadakis MA. Current Medical Diagnosis & Treatment. New York, NY: McGraw-Hill; 2001.

Veronesi R. Doencas infecciosas e parasitarias. 5th ed. Guanabara Koogan; Rio de Janeiro, 1972.

Walson JL, Herrin BR, John-Stewart G. Deworming helminth co-infected individuals for delaying HIV disease progression. Cochrane Database Syst Rev. 2009;3:CD006419.

References by Disease

Amebiasis

Chavez-Tapia NC, Hernandez-Calleros J, Tellez-Avila FI, Torre A, Uribe M. Image-guided percutaneous procedure plus metronidazole versus metronidazole alone for uncomplicated amoebic liver abscess. Cochrane Database Syst Rev. 2009;1:CD004886.

Gonzales MLM, Dans LF, Martinez EG. Antiamoebic drugs for treating amoebic colitis. Cochrane Database Syst Rev. 2009;2:CD006085.

Haque R, Huston CD, Hughes M, Houpt E, Petri WA Jr. Amebiasis. N Engl J Med. 2003;348(16):1565–1573.

Branchereau B. Regarding a Case of Intestinal Amebiasis Sexually Transmitted to a Male Homosexual [dissertation]. Paris, France: Lariboisiere Saint-Louis; 1983.

Meunier YA. Sexually transmitted intestinal amebiasis: apropos of 2 cases. Sem Hop Paris. 1983;45:3137–3139.

Meunier YA. Amebic liver abscesses in temperate climate countries. One case report. Sem Hop Paris. 1984;41:2911–2913.

Bonstein U. Amebic Liver Abscesses: Regarding 2 Cases Seemingly Autochthonous [dissertation]. Paris, France: Saint Antoine Faculty of Medicine; 1984.

Stanley SL Jr. Amoebiasis. Lancet. 2003;361(9362):1025–1034.

Ximénez C, Cerritos R, Rojas L, et al. Human amebiasis: breaking the paradigm? Int J Environ Res Public Health. 2010;7(3):1105–1120.

Petri WA Jr, Singh U. Diagnosis and management of amebiasis. Clin Infect Dis. 1999;29(5):1117–1125.

Ancyclostomiasis

Meunier YA. Dyspeptic disorders and eosinophilia due to ancylostomiasis: a case report. Asian Pac J Trop Med. 2009;2(1):76–77.

Ascariasis

Khuroo MS. Ascariasis. Gastroenterol Clin North Am. 1996;25(3):553–577.

Massara CL, Enk MJ. Treatment options in the management of Ascaris lumbricoides. Expert Opin Pharmacother. 2004;5(3):529–539.

Meunier YA. Loeffler's syndrome: unusual symptoms and signs of ascariasis. A case report. Asian Pac J Trop Med. 2008;1(1):27–29.

Blastomycosis (South American)

da Mota Menezes V, Soares BGO, Fontes CJF. Drugs for treating paracoccidioidomycosis. Cochrane Database Syst Rev. 2006;2:CD004967.

Chagas Disease

Coura JR. Chagas disease: what is known and what is needed—a background article. Memórias do Instituto Oswaldo Cruz. 2007;102(suppl 1):113–122.

Lutje V, Seixas J, Kennedy A. Chemotherapy for second-stage human African trypanosomiasis. Cochrane Database Syst Rev. 2010;8:CD006201.

Meunier YA. Chagas disease. 2nd chapter Parasitic Diseases, pp 120–125. In: Gentilini M, Duflo B, eds. Medecine tropicale. 4th ed. Paris, France: Flammarion; 1986.

Morel CM, Lazdins J. Chagas disease. Nat Rev Microbiol. 2003;1(1):14–15.

Tarleton RL, Reithinger R, Urbina JA, Kitron U, Gürtler RE. The challenges of Chagas disease—grim outlook or glimmer of hope. PLoS Med. 2007;4(12):e332.

Vallejo M, Reyes PPA. Trypanocidal drugs for late stage, symptomatic Chagas disease (Trypanosoma cruzi infection). Cochrane Database Syst Rev. 2005;4:CD004102.

Villar JC, Villar LA, Marin-Neto JA, Ebrahim S, Yusuf S. Trypanocidal drugs for chronic asymptomatic *Trypanosoma cruzi infection*. Cochrane Database Syst Rev. 2002;1:CD003463.

Cholera

Graves PM, Deeks JJ, Demicheli V, Jefferson T. Vaccines for preventing cholera: killed whole cell or other subunit vaccines (injected). Cochrane Database Syst Rev. 2010;8:CD000974.

Meunier YA, Felix H. Struggle strategy against cholera. 10th International Congress on Tropical Medicine and Malaria. Manila, Philippines, November 9–15, 1980.

Musekiwa A, Volmink J. Oral rehydration salt solution for treating cholera: ≤270 mOsm/L solutions vs ≥310 mOsm/L solutions. Cochrane Database Syst Rev. 2011;12:CD003754.

Sinclair D, Abba K, Zaman K, Qadri F, Graves PM. Oral vaccines for preventing cholera. Cochrane Database Syst Rev. 2011;3:CD008603.

Cysticercosis

Abba K, Ramaratnam S, Ranganathan LN. Anthelmintics for people with neurocysticercosis. Cochrane Database Syst Rev. 2010;3:CD000215.

Dengue Fever

Panpanich R, Sornchai P, Kanjanaratanakorn K. Corticosteroids for treating dengue shock syndrome. Cochrane Database Syst Rev. 2006;3:CD003488.

Schiøler KL, McCarty CW. Vaccines for preventing dengue infection (protocol). Cochrane Database Syst Rev. 2003;4:CD004613.

Drancunculiasis

Meunier YA. Leg edema and painful gait in a western African due to dracunculiasis: a case report. Asian Pac J Trop Med. 2009;2(2):72–73.

Ebola Virus

Groseth A, Feldmann H, Strong JE. The ecology of Ebola virus. Trends Microbiol. 2007;15(9):408–416.

Leach M. Time to put Ebola in context. Bull WHO. 2010;88(7):488–489.

Leroy EM, Epelboin A, Mondonge V, et al. Human Ebola outbreak resulting from direct exposure to fruit bats in Luebo, Democratic Republic of Congo, 2007. Vector Borne Zoonotic Dis. 2009;9(6):723–728.

Pourrut X, Kumulungui B, Wittmann T, et al. The natural history of Ebola virus in Africa. Microbes Infect. 2005;7(7–8):1005–1014.

Filariasis

Ottesen EA. Major progress toward eliminating lymphatic filariasis. N Engl J Med. 2002;347(23):1885–1886.

Witt C, Ottesen EA. Lymphatic filariasis: an infection of childhood. Trop Med Int Health. 2001;6(8):582–606.

Giardiasis

Buret AG. Pathophysiology of enteric infections with Giardia duodenalis. Parasite. 2008;15:261.

Escobedo AA, Almirall P, Robertson LJ, et al. Giardiasis: the ever-present threat of a neglected disease. Infect Disord Drug Targets. 2010;10(5):329–348.

Gardner TB, Hill DR. Treatment of giardiasis. Clin Microbiol Rev. 2001;14(1):114–128.

Lalle M. Giardiasis in the post-genomic era: treatment, drug resistance and novel therapeutic perspectives. Infect Disord Drug Targets. 2010;10(4):283–294.

Meunier YA, Hole MK. Apyretic gastrointestinal disorders due to giardiasis contracted in Morocco. Clinics and Practice. 2011:1:e40.

Ortega YR, Adam RD. Giardia: overview and update. Clin Infect Dis. 1997;25(3):545–549.

Hendra Virus

World Health Organization. Hendra virus. Fact sheet 329, July 2009. Accessed on 3/21/13 http://www.who.int/mediacentre/factsheets/fs329/en/index.html.

Hepatitis

Meunier YA. Isolated asthenia in a frequent traveler due to hepatitis E. Reviews in Infection. 2010;1(1):29–30.

Meunier YA. Hepatitis B: who must be immunized? Panorama du Medecin. 1984;vol 1909:18.

Histoplasmosis

Meunier YA. Oozing sub-cutaneous masses due to histoplasmosis in a patient from Mali: a case report. Asian Pac J Trop Med. 2010;3(2):158–159.

HIV/AIDS

Cousin J. Analysis of Cotrimoxazole and Pentamidine Side Effects in the Treatment of 21 AIDS Patients with PCP [dissertation]. Paris, France: Necker Enfants Malades Faculty of Medicine, Paris, 1986.

Meunier YA. Do...don't...when AIDS is suspected. Contracept Fertil Sex. 1984;3:536–537.

Meunier YA. The HIV/AIDS pandemic: failures and questions. PloS Med. 2007;4(12).:http://www.plosmedicine.org/annotation/listThread.action;jsessionid=623D561218053F8A2263FAE0A7956364?root=8045

Meunier YA. What must be done when AIDS is suspected. Rev Bras Med Trop. 1984;17:107–108.

Meunier YA, Rozenbaum W, Duflo B, Danis M, Gentilini M. Treatment of pneumocystis pneumonia (PCP) in the acquired immunodeficiency syndrome (AIDS): cotrimoxazole can be continued with efficacy despite side effects, which often regress spontaneously. ICAAC Meeting, December 5, 1985, Paris, France.

World Health Organization. HIV/AIDS. http://www.who.int/hiv/data/en/. Accessed on 3/25/13.

Hookworm

Hotez PJ, Brooker S, Bethony JM, Bottazzi ME, Loukas A, Xiao S. Hookworm infection. N Engl J Med. 2004;351(8):799–807.

Sarinas PS, Chitkara RK. Ascariasis and hookworm. Semin Respir Infect. 1997;12(2):130–137.

Stoltzfus RJ, Dreyfuss ML, Chwaya HM, Albonico M. Hookworm control as a strategy to prevent iron deficiency. Nutr Rev. 1997;55(6):223–232.

Hydatidosis

Meunier YA. Muscular hydatidosis: presentation of 2 cases. Sem Hop Paris. 1983;40:2785–2786.

Nasseri-Moghaddam S, Abrishami A, Taefi A, Malekzadeh R. Percutaneous needle aspiration, injection, and re-aspiration with or without benzimidazole coverage for uncomplicated hepatic hydatid cysts. Cochrane Database Syst Rev. 2011;1:CD003623.

Kala-Azar

Meunier YA, Hole MK. Kala azar in a Brazilian child. Clinics and Practice. 2011;1:e27.

Lassa Fever

Fichet-Calvet E, Rogers DJ. Risk maps of Lassa fever in West Arica. PLoS Negl Trop Dis. 2009;3(3):e388.

Leishmaniasis

Alvar J, Yactayo S, Bern C. Leishmaniasis and poverty. Trends Parasitol. 2006;22(12):552–557.

Desjeux P. Leishmaniasis. Public health aspects and control. Clin Dermatol. 1996;14(5):417–423.

González U, Pinart M, Rengifo-Pardo M, Macaya A, Alvar J, Tweed JA. Interventions for American cutaneous and mucocutaneous leishmaniasis. Cochrane Database Syst Rev. 2009;2:CD004834.

González U, Pinart M, Reveiz L, Alvar J. Interventions for Old World cutaneous leishmaniasis. Cochrane Database Syst Rev. 2008;4:CD005067.

Herwaldt BL. Leishmaniasis. Lancet. 1999;354(9185):1191–1199.

Murray HW. Treatment of visceral leishmaniasis in 2004. Am J Trop Med Hyg. 2004;71(6):787–794.

Leprosy

Reinar LM, Forsetlund L, Bjørndal A, Lockwood D. Interventions for skin changes caused by nerve damage in leprosy. Cochrane Database Syst Rev. 2008;3:CD004833.

Van Veen NHJ, Lockwood DNJ, van Brakel WH, Ramirez J Jr, Richardus JH. Interventions for erythema nodosum leprosum. Cochrane Database Syst Rev. 2009;3:CD006949.

Van Veen NHJ, Nicholls PG, Smith WCS, Richardus JH. Corticosteroids for treating nerve damage in leprosy. Cochrane Database Syst Rev. 2007;2:CD005491.

Van Veen NHJ, Schreuders TAR, Theuvenet WJ, Agrawal A, Richardus JH. Decompressive surgery for treating nerve damage in leprosy. Cochrane Database Syst Rev. 2012;12:CD006983.

Leptospirosis

Brett-Major DM, Coldren R. Antibiotics for leptospirosis. Cochrane Database Syst Rev. 2012;2:CD008264.

Brett-Major DM, Lipnick RJ. Antibiotic prophylaxis for leptospirosis. Cochrane Database Syst Rev. 2009;3:CD007342.

Loaisis

Meunier YA, Hole MK. Transient wrist and ankle edema, erratic skin lesions, and eosinophilia secondary to loiasis: a case report. Case Study Case Rep. 2011;1(2):74–76.

Lymphatic Filariasis

Addiss D, Gamble CL, Garner P, Gelband H, Ejere HOD, Critchley JA; International Filariasis Review Group. Albendazole for lymphatic filariasis. Cochrane Database Syst Rev. 2005;4:CD003753.

Adinarayanan S, Critchley JA, Das PK, Gelband H. Diethylcarbamazine (DEC)–medicated salt for community-based control of lymphatic filariasis. Cochrane Database Syst Rev. 2007;1:CD003758.

Malaria

Ben Slama L. Malaria Auto-Immunity. Study of Anti-Nuclear and Anti-Smooth Muscle Antibodies in Relation to Anti-Malarial Immunity [dissertation]. Paris, France: Pitie-Salpetriere Faculty of Medicine; 1982.

Bouland P. Production of Plasma Interferon in Man in Response to Malaria [dissertation]. Paris, France: Saint-Antoine Faculty of Medicine; 1982.

Chatap C. Plasmodium falciparum Malaria Epidemiological Problems. Regarding a Parisian Case Seemingly Autochthonous [dissertation]. Paris, France: Lariboisiere Saint-Louis Faculty of Medicine; 1981.

Mathe D. Treatment of Drug Resistant Malaria: A Clinical Trial with Mefloquine in Paris [dissertation]. Paris, France: Pierre and Marie Curie University, Saint-Antoine Faculty of Medecine; 1984.

Meunier YA. Report: technical update on malaria. International Center for Childhood/WHO, WHO publisher, 1985.

Marburg Virus

Hartman AL, Towner JS, Nichol ST. Ebola and Marburg hemorrhagic fever. Clin Lab Med. 2010;30(1):161–177.

Peterson AT, Lash RR, Carroll DS, Johnson KM. Geographic potential for outbreaks of Marburg hemorrhagic fever. Am Trop Med Hyg. 2006;75(1):9–15.

Peters CJ. Marburg and Ebola—arming ourselves against the deadly filoviruses. N Engl J Med. 2005;352(25):2571–2573.

Nipah Virus

World Health Organization. Nipah virus. Fact sheet 262, revised July 2009. Accessed on 3/21/13. http://www.who.int/mediacentre/factsheets/fs262/en/. Accessed on 3/25/13.

Onchocerciasis

Ejere HOD, Schwartz E, Wormald R, Evans JR. Ivermectin for onchocercal eye disease (river blindness). Cochrane Database Syst Rev. 2012;8:CD002219.

Meunier YA, Wright ZJ, Hole KH. Onchocerciasis contracted in Togo: Apropos of one clinical case. WebmedCentral: Tropical Medicine. 2011;2(12): WMC002712.

Rift Valley Fever

Jost CC, Nzietchueng S, Kihu S, et al. Epidemiological assessment of the Rift Valley fever outbreak in Kenya and Tanzania in 2006 and 2007. Am J Trop Med Hyg. 2010;83(suppl 2):65–72.

Pepin M, Bouloy M, Bird BH, Kemp A, Paweska J. Rift Valley fever virus (Bunyaviridae: Phlebovirus): an update on pathogenesis, molecular epidemiology, vectors, diagnostics and prevention. Vet Res. 2010;41(6):61.

Salmonellosis

Odey F, Okomo U, Oyo-Ita A. Vaccines for preventing invasive *Salmonella* infections in people with sickle cell disease. Cochrane Database Syst Rev. 2009;4:CD006975.

Onwuezobe IA, Oshun PO, Odigwe CC. Antimicrobials for treating symptomatic non-typhoidal *Salmonella* infection. Cochrane Database Syst Rev. 2012;11:CD001167.

SARS

Hui DS, Chan PK. Severe acute respiratory syndrome and coronavirus. Infect Dis Clin North Am. 2010;24(3):619–638.

Leung GM, Ho LM, Lam TH, Hedley AJ. Epidemiology of SARS in the 2003 Hong Kong epidemic. Hong Kong Med J. 2009;15(suppl 9):12–16.

Scabies

Strong M, Johnstone P. Interventions for treating scabies. Cochrane Database Syst Rev. 2007;3:CD000320.

Schistosomiasis

Blanchard TJ. Schistosomiasis. Travel Med Infect Dis. 2004;2(1):5–11.

Danso-Appiah A, Olliaro PL, Donegan S, Sinclair D, Utzinger J. Drugs for treating Schistosoma mansoni infection. Cochrane Database Syst Rev. 2013;2:CD000528.

Danso-Appiah A, Utzinger J, Liu J, Olliaro P. Drugs for treating urinary schistosomiasis. Cochrane Database Syst Rev. 2008;3:CD000053.

Elliott DE. Schistosomiasis. Pathophysiology, diagnosis, and treatment. Gastroenterol Clin North Am. 1996;25(3):599–625.

Gryseels B, Polman K, Clerinx J, Kestens L. Human schistosomiasis. Lancet. 2006;368(9541):1106–1118.

Meunier YA. Intestinal schistosomiasis acquired in Cameroon: a case report. Internet Journal of Tropical Medicine. 2010;6(2). http://archive.ispub.com/journal/the-internet-journal-of-tropical-medicine/volume-6-number-2/intestinal-schistosomiasis-acquired-in-cameroon-a-case-report.html#sthash.2ilJ2bbD.dpbs

Meunier YA, Gentilini M, Duflo B, Richard-Lenoble D. Assessment of 35972 RP (Oltipraz): a new antischistosomal compound against Schistosoma hematobium, S. mansoni and S. intercalatum. Acta Trop. 1980;37:271–274.

Meunier YA, Intestinal schistosomiasis acquired in Cameroon: A case report. Internet Journal of Tropical Medicine. 2010;6(2).

Shigellosis

Christopher PRH, David KV, John SM, Sankarapandian V. Antibiotic therapy for Shigella dysentery. Cochrane Database Syst Rev. 2010;8:CD006784.

Snake Bites

Nuchprayoon I, Garner P. Interventions for preventing reactions to snake antivenom. Cochrane Database Syst Rev. 1999;4:CD002153.

Strongyloidiasis

Concha R, Harrington W Jr, Rogers AI. Intestinal strongyloidiasis: recognition, management, and determinants of outcome. J Clin Gastroenterol. 2005;39(3): 203–211.

Meunier YA. Strongyloidiasis: one case report with its lessons and rare facts about the disease. Asian Pac J Trop Med. 2008;1(1):29–31.

Zaha O, Hirata T, Kinjo F, Saito A, Fukuhara H. Efficacy of ivermectin for chronic strongyloidiasis: two single doses given 2 weeks apart. J Infect Chemother. 2002;8(1):94–98.

Syphilis

Bai ZG, Wang B, Yang K, et al. Azithromycin versus penicillin G benzathine for early syphilis. Cochrane Database Syst Rev. 2012;6:CD007270.

Walker GJA. Antibiotics for syphilis diagnosed during pregnancy. Cochrane Database Syst Rev. 2001;3:CD001143.

Toxocariasis

Finsterer J, Auer H. Neurotoxocariasis. Rev Inst Med Trop Sao Paulo. 2007;49(5):279–287.

Trachoma

Ejere HOD, Alhassan MB, Rabiu M. Face washing promotion for preventing active trachoma. Cochrane Database Syst Rev. 2012;4:CD003659.

Evans JR, Solomon AW. Antibiotics for trachoma. Cochrane Database Syst Rev. 2011;3:CD001860.

Rabiu M, Alhassan MB, Ejere HOD, Evans JR. Environmental sanitary interventions for preventing active trachoma. Cochrane Database Syst Rev. 2012;2:CD004003.

Yorston D, Mabey D, Hatt SR, Burton M. Interventions for trachoma trichiasis. Cochrane Database Syst Rev. 2006;3:CD004008.

Trichuriasis

Meunier YA. Treatment of trichuriasis: a single drug is efficient and available in France: Fluvermal. Panorama du Medecin. 1983;1679:11.

Trypanosomiasis

Barrett MP, Burchmore RJ, Stich A, et al. The trypanosomiases. Lancet. 2003;362(9394):1469–1480.

Pépin J, Méda HA. The epidemiology and control of human African trypanosomiasis. Adv Parasitol. 2001;49:71–132.

Smith DH, Pepin J, Stich AH. Human African trypanosomiasis: an emerging public health crisis. Br Med Bull. 1998;54(2):341–355.

Stich A, Abel PM, Krishna S. Human African trypanosomiasis. BMJ. 2002;325(7357):203–206.

For reprints that cannot be found, please e-mail your request(s) to: ymeuniermd@gmail.com

Index

African eyeworm (or Loiasis), 70–72
African Histoplasmosis, 120–122
air travel, 297
allergic reactions, to cats, 256
Amebiasis
   Ameboma, 24–25
   geographic distribution, 22, 26
   historical background, 22
   intestinal, 22–24
   liver, 24
American Histoplasmosis. See Histoplasmosis (American or Darling disease)
Ancylostomiasis (Hookworm infection), 27–29
Angiostrongyliasis, 89–90
animal-induced diseases
   bees and hymenoptera-induced diseases, 253–254
   butterfly-induced diseases, 254
   cat-induced diseases, 256–260
   centipede-induced diseases, 260
   dog-induced diseases, 260–265
   fish-induced diseases, 265
   flea-induced diseases, 266–268
   jellyfish-induced diseases, 269
   leech-induced diseases, 269–270
   lice-induced diseases, 270–273
   mollusk-induced diseases, 274
   Muraenae (or Moray eel)-induced diseases, 274–275
   physaliae-induced diseases, 269
   rat-induced diseases, 275–276
   scorpion-induced diseases, 276–277
   sea anemone-induced diseases, 269
   snake-induced diseases, 277–278
   spider-induced diseases, 278–279
   tick-induced diseases, 279–281
   Trombiculidae, 282–283

Anthrax, 139–141
antibiotic resistance, 299–301
Arboviral diseases, 235–236, 279
Arenaviral diseases
   Lassa fever, 239
   Tacaribe complex, 237–238
Ascariasis, 30–31

bacterial diseases
   Anthrax, 139–141
   Bartonellosis (or Carrion Disease), 141–142
   Bejel (or Endemic syphilis), 143
   Buruli ulcers (or Bairsndale, Daintree, Mossman, or Searls ulcer or Mycoburuli ulcers), 144–145
   Chancroid (or Soft chancre or Ulcus molle), 146
   Cholera, 146–148
   Diphtheria, 152–153
   Gonorrhea (or Clap), 153–155
   Granuloma inguinale (or Donovan disease), 155–158
   Leprosy (or Hansen disease), 159–162
   Leptospirosis (or Weil disease or Nanukayami fever), 162–163
   Melioidosis (or Whitmore disease), 163–166
   Meningococcal meningitis, 167–169
   Pertussis (or Whooping cough), 170–171
   Pinta (or Carate), 171–173
   Plague (or Black death), 174–176, 268
   Pneumococcal disease, 177–182
   Salmonellosis (Salmonella gastroenteritis), 187

bacterial diseases (*Cont.*)
  Salmonellosis (Typhoid fever or Enteric fever and Paratyphoid fever), 182–186
  Shigellosis, 188–189
  Syphilis (or Hard chancre), 190–192
  Tuberculosis, 192–195
  Yaws (Pian, Parangi, Paru, or Frambesia tropics), 195–196
Bairnsdale disease (or Buruli ulcers), 144–145
Balantidiasis (Balantidiosis), 35
Bartonellosis (or Carrion disease), 141–142
Basidiobolomycosis, 107–108
Beaver fever (or Giardiasis), 39–40
bees and hymenoptera-induced diseases, 253–254
Bejel (or Endemic syphilis), 143
Biliary/liver or Biliary/liver fluke infection (or Distomatosis)
  Fascioliasis, 32–33–36
  Opisthorchiasis, 35–34
Black death. See Plague (or Black death)
Black vomit (or Yellow fever), 232–234
Blackwater fever. See Malaria (Blackwater fever)
Blastomycosis (North American or Gilchrist disease or Chicago disease), 109–110
Blastomycosis (South American or Lutz-Splendore-Almeida disease), 110–112
blood and lymphatic system
  Filariasis (lymphatic), 1–3
  Leishmaniasis (visceral, Kala-azar, Dum dum disease), 4–6
  Malaria (Blackwater fever), 7–14, 293, 294
  Trypanosomiasis (African, or Sleeping sickness), 15–18
  Trypanosomiasis (American, or Chagas disease), 19–21
Body lice (Pediculosis corporis), 80, 272
Breakbone fever. See Dengue fever (or Breakbone fever)
Bunyaviral diseases, 239–240
Buruli ulcers (or Bairnsdale, Daintree, Mossman, or Searls ulcer or Mycoburuli ulcers), 144–145
butterfly-induced diseases, 254

Candidiasis (Moniliasis)
  geographic distribution, 52, 55, 58
  preventive measures, 52, 56, 58
  symptoms, 52, 55–56, 58
  treatment, 52, 56, 58
Carate (or Pinta), 171–173
Carrion disease (or Bartonellosis), 141–142
Cat scratch disease, 257
cat-induced diseases, 256–260
centipede-induced diseases, 260
Cenurosis, 91
Chagas disease (or Trypanosomiasis-American), 19–21
Chancroid (or Soft chancre or Ulcus molle), 146
Chicago disease (or Blastomycosis-North American), 109–110
Chikungunya virus disease, 250–251
chlamydial diseases
  Lymphogranuloma venereum (or Nicholas-Favre-Durand disease), 196–198
  Trachoma (or Granular conjunctivitis or Egyptian ophthalmia), 199–200
  Urethritis and cervicitis, 201–202
Cholera
  geographic distribution, 149, 150, 148
  historical background, 147
  new problems, 147
  preventive measures, 149
  treatment, 149
Chromomycosis, 113–114
Clap (or Gonorrhea), 153–155
climate adjustment, 295
Coccidioidomycosis (or Posadas-Wernicke, or Posadas-Rixford disease), 115–117
Cold sore (or Herpes simplex), 215–216
common cold, 293
Conidiobolomycosis, 118–119
contact card, 297
Coronaviral Disease Sever Acute Respiratory Syndrome (S.A.R.S.), 242–243
Crabs (Pthiriasis), 54, 272
Creeping eruption (or Larva | migrans-cutaneous), 99, 260
Cysticercosis, 91–92

Daintree disease (or Buruli ulcers), 144–145
Darling disease. See Histoplasmosis (American or Darling disease)

deep fungal diseases. *See* fungal diseases
Dengue fever (or Breakbone fever)
  geographic distribution, 206, 207
  historical background, 205–206
  new problems, 206
  preventive measures, 207
  symptoms, 206–207
  treatment, 207
Dermatophytosis
  geographic distribution, 59
  preventive measures, 59
  symptoms, 53, 59
  treatment and prevention, 53, 59
digestive tract
  Amebiasis, 22–26
  Ancylostomiasis (Hookworm infection), 27–29
  Ascariasis, 30–31
  Balantidiasis (Balantidiosis), 35
  Distomatosis (intestinal), 37–38
  Fascioliasis, 32–33–36
  Giardiasis (Beaver fever), 39–40
  Schistosomiasis (intestinal), 40–45
  Strongyloidiasis, 46–48
  Trichuriasis (Whipworm infection), 49
Diphtheria, 152–153
diseases. *See also* Disease Index
Distomatosis (Biliary/liver or Biliary/liver fluke infection)
  Fascioliasis, 32–33–36
  Opisthorchiasis, 35–34
Distomatosis (intestinal), 37–38
dog-induced diseases, 260–265
Donovan disease (or Granuloma inguinale), 155–158
Dracontiasis (or Dracunculiasis), 60–62
Dracunculiasis (Guinea worm disease, Guinea worm infection, or Dracontiasis), 60–62
Dum dum disease (Visceral Leishmaniasis), 4–6

Ebola virus disease, 243–244
Egyptian ophthalmia (or Trachoma), 199–200
Endemic syphilis (or Bejel), 143
Enteric fever. *See* Salmonellosis (Typhoid fever or Enteric fever and Paratyphoid fever)
Epidemic louse-borne typhus, 270–271

Fascioliasis, 32–33–36
Fever sore (or Herpes simplex), 215–216
Filariasis (lymphatic), 1–3
Filoviral diseases
  Ebola virus disease, 243–244
  Marburg virus disease, 244–245
first aid supplies, 296
fish poisoning, 287–288
fish-induced diseases, 265
Flaviviral diseases, 245–246
flea-induced diseases, 266–268
Flu (or Influenza), 225–227
food poisoning
  Ciguatera, 284–286
  fish poisoning, 287–288
  geographic distribution, 284, 286
  Ichthyosarcotoxisms, 287
  mushroom poisoning, 288–289
  precautions to take to prevent, 294–295
  preventive measures, 284–285
  symptoms, 284
  treatment, 284
Frambesia tropics (Yaws), 195–196
fungal diseases
  Basidiobolomycosis, 107–108
  Blastomycosis (North American or Gilchrist disease or Chigcao disease), 109–110
  Blastomycosis (South American or Lutz-Splendore-Almeida disease), 110–112
  Chromomycosis, 113–114
  Coccidioidomycosis (or Posadas-Wernicke, or Posadas-Rixford disease), 115–117
  Conidiobolomycosis, 118–119
  Histoplasmosis (African), 120–122
  Histoplasmosis (American or Darling disease), 123–126
  Lobomycosis (or Jorge Lobo disease), 127–128
  Mycetoma (or Madura foot disease), 129–131
  Pythiosis, 132–133
  Rhinosporidiosis, 134–135
  Scytalidiosis, 136–137

Giardiasis (Beaver fever), 39–40
Gilchrist disease (or Blastomycosis-North American), 109–110
Gnathostomiasis, 94
Gonorrhea (or Clap), 153–155
Granular conjunctivitis (or Trachoma), 199–200

Granuloma inguinale (or Donovan disease), 155–158
Guinea worm disease/infection (or Dracunculiasis), 60–62

hair. See nails and hair
Hansen disease. See Leprosy (or Hansen disease)
Hantaan virosis, 240–241
Hard chancre (or Syphilis), 190–192
Head lice (Pediculosis capitis), 53, 272
Head ringworm (Tinea capitis), 54–55
health kit, 295–297
Heat asthenia (or Tropical anhidrotic asthenia), 290
Heat exhaustion, 290–291
Heat stroke, 291–292
heat-related illnesses
    Heat asthenia (or Tropical anhidrotic asthenia), 290
    Heat exhaustion, 290–291
    Heat stroke, 291–292
    Milaria (or Prickly heat), 292
Hendra virosis, 246–247
Hepatitis
    geographic distribution, 209–210, 213, 214
    preventive measures, 211–212
    symptoms, 210
    treatment, 210–211
Herpes simplex (or Cold or Fever sore), 215–216
Histoplasmosis (African), 120–122
Histoplasmosis (American or Darling disease)
    geographic distribution, 123, 126
    preventative measures, 124–125
    symptoms, 123
    treatment, 123–124
His-Werner disease (or Trench fever), 272
HIV/AIDS
    geographic distribution, 216–217
    historical background, 216
    preventive measures, 224–225
    symptoms, 217–222
    treatment, 222–224
Hookworm infection (or Ancylostomiasis), 27–29
Hydatidosis, 96–97
hygiene, general, 295

Ichthyosarcotoxisms, 287
immunizations, 294
Influenza (or Flu), 225–227

insurance, medical, 297
integumentary system. See skin and integumentary system

jellyfish-induced diseases, 269
Jorge Lobo disease (or Lobomycosis), 127–128

Kala-azar (Visceral Leishmaniasis) or Dum dum disease, 4–6

Larva migrans (cutaneous, or Creeping eruption), 99, 260
larval diseases. See parasitic dead ends and larval diseases
Lassa fever, 239
leech-induced diseases, 269–270
Leishmaniasis (cutaneous)
    geographic distribution, 63, 66, 68, 69
    symptoms, 63–64
    treatment, 64–65
Leishmaniasis (mucocutaneous), 67–69
Leishmaniasis (visceral, Kala-azar, Dum dum disease), 4–6
Leprosy (or Hansen disease)
    geographic distribution, 159
    preventive measures, 162
    symptoms, 159–161
    treatment, 161–162
Leptospirosis (or Weil disease or Nanukayami fever), 162–163
lice-induced diseases, 270–273
Linguatulosis, 99, 260
Lobomycosis (or Jorge Lobo disease), 127–128
Loiasis (African eyeworm), 70–72
Lung fluke infection (Paragonimiasis), 49–51
lungs
    Paragonimiasis (Lung fluke infection), 49–51
Lutz-Splendore-Almeida disease (or Blastomycosis-South American), 110–112
lymphatic system. See blood and lymphatic system
Lymphogranuloma venereum (or Nicholas-Favre-Durand disease), 196–198
Lyssavirus disease, 250

Madura foot disease (or Mycetoma), 129–131
Malaria (Blackwater fever)

geographic distribution, 8, 14
historical background, 7
immunizations for, 294
morbidity from, 293
preventive measures,
  11, 13
problems, new, 7–8
symptoms, 8–9
treatment, 9–11, 12
Malasseziosis (Pityriasis versicolor), 73
maps. See Map and Table Index
Marbug virus disease, 244–245
Measles, 227–229
medicine kit, 295
Melioidosis (or Whitmore disease)
  geographic distribution, 164, 166
  historical background, 163
  new problems, 164
  preventive measures, 165
  symptoms, 164
  treatment, 164–165
Meningococcal meningitis
  geographic distribution, 167, 169
  historical background, 167
  new problems, 167
  preventive measures, 168
  symptoms, 167–168
  treatment, 168
Milaria (or Prickly heat), 292
mollusk-induced diseases, 274
Moniliasis. See Candidiasis (Moniliasis)
morbidity, 293–294
mortality, 292–293
mosquito bites, 294
Mossman disease (or Buruli ulcers),
  144–145
Mossuril virus disease, 249
Muraenae (or Moray eel)-induced diseases, 274–275
Murine typhus, 266–267
mushroom poisoning, 288–289
Mycetoma (or Madura foot disease),
  129–131
Mycoburuli ulcers (or Buruli ulcers),
  144–145
Mycoses
  from cats, 257
  from dogs, 260
Myiasis (Tumba fly), 73–75

nails and hair
  Candidiasis (Moniliasis), 52–53, 56,
    58
  Dermatophytosis, 52, 53, 59
  Pediculosis capitis (Head lice), 53,
    272

Pthiriasis (Crabs), 54, 272
Tinea capitis (Head ringworm),
  54–55
Nanukayami fever (or Leptospirosis),
  162–163
Nicholas-Favre-Durands disease
  (or Lymphogranuloma
  venereum), 196–198
Nipah virosis, 247
Norwegian Itch. See Scabies
  (Norwegian Itch)

Onchocerciasis (River blindness),
  76–78
Opisthorchiasis, 35–34

Paragonimiasis (Lung fluke infection),
  49–51
Paramyxoviral diseases
  Hendra virosis, 246–247
  Nipah virosis, 247
Parangi (Yaws), 195–196
parasitic dead ends and larval diseases
  Angiostrongyliasis, 89–90
  Cenurosis, 91
  Cysticercosis, 91–93
  Gnathostomiasis, 94–95
  Hydatidosis, 96–98
  Larva migrans (cutaneous, or
    Creeping eruption), 99
  Linguatulosis, 100
  Porocephalosis, 100–101
  Sparganosis, 101–102
  Toxocariasis (Toxocarosis, Visceral
    larva migrans or Roundworm
    infection), 103–104
  Trichinosis (Trichinellosis), 104–105
parasitic diseases
  adult parasitic locations, 1–88
  Distomatosis (Biliary/liver or Biliary/
    liver fluke disease), 35–36
  parasitic dead end and larval diseases, 89–105
Paratyphoid fever. See Salmonellosis
  (Typhoid fever or Enteric fever
  and Paratyphoid fever)
Paru (Yaws), 195–196
patient cases. See Patient Cases Index
Pediculosis capitis (Head lice), 53, 272
Pediculosis corporis (Body lice), 80,
  272
Pertussis (or Whooping cough),
  170–171
physaliae-induced diseases, 269
Pian (Yaws), 195–196
Pinta (or Carate), 171–173

Pityriasis versicolor (Malasseziosis), 73
Plague (or Black death)
   from fleas, 268
   geographic distribution, 174, 176
   historical background, 174
   new problems, 174
   preventive measures, 175
   symptoms, 174–175
   treatment, 175
Pneumococcal disease
   geographic dtsirbution, 177
   preventive measures, 180–182
   symptoms, 177–179
   treatment, 179–180
Poliomyelitis (or Polio), 229–231
Porocephalosis, 99–100
Posadas-Rixford disease (or Coccidioidomycosis), 115–117
Posadas-Wernicke disease (or Coccidioidomycosis), 115–117
precautions to take before, during, and after traveling, 294–297
preexisting medical conditions, 295
Prickly heat (or Milaria), 292
Prion disease (Variant Creutzfeldt-Jakob disease), 202–204
Pthiriasis (Crabs), 54, 272
Pythiosis, 132–133

Rabies
   geographic distribution, 257, 261, 263
   prevention measures, 262
   preventive measures, 257
   symptoms, 261
   treatment, 261–262
Rat bite fever (Sodoku), 275–276
rat-induced diseases, 275–276
Regional relapsing fever
   geographic distribution, 279, 282
   preventive measures, 281
   symptoms, 280
   treatment, 281
Reoviral diseases, 247–248
Rhabdoviral diseases
   Lyssavirus disease, 250
   Mossuril virus disease, 249
Rhinosporidiosis, 134–135
Rift Valley fever, 242
River blindness (Onchocerciasis), 76–78
Rotavirus disease, 248–249
Roundworm infection (Toxocariasis), 103–104, 260, 265

Salmonellosis (Salmonella gastroenteritis), 187
Salmonellosis (Typhoid fever or Enteric fever and Paratyphoid fever)
   geographic distribution, 182, 186
   historical background, 182
   new problems, 182
   preventive measures, 185
   symptoms, 183
   treatment, 183–184
S.A.R.S. (Coronaviral Disease Sever Acute Respiratory Syndrome), 242–243
Scabies (Norwegian Itch)
   from cats, 257
   from dogs, 264
   geographic distribution, 80
   preventive measures, 81–82
   symptoms, 80–81
   treatment, 81
Schistosomiasis (intestinal)
   complications, 41
   geographic distribution, 40, 44, 45
   historical background, 40
   preventive measures, 41–42
   symptoms, 40–41
   treatment, 41
Schistosomiasis (urinary), 85–88
scorpion-induced diseases, 276–277
Scrub typhus, 282–283
Scytalidiosis, 136–137
sea anemone-induced diseases, 269
Searls ulcer (or Buruli ulcers), 144–145
senior travelers, 294
sexual organs
   Candidiasis (Moniliasis), 55–56
   Trichomoniasis, 56–57
sexually transmitted dieases
   morbidity from, 293
Shigellosis, 188–189
skin and integumentary system
   Candidiasis (Moniliasis), 52, 55–56, 58–59
   Dracunculiasis (Guinea worm disease, Guinea worm infection, Dracontiasis), 59–62
   Leishmaniasis (cutaneous), 63–66, 68, 69
   Leishmaniasis (mucocutaneous), 67–69
   Loiasis (African eyeworm), 70–72
   Malasseziosis (Pityriasis versicolor), 73
   Myiasis (Tumba fly), 73–75
   Onchocerciasis (River blindness), 76–78

Pediculosis corporis (Body lice), 80, 272
Scabies (Norwegian itch), 80–82, 257, 264
Tinea nigra palmis (plantaris), 82
Tungiasis, 82–84, 268
Sleeping sickness (or Trypanosomiasis-African), 15–18
snake-induced diseases, 277–278
Sodoku (Rat bite fever), 275–276
Soft chancre (or Chancroid) or Ulcus molle, 146
Sparganosis, 100
spider-induced diseases, 278–279
Strongyloidiasis, 46–48
symptoms. See Symptom Index
Syphilis (or Hard chancre), 190–192

tables. See Map and Table Index
Tacaribe complex, 237–238
Taeniasis
  from cats, 257
  from fleas, 268
Tetanus
  from cats, 260
  geographic distribution, 264
  preventive measures, 265
  symptoms, 264
  treatment, 264
Toxoplasmosis, 258–259
tick-induced diseases, 279–281
Tinea capitis (Head ringworm), 54–55
Tinea nigra palmis and plantaris, 82
Togaviral diseases, 250
Toxocariasis (toxocarosis, visceral larva migrans or roundworm infection), 103–104, 260, 265
Trachoma (or Granular conjunctivitis or Egyptian ophthalmia), 199–200
travel medicine kit, 295
travelers and tropical diseases, 292–294
Traveler's diarrhea (Turista), 293, 297–299
Trench fever (or His-Werner disease), 272
Trichinellosis (Trichinosis), 104–105
Trichinosis (Trichinellosis), 104–105
Trichomoniasis, 56–57
Trichuriasis (Whipworm infection), 49
Trombiculidae, 282–283
Tropical anhidrotic asthenia (or Heat asthenia), 290
Trypanosomiasis (American, or Chagas disease), 19–21
Trypanosomiasis (African, or Sleeping sickness)
  geographic distribution, 15, 18
  historical background, 15
  preventive measures, 16–17
  symptoms, 15–16
  treatment, 16
Tuberculosis
  geographic distribution, 193
  historical background, 192–193
  new problems, 193
  preventive measures, 195
  symptoms, 193–194
  treatment, 194–195
Tumba fly (Myiasis), 73–75
Tungiasis
  from fleas, 268
  geographic distribution, 82, 84
  preventive measures, 83
  symptoms, 82
  treatment, 82
Turista (Traveler's diarrhea), 293, 297–299
Typhoid fever. See Salmonellosis (Typhoid fever or Enteric fever and Paratyphoid fever)

Ubiquitous relapsing fever, 272–273
Ulcus molle (or Chancroid), 146
Urethritis and cervicitis, 201–202
urinary tract
  Schistosomiasis (urinary), 85–88

Variant Creutzfeld-Jakob disease, 202–204
viral diseases
  Arboviral diseases, 235–236, 279
  Arenaviral diseases, 237–239
  Bunyaviral diseases, 239–240
  Chikungunya virus disease, 250–251
  Coronaviral Disease Sever Acute Respiratory Syndrome (S.A.R.S.), 242–243
  Dengue fever (or Breakbone fever), 205–207
  Filoviral diseases, 243–245
  Flaviviral diseases, 245–246
  Hantaan virosis, 240–241
  Hepatitis, 209–214
  Herpes simplex (or Cold or Fever sore), 215–216
  HIV/AIDS, 216–225
  Influenza (or Flu), 225–227
  Measles, 227–229
  Paramyxoviral diseases, 246–247
  Poliomyelitis (or Polio), 229–231
  Reoviral diseases, 247–248
  Rhabdoviral diseases, 249–250

viral diseases (*Cont.*)
  Rift Valley fever, 242
  Rotavirus disease, 248–249
  Togaviral diseases, 250
  Yellow fever (or Black vomit), 232–234
Visceral larva migrans (Toxocariasis), 103–104, 260, 265

Weil disease (or Leptospirosis) or Nanukayami fever, 162–163

Whipworm infection (Trichuriasis), 49
Whitmore disease. See Melioidosis (or Whitmore disease)
Whooping cough (or Pertussis), 170–171

Yaws (Pian, Parangi, Paru, or Frambesia tropics), 195–196
Yellow fever (or Black vomit), 232–234

www.ingramcontent.com/pod-product-compliance
Ingram Content Group UK Ltd.
Pitfield, Milton Keynes, MK11 3LW, UK
UKHW021257180426
11947UKWH00015B/896